Community Psychiatric

Nursing

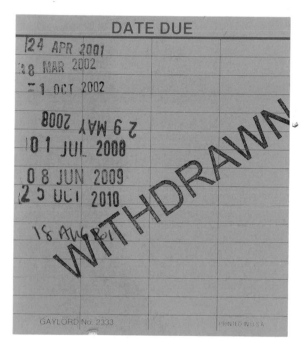

Community Psychiatric Nursing

A research perspective

Edited by

CHARLES BROOKER BA(Hons), MSc, RMN,
DipNEd, RNT

Senior Research Fellow
Department of Nursing
University of Manchester

Chapman and Hall

London · New York · Tokyo · Melbourne · Madras

UK   Chapman and Hall, 11 New Fetter Lane, London EC4P 4EE

USA   Chapman and Hall, 29 West 35th Street, New York NY10001

JAPAN   Chapman and Hall Japan, Thomson Publishing Japan, Hirakawacho
              Nemoto Building, 7F, 1–7–11 Hirakawa-cho, Chiyoda-ku, Tokyo 102

AUSTRALIA   Chapman and Hall Australia, Thomas Nelson Australia, 480 La Trobe
              Street, PO Box 4725, Melbourne 3000

INDIA   Chapman and Hall India, R. Seshadri, 32 Second Main Road, CIT East,
              Madras 600 035

First edition 1990

© 1990 Chapman and Hall

Typeset in 10/12pt Times
by Leaper & Gard Limited, Bristol

Printed in Great Britain by
T.J. Press (Padstow) Ltd, Padstow, Cornwall

ISBN 0 412 34790 3

British Library Cataloguing in Publication Data

Community psychiatric nursing research
  1. Great Britain. Psychiatric
  patients. District nursing
  I. Brooker, Charlie
  610.73680941

ISBN 0-412-34790-3

Library of Congress Cataloging-in-Publication Data

Available

Contents

Contents

Contributors

Chris Atha
Community Psychiatric Nurse – Research
The General Infirmary at Leeds
Leeds

Charles Brooker
Senior Research Fellow
Department of Nursing
University of Manchester
Manchester

Chris Drinkwater
Senior Lecturer
Division of Primary Health
University of Newcastle
Newcastle-upon-Tyne

Don Foster
Senior Lecturer
Division of Community Medicine
University of Newcastle
Newcastle

Maura Hunt
Regional Research Nurse
S.E.T.R.H.A.
Thrift House
Bexhill-on-Sea
East Sussex

Jan Illing
Research Student
Department of Social Policy
The University
Newcastle-Upon-Tyne

Helen Lee
Psychotherapist
Nottingham Psychotherapy Unit
Nottingham

Contributors

John Mangen   Acting Unit General Manager
                             All Saints' Hospital
                             Chatham
                             Kent

Liz Matthew   Clinical Nurse Specialist
                             Community Psychiatry and Elderly Services
                             Tameside

Rachel Munton   Clinical Nurse Manager (community)
                             North Nottingham and Hucknall Sector Team
                             Nottingham Health Authority

Linda Pollock   Director of Nursing Services
                             Mental Health Services Unit
                             Royal Cornhill Hospital
                             Aberdeen

Tony Rogerson   Lecturer in Nursing Studies
                             Newcastle Polytechnic
                             Newcastle-upon-Tyne

Peter Rutherford   Manager of a community health centre
                             Newcastle-upon-Tyne

Sue Simmons   Senior Lecturer
                             Division of Health Studies
                             Polytechnic of East London
                             London

Edward White   Senior Research Fellow
                             Department of Nursing
                             University of Manchester
                             Manchester

Phil Wolsey   Trainer
                             Organisational and Personal Development
                             Consultants
                             2 Camp Road
                             West Coker
                             Somerset

Foreword

by Tony Butterworth

COMMUNITY PSYCHIATRIC NURSING RESEARCH – ITS RELEVANCE TO PRACTICE

Community psychiatric nursing has been a significant force in the struggle to give mental health issues a meaningful place in the nursing profession of the United Kingdom. Few professional groups have moved with such commendable speed to change their ideology, clinical practices, education and systems of management.

This shift of focus has had its difficulties, as new interprofessional boundaries have been negotiated and the client group has moved to centre stage and taken more self control of their care. But it is possible to hypothesize that community psychiatric nursing has developed, from an uncertain beginning, through a period of gauche, confident adolescence to a current state of more mature adulthood.

Fortunately, there have been some individuals on hand who, through research effort have recorded, shaped and experimented upon this process. This is a vital ingredient in the development of good practice. The contributors to this book are therefore to be applauded for their research activities in the field of community psychiatric nursing.

The text is a reflection of some of the central concerns of nursing activity, namely, clinical practice, management and education.

The clinical practice of community psychiatric nurses has raised a number of debating points and some commentators have suggested that the focus of their work has moved away from involvement with those with long-term mental illnesses to the so called 'worried well'. There is ample evidence throughout this book that the chronically mentally ill remain a central concern for community psychiatric nurses and pointers to improving practice in this area of work are plentiful.

It should also be pointed out that significant attention is paid to those providing informal care in community settings. This, of course, is a most worthy area of study which can only grow in importance.

The chapters on the management and organization of services has produced interesting research which is reflected in the second part of the book. The type of work undertaken by CPNs, the referral process and the appropriate permissions to practise in a responsible and independent way are all matters which have preoccupied those who organize and manage services. Some most important initial descriptions and evaluative studies are to be found here.

The proper educational preparation for clinical practice is an issue which has been constantly evolving in community psychiatric nursing. A constantly revised curriculum has been available since 1974 but little research has been carried out on those nurses who have attended such post-basic courses. This final section contains invaluable new insights into this important field.

Overall, the book is another crucial stepping stone in the development of community psychiatric nursing. It should be read by all nurses working in the specialty and will help them considerably to illuminate their practice. Equally, it should be read by any nurse with an involvement in mental health nursing or research *per se*. The lessons to be learned from it are essential.

Introduction

To paraphrase Sidney Webb, gradualness has a certain inevitabilty, and advances in community psychiatric nursing research over the last decade have certainly seemed to be gradual but also somehow inevitable. In 1982 when I first began community psychiatric nursing, research efforts seemed few and far between. The Springfield study, led by Paykel, had been completed and was near to publication. A significant watershed, as it was to be the first comparative research study to examine CPN outcome prospectively.

I remember visiting Hastings on a cold and blustery morning to hear about research being conducted by Edward White in relation to general practitioners and their referral patterns to CPNs. I can also recall a trip to Manchester Polytechnic, accompanied by Sue Simmons, to look at students' research projects completed while attending the ENB 810 course in community psychiatric nursing. The Manchester CPN course had an excellent reputation and notable luminaries in the field such as Paddy Carr and Tony Butterworth were responsible for its leadership.

Important though these efforts were they did not satisfy the appetite completely. Surely, the activity of community psychiatric nursing needed a far more systematic and substantial research base than this? I became convinced personally that this was the direction in which my own career would develop and fortuitously was approached and asked to become the Research Officer to the Community Psychiatric Nurses' Association. The immediate task that beset me in this new undertaking was the design and conduct of the Second Quinquennial National CPN Survey. To carry out this work, in tandem with my role as a practising CPN, would have been onerous without a sympathetic employer.

I was extremely fortunate because at that time I worked in the Bloomsbury Health Authority where Paul Beard was my immediate manager and Christine Hancock the District Nursing Officer. Their recognition and help was invaluable and I happily acknowledge that Paul Beard, in particular, is a person whose enthusiasm, drive, and support through the years must bear a great deal of the responsibility for the ultimate production of this book.

The National Survey was finally published in 1985 and in concert with the 1980 CPN survey, produced by David McKendrick, provided a picture of change over a 5 year period of various salient aspects of community psychiatric nursing practice. It was established, for example, that the CPN workforce had increased dramatically; that CPN specialization was far more prevalent than anyone had previously imagined; that referrals from psychiatrists were diminishing whereas referrals from GPs were on the increase. In summary, for the first time, this comparative longitudinal snapshot view allowed those involved with the development of community psychiatric nursing, to peer through the fog and gain some idea of the ways in which this branch of nursing was evolving.

It is a source of some pleasure to me that this series of data is now in the process of being extended. The English National Board has now funded the Third Quinquennial Survey of community psychiatric nursing, full time research which is being undertaken by Edward White, the current research officer of the CPNA, in the Department of Nursing at the University of Manchester. This work will undoubtedly extend our knowledge of developments in CPN practice much further.

However, the 1985 survey was only the first faltering step down the long road of research involving the activities of CPNs. In the last five years many projects have been undertaken and this book contains a good sample of these. Broadly, the research presented here covers three main areas: management, clinical practice, and education, and different motives have prompted all the chapter authors to frame their research question in a particular way. For example, Helen Lee, Rachel Munton and Liz Matthew's contributions have been responses to local problems/issues which have generated findings with a relevance for CPN's day to day practice. John Mangen and Maura Hunt describe research which has been implemented throughout an entire Regional Health Authority. Phil Wolsey, Sue Simmons, Linda Pollock and Edward White have individually examined substantive areas with important implications for community psychiatric nursing as part of their registration for higher degrees. On the other hand, Jan Illing and Chris Atha have collaborated in multidisciplinary research which has been externally funded.

This book, however, can only be a signpost down the long road that was mentioned earlier. Perhaps the most encouraging marker that the journey is now well and truly underway is the interest that has been demonstrated recently by the Department of Health in centrally funding a wide range of CPN orientated research work. These projects are examining: the training of CPNs in psychosocial intervention strategies; the work undertaken by CPNs in the primary health care setting and the CPN's role with the elderly person suffering from depression. The CPN's role is also being examined within schemes looking at aspects of innovative multidisciplinary team-work, for example the Early Intervention Scheme and the Daily Living Project.

It has been a decade in which many changes have occurred. The Health Service has been substantially reorganized, and care in the community will radically alter in the next few years as social service departments become the lead agency in the delivery of care. In the midst of all this change, CPNs continue to offer the best care they possibly can to people who are beset by mental health problems.

My hope is that this book also demonstrates that the past decade has witnessed an upsurge in credible community psychiatric nursing research which, ultimately, will inform this delivery of care.

Charles Brooker
University of Manchester

CHAPTER ONE

The role of the CPN with clients who deliberately harm themselves

Chris Atha

SUMMARY

For a number of years there has been an interest in the value of community psychiatric nurses (CPNs) working in the emergency setting. It was originally mentioned in the document published by the Department of Health and Social Security (DHSS, 1981) as an area in which CPNs would work in the future. Despite this statement from the DHSS very little development in this area has taken place. Since this publication other considerations have been taken into account the first being that of current political policy of shifting care of the mentally ill into the community and closure of large psychiatric hospitals. One of the results of this change in policy is to leave the psychiatric population with an inadequate community service. A likely outcome of this is that the Accident and Emergency (A&E) department will be the only easily available facility providing 24-hour care for those with psychiatric problems, including a growing number of disturbed former in-patients. In the future patients who normally receive care on a 24-hour basis as in-patients in psychiatric hospitals will no longer have this available to them. For many of these individuals the A&E department will represent the only medical facility available to them on demand. Thus, in the absence of alternative care A&E departments will understandably have increasing demands made on them by this client group.

Whilst it may be a little unusual for a CPN to be based within an A&E department I hope to show its importance as a point of referral for patients who are having psychological difficulties and who are discharged into the community. In this chapter the involvement of CPNs as a way of delivering care to this group in the community will be described.

The research was developed from the individual demands of patients but many of the ideas for clinical research came from the nurses working in the emergency setting. The ideas were generated by nurses' interest in what happened to patients after discharge from hospital. Here are some examples of questions they seemed to require answers for: Why does a particular patient return so often? What has happened to that lady? Was he depressed? It was the nurses inquiring about clinical practice that inspired this work. We need to develop and examine more closely the most appropriate type of nursing care to give to our patients. When looking at future roles in nursing the opportunity should be taken to do this in a scientific way. This is what we set out to achieve with our research.

BACKGROUND

First we have to examine the setting in which the study took place. The research CPN was attached to the psychiatric liaison team which comprises a 16-bedded in-patient facility and a psychiatric medical team consisting of two social workers, a clinical psychologist, a CPN and an occupational therapist. The majority of the team's clinical time is spent dealing with referrals from general wards and assessment of self-harm patients. Whilst working closely with the general medical facility the liaison team forms part of an integral service with other psychiatric teams within the Leeds Western Health Authority. Other psychiatric services tend to cover a defined geographical area, with the exception of the more specialized services.

One important feature of the liaison unit and the A&E department is the close working relationship that has been developed over a number of years through sharing ideas and mutual interest in nursing research. The A&E department catchment area covers mainly the inner city area served by Leeds Western Health Authority. The population it serves is around 400000 people. The A&E department deals with an average of about 350 patients per day. As a result of this work-load a computerized based A&E record system (CAER) has been introduced in recent years. Since the introduction of this system it is much easier to access information and records. One benefit of this type of system is that you can 'flag' patients for future attendances or alert the appropriate services. The CAER system can be used in a similar way to the 'at risk' register for children with non accidental injury. This enabled us to keep track of patients during the study without the laborious task of searching through endless records.

As the working relationships of the liaison unit and the A&E department developed, ideas about future care and treatment began to emerge. One proposal put forward was to place a CPN in the A&E department, this idea gave the opportunity not only to look at the type of involvement a CPN could have, but also to develop a research project looking into the effectiveness of a CPN attached to the A&E department. A number of questions needed to be addressed, however, before this could occur. Was there any value in placing a CPN in the A&E department? Would the patients benefit from such an arrangement? Should we alter already existing clinical practice? Many of these dilemmas were to become part of the research process that we would need to grapple with.

EXPLORATORY WORK

The obvious starting point for the study was to measure existing practice. Therefore a CPN began to take referrals from the emergency team. These were made on the assumption that patients would benefit from psychological help delivered by the CPN. After collecting data over an 18 month period the referrals were divided into two groups of patients. The first group consisted of patients identified as having formal psychiatric problems, i.e. those with psychiatric diagnoses and histories. In the second group were patients who seemed to frequently return to the department, mainly with minor physical complaints. The emergency team noticed that despite medical treatment the more incapacitating psychological problems remained.

After the initial attendance we began to collect data on both these groups of patients. We measured the amount of National Health Service (NHS) use of both groups six months prior to CPN intervention. We collected the same data during the six month treatment period (although treatment only lasted on average six to eight weeks) and the six month follow-up period. Treatment was carried out at home. Some involvement of family members, general practitioners (GPs) and local resources took place. Behavioural techniques were used when appropriate and referrals made to other specialist services when the need arose. We therefore collected data over an 18 month period consisting of a general count up of service use. Whilst this type of measurement is crude in terms of research, it gave us an important indication about the CPNs effect during clinical practice and the follow-up period.

As Figures 1.1 and 1.2 show, a clear pattern began to emerge from this pilot work. The results show that it is possible that the CPN is effecting a considerable change in patients referred. The major consequence being a reduction in their demands on NHS facilities and emergency services. Over the 18-month period in which data was collected there was a substantial drop in the use of NHS facilities, when compared to the pre-treatment stage. One of the differences emerging from the two groups of data was the increase in service use by the group with no previous psychiatric history. As shown in Figure 1.2 this took place immediately after CPN intervention. This was accounted for by the CPN making new referrals to psychiatric out-patient clinics, day hospitals and other psychiatric services.

The psychiatric history group shows, in Figure 1.2, a gradual reduction

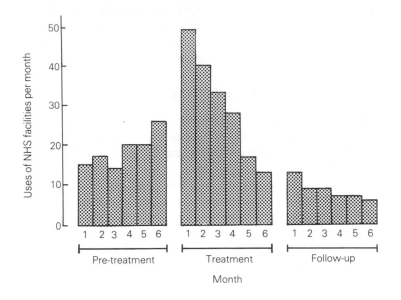

Figure 1.1 Patients with no previous psychiatric history (*n*=58).

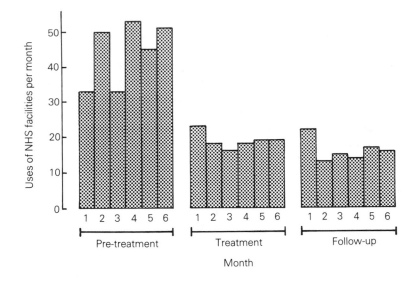

Figure 1.2 Patients with previous psychiatric history (*n*=41).

of service use during the treatment period which is maintained at follow-up. These results are very interesting but we could not tell if individuals had made any improvements although we suspect from the results that it might be so. However, it may be that they are staying away from the services and are being distressed at home.

Therefore, one of the ways in which we chose to answer this question more fully was to carry out a controlled trial on a similar group of patients. The comparison we wanted to make was between the effectiveness of treatment delivered by a CPN and that of existing treatment. This obviously had wider implications for clinical practice and the feasibility of research in this busy setting. We already had some important information gained from the pilot work. Gathering further information was difficult because the subject area is largely new and very little has been described as far. A major part of the study would have to be experimental both in terms of research design and approach to treatment.

Our first task was to define the research more clearly from the earlier work and in consultation with the A&E staff our ideas emerged.

The assumptions were that:

1. Non essential attendance may result in poor efficiency of the A&E department.
2. Psychological factors may operate in the patients' decision to attend the A&E department.
3. Early detection and treatment of the psychological difficulties may lead to more efficient use of NHS facilities.

Once our assumptions were formulated we then looked at a systematic way of developing our research. Before this could take place, we needed to be more explicit about who was going to be treated than we had been in our previous work. Our proposed treatment had to have flexibility, because if it showed that a large number of people attend with yet undetected psychological difficulties then the treatment would have to be adjusted to take this into account.

An important aspect of this work is to look at the questions which are relevant to clinical work and to do this in a systematic way. As shown in Table 1.1 we were examining both theoretical and practical issues, which is important when carrying out any research of this kind.

Our first practical task in Study 1 was to answer the question: how many people were attending the A&E department with psychological difficulties and could we easily identify who these people were? Another consideration was could we identify people that may benefit from CPN intervention rather than leaving the choice about which patients to refer to the A&E staff, as happened in the pilot study. We chose to use a large sub-sample of patients attending the A&E department (obviously we could not take

Table 1.1 Research and clinical questions for the A&E research project

Research questions	Practical issues
Study 1	
What is the incidence of psychiatric disturbance in A&E amongst non-psychiatric attenders?	How big a problem is there?
Study 2	
Is the disturbance transient (lasts less than one month after A&E attendance)?	Do patients really need treatment?
Study 3	
Can this be simply predicted?	Will it be easy to choose patients for treatment?
Study 4	
Is a time limited, problem solving treatment effective with other patients attending A&E for apparently non-psychiatric reasons?	How cost-effective is it to have a CPN working in A&E?
Study 5	
Is a time limited, problem solving treatment effective in preventing repeat overdoses in a group at very high risk of repeat?	How can we best combine a CPN's work with existing facilities to deal with a major continuing clinical problem?

everybody because of the large number of patients attending in any one week). This would give us details on the difficulties patients were having and the type of help a CPN could hope to provide.

Study 1 What is the incidence of psychiatric disturbance in A&E amongst non-psychiatric attenders?

A series of screening studies were designed in an attempt to answer this particular question. The screening studies were carried out over six-hour periods on different days in the week. All attenders at the A&E department were requested to complete a series of questionnaires before receiving medical attention.

Patients were excluded if they (a) were too ill to complete question-naires, (b) under 16 years of age or over 65, (c) intoxicated with drugs or alcohol or (d) attending for psychiatric reasons. In this part of the screening process we used three scales. 1. The Goldberg General Health Question-naire (GHQ) (Goldberg and Hillier, 1979) which has been widely used to detect psychiatric disturbance within the general population. 2. The Hospital Anxiety and Depression scale (HAD) (Zigmond and Snaith, 1983), which is a similar scale but more extensively used in the medical out-patient clinics. 3. We designed our own nine item Health Care Questionnaire (HCQ) with 'true' or 'false' responses. Our reason for developing a separate scale was to devise a simple questionnaire, that would predict the more severe cases identified by the other two assessment schedules. The majority of patients screened at this time attended with minor physical complaints. Often these people are commonly known as the 'walk in' cases. Included in the screening studies were acute medical and surgical cases that arrived by the emergency services. A full explanation and help were both given on request. We had only one refusal on the initial screening and the majority found it useful whilst waiting to receive medical help, which at times can be a lengthy process in an A&E department. Table 1.2 gives the results from our initial screening study.

FREQUENT ATTENDERS

Our screening study shows that there is a higher proportion of patients with psychological problems found in the A&E department compared with the general population. Over 25% were picked out as having some psycho-logical difficulties such as panic disorder and depression on both the GHQ and HAD scales. As part of the screening procedure we excluded people attending for overt psychiatric consultation, i.e. for acute psychosis, drug abuse and parasuicide attempt. If we include this group and the 25% identified by the GHQ and HAD scales then the potential number of referrals over a year could be enormous.

Table 1.2 Results of the initial screening study (143 patients screened; follow-up rate 93%)

	GHQ	HAD depression	HAD anxiety
Index attendance (%)	24	8	28
Follow-up at one month (%)	26	13	34

Study 2 Is the psychological disturbance transient?

As part of the design of study we repeated the screening one month later.

It is possible that our results could have been explained by psychological problems arising from physical trauma which would remit once the physical problems had been treated. To answer this particular question we repeated the screening a month after the index visit to the A&E department, with the identical group of patients. This was done by post, a reminder letter was sent, followed by a home visit if no response had been received. This method allowed us to receive a completed follow-up rate of 93%, although our sample did not include people of no fixed abode.

As the results show in Table 1.1, taking their problems to the A&E department did not solve them. In some cases the difficulties worsened as seen on the measures during the follow-up period. These results demonstrated the types of patients that would be more suitable for treatment. These fell into two groups:

1. The injury is secondary to an existing psychological problem.
2. The injury may give rise to the psychological problem but it persists.

There was no difficulty in identifying groups of people with severe psychological problems by using questionnaires, although it was a time consuming practice. We therefore had to design a way in which psychological assessment could be integrated into routine patient care without interfering with the efficiency of a busy A&E department. We examined our data from our screening studies in an attempt to try and solve this difficulty.

Study 3 Can the psychological disturbance be simply predicted?

At this stage in the research it was felt important to be able to identify patients with psychological problems who would accept treatment using our screening measures without interfering with the overall efficiency of a busy A&E department.

Interestingly, the HCQ correlated significantly with high scores on the GHQ and the HAD in two important areas where patients made positive responses.

1. Do you feel that it would be useful to talk to someone from the hospital about your worries after you go home?
2. Do you have any problems which make coping with everyday life difficult?

The results demonstrated (a) that these patients had difficulty in coping and (b) that they were willing to accept treatment/intervention. We there-fore used the CAER to 'flag' up a small group of these patients ($n=15$) and compared them with an identical number of matched controls. We found that the 'predicted patients' attended the A&E department a total of 19 times compared with three visits by the comparison group over the next three months. This study was repeated using a larger sample and similar results were found which were statistically significant ($p < 0.005$). Also the scores that were achieved on the measurement scales indicated that we had picked a particularly severe client group.

DEVELOPMENT OF A CPN'S ROLE

It is not clear until you have examined things in a systematic way, for example identified the patient groups and assessed the amount of service involvement (as done in this study), that you can begin to develop the CPN role in this type of setting. This needs to be understood before any inter-vention programme can begin.

The results of the screening studies showed that any CPN involvement with the A&E team would be potentially difficult. If we assume that the CPN would be expected also to deal with the patients who attend for psychiatric reasons (such as the self-harm group) and the people with undetected psychological problems found in our screening studies then the potential numbers are considerable. We then have to look at the role closely in order to define the way a CPN can expect to reasonably operate. If inappropriate tasks, such as engaging in any long-term psychotherapy, psychiatric rehabilitation or monitoring injections, were excluded the most appropriate use of CPN skills that could be carried out in the emergency department are as follows:

1. To act as a resource for the emergency department staff; as the majority of patients are discharged home, it is helpful for staff to be able to consult with the CPN about what community mental health services are available.
2. To provide a liaison between psychiatric teams and the A&E depart-ments. In our team the CPN is able to refer to other specialities within the multidisciplinary psychiatric team and use in-patient facilities if necessary, such as addiction and alcohol services.
3. To offer support (informally and formally) with respect to psycho-logical difficulties with patients when they arise. A&E is a very stressful area in which to work and burn-out rates amongst nurses have been shown to be high.
4. To act as an educator for A&E staff with respect to the assessment of and help they provide to patients with psychological difficulties. In

some cases this may mean an element of therapy supervision for the A&E staff.

5. To carry out brief time limited treatment interventions; these might include:

    (a) crisis intervention and crisis counselling for people who have chronic coping difficulties, based on cognitive–behavioural problem solving intervention;

    (b) time limited cognitive–behavioural intervention for neurotic conditions such as anxiety disorders (for example panic attacks being a frequent reason for attendance at A&E).

When CPN developments of a similar nature take place consideration will have to be given to existing psychiatric service provision. Once a role definition has been developed within this context then the next priority becomes deciding on the type of appropriate intervention.

Type of intervention used in Studies 4 and 5

Intervention had to be chosen bearing in mind the difficulties in resources already outlined. We had to develop a treatment that would be flexible, that had a great deal of structure and could be applied to a wide range of patient problems. It also needed to have a time limit to it and to be learned by those with a more general training in psychological treatment. The intervention that met these requirements was problem solving therapy. It has been demonstrated by others that the patients such as those we had targeted have a deficit in their ability to solve problems (Schotte and Clum, 1987). Problem solving therapy had been successfully used with psychiatric patients (Linehan *et al.*, 1987) and also in general practice (Gath and Catalan, 1986). We therefore structured the intervention model around a problem solving approach. As part of the intervention we used a wide range of cognitive strategies in the package. Intervention was limited to five hourly sessions, with agreement from the patient. Homework was used between sessions as part of a collaborative process. Members of the family occasionally joined therapy sessions if it was thought to be of therapeutic value. All treatment took place in the patient's home unless it was felt inappropriate. This allowed a more realistic view of the patient's problems and improved the likely efficiency of intervention.

The battery of measurements shown in Table 1.3 were used in both intervention studies with the exception of the Beck Suicidal Ideation Scale which was only used in the self-harm trial. First measure took place immediately after referral and during the assessment procedure before the patient was discharged. During the assessment a problem list was compiled between the CPN and patient. This was then ranked in order of severity

Table 1.3 Measures used in intervention studies

Scale	Description
Beck Suicidal Ideation Scale[a]	Structured interview which measures thoughts, plans and attitudes related to future suicide.
Profile of Mood States[b]	Short self-rating scale, giving scores for depression, vigour, anger, tension, fatigue.
Beck Depression Inventory [c]	Short self-rating scale which measures the severity of depressive symptoms.
Beck and Weissman Hopelessness Scale[d]	Short questionnaire (true/false) measuring degree of hopelessness about the future.
Personal Questionnaire Rapid Scaling Technique[e]	A questionnaire in which the items are generated by the patient as a problem list in the initial interview. Although the problems are personalized, the ratings of each problem are standard, and the use of paired comparisons allows a check of consistency to be made for each item every time it is scored.

[a] Beck, Kovacs and Weissman (1979)
[b] McNair and Lorr (1964)
[c] Beck *et al.* (1961)
[d] Beck *et al.* (1974)
[e] Mulhall (1977)

and rated on the Personal Questionnaire Rapid Scaling Technique (PQRST). This problem list then became the focus for the problem solving intervention in both studies. Assessment and measures were completed on the index day and at the follow-ups after one week, one month, three months, six months and one year.

Study 4 Intervention study

Patients attending the A&E department were screened using a short questionnaire. The first question was: 'Do you feel it would be useful to talk to someone from the hospital about your worries after you go home?' Any positive response to this question would mean they would be willing to accept treatment in the home setting, if it was offered. The second question was: 'Do you have any problems which make coping with everyday life difficult?' A positive reply to this suggested that problem solving therapy with a cognitive component was going to be acceptable and suitable. The effectiveness of these screening questions became more apparent when results were examined as no patients refused intervention or dropped out of the two studies. We chose to incorporate the two questions as part of the A&E nurses' general assessment of the patients. Selection into Study 4 was based on the patients' positive response to the simple predictive questions. Referral then took place before allocation into intervention group or control group. Using this approach increased the level of awareness of psychiatric problems, both overt and undetected. We developed a video teaching package that incorporated work on psychological assessment. As we were unable to take large numbers of nurses out of the department for teaching this seemed the most appropriate method. Further work is needed to assess the validity of this method of teaching.

COMPARING INTERVENTION

In the earlier pilot study we looked at substantial change using a longer series of measurements. The results were not sufficient to conclude that any change was due to intervention alone. The only way we could determine whether or not the intervention was effective was to compare the results with those from a group that was assessed and dealt with in the same way. One group receiving treatment in the 'usual way', i.e. a control group, was compared with the experimental intervention group. A controlled trial was therefore designed. All patients gave consent before being randomly allocated to either 'treatment as usual' group or to the experimental intervention group. We decided that a follow-up period of one year was a reasonable length of time to measure any changes that might take place. This is considered an appropriate length of time in studies of this kind. Seventeen intervention and 16 control patients were randomly allocated to this study.

Study 5 Treatment study (self-harm group)

A DHSS document was published in 1984 stating:

> . . . research is needed to establish the most effective patterns of care for patients who deliberately harm themselves, whilst at the same time making better use of scarce resources
>
> (DHSS, 1984).

The resource most in demand by the self-harm group of patients is nurse–patient contact. Research has shown that experienced, trained nurses are as effective in carrying out the assessment and management of self-poisoning as the psychiatrist (Hawton *et al.*, 1981). This increased the value of using scarce resources such as CPNs. The CPN would be the most obvious member of the psychiatric team to effectively and economically manage the self-harm group of patients both in hospital and after discharge into the community. As in Study 4, consideration had to be given to the potential number of referrals. Again, we did this before the research took place. In an average year between 650–800 self-harm referrals are made to the department. As seen in the other study, this creates difficulties for the CPN and resources have to increase to meet this demand. The most appropriate group to study would be a small but high-service user group that makes excessive demands on health resources. This suggests that the obvious choice would be the repeat self-poisoning group of patients.

The selection criteria used in Study 5 are listed below. Several studies have noted that patients fulfilling such criteria have a 50% chance of a repeated attempt of self-poisoning within six months of attendance (Buglass and Horton, 1974).

1. Previous psychiatric care;
2. alcohol related problems (includes excessive drinking);
3. two or more parasuicide admissions;
4. sociopathy (predominant distress of patient's situation falls on society);
5. not living with a relative.

Patients had to fulfil at least 3 of the above criteria before allocation into Study 5 could take place.

Some patient exclusions took place and these were based on: (a) usual age categories, (b) not living within the catchment area, (c) inability to complete rating scales.

The population we chose was a particularly high risk group. Many psychiatrists and nurses would regard this group as 'no hopers', believing that they would not respond to treatment. We wanted to know if treatment would have any affect in reducing overdose rates, although this posed substantial methodological problems. We chose this difficult group hoping to demonstrate any differences in response between these changes on the 'first timers' (people who only take one overdose) who often spontaneously improve. The 'first timers' often show no significant change on self-rating scales. This is because their problems are part of a temporary situation which will quickly resolve itself regardless of whether or not they receive treatment.

After the psychiatrist had completed the routine screening assessment, making sure that the patient was not requiring psychiatric admission or out-patient treatment, patients who then fulfilled the sample criteria were randomly allocated into one of the two groups. The study was designed in an identical manner to Study 4, we were comparing our five hourly sessions of problem solving intervention to an already existing service. Twelve intervention and eight control patients were randomly allocated to Study 5. All intervention, measurement and assessment times were identical to Study 4.

The results for both studies were analysed during a repeated measure analysis of covariance, with intervention as the group factor. The characteristics of both studies can be seen in Tables 1.4 and 1.5.

Results for Study 4

Table 1.4 Characteristics of Study 4

Variable	Intervention group		Control group	
	Men	Women	Men	Women
n	7	9	11	5
Age	32.2	30.0	29.3	27.8
Marital status (single : marr. : sep. : div.)	4:2:0:1	5:2:1:1	5:3:2:1	2:1:2:0
Previous A&E attendances (12 months)	21	24	30	13

Interview-based measure

Personal Questionnaire Rapid Scaling Technique. During the index assessment the three main problems were identified and analysed. The effects of treatment on the first rated problem were not found to be significant. However on the second rated problem there was a significant 'time × group interaction' effect ($p < 0.05$), indicating a more rapid decrease in problems occurring with the intervention group. The third rated problem did not show any statistical significance.

Self-rating

a) Beck Depression Inventory. This scale showed the importance of the selection criteria in that the means for the whole group was 27.4 which is well into the clinical depressed range. However, there was no evidence of any intervention effect. The one-year follow-up mean depression score of 21.2 indicates the lack of any intervention effect.

b) Beck and Weissman Hopelessness Scale. Hopelessness scores revealed a significant 'group' × sex' interaction ($p < 0.05$) indicating that intervention had the effect of reducing hopelessness in women but not in men. None of the other interactions approached significance.

c) Profile of Mood States. The Profile of Mood States showed no significant main effects or interactions for the anxiety, fatigue and tension sub-scales. The vigour sub-scale showed a significant group effect ($p < 0.05$) with the treated group showing higher vigour scores.

d) Re-attendance at A&E. In the treated group 30.9% of the patients returned for further consultation compared with 56% of the control group. This difference was statistically significant ($p < 0.05$).

Results for Study 5

Table 1.5 Characteristics of Study 5

Variable	Intervention group	Control group
n	12	8
Mean age (s.d.)	26.42 (5.95)	28.5 (7.91)
Sex ratio (Male:female) (%female)	5:7 (58%)	5:3 (38%)
Marital status (single:marr.:sep.:div.)	6:3:1:2	2:3:0:3

Interview-based measures

a) Beck Suicidal Ideation Scale. In Study 4 the suicidal ideation sub-scale I (which measures attitude towards living/dying) showed no group effect or group × time effect.

For scale II (measures control over suicidal action/acting-out wish) there was a significant group effect ($p < 0.025$), but no group × time effect. No significant effects were found on the remaining sub-scale.

b) Personal Questionnaire Rapid Scaling Technique. As in Study 4 the three main problems were analysed. The means for these main problems are shown in Figure 1.3.

There was a significant group effect for problem 1 ($p < 0.005$), but the group × time effect was not significant. For problem 2 the group effect was also significant ($p > 0.001$) but as with problem 1 there was not a group × time effect. The third rated problem also showed significance for group effect ($p < 0.005$) while the group × time effect again was not significant. Therefore the problem solving intervention group showed significantly better overall results on their three main problems compared to the group that received 'treatment as usual'.

Self-rating scales

a) Beck Depression Inventory. The initial index scores show very high levels of depression for the intervention group 31.7 and for the control

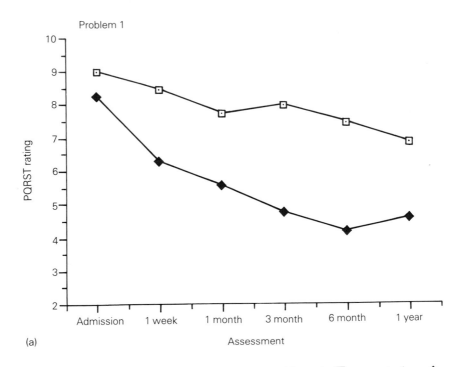

(a)

Figure 1.3 PQRST ratings of the three main problems (—☐— , controls; —◆— , treated).

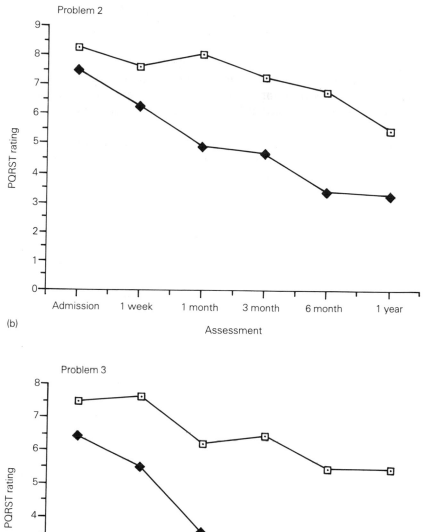

Problem 2

(b)

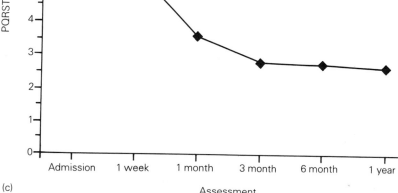

Problem 3

(c)

group 30.3. The cut-off for clinical depression is 12 on the Beck Depression Inventory. The results show a main group effect ($p < 0.005$) but no group × time interaction.

b) Beck and Weissman Hopelessness Scale. The hopelessness scale also showed a significant main effect on post-intervention hopelessness scores ($p > 0.01$) with group × time effect not being significant.

c) Profile of Mood States. Significant group effects were found for depression ($p < 0.001$) and fatigue ($p < 0.05$) on these sub-scales, and a significant group × time interaction was found for tension ($p < 0.01$).

d) Re-attendance at A&E. This is shown in Table 1.6 for the first six months after the indexed suicide attempt. The difference between proportions of patients repeating a suicide attempt in the six months after the index attempt was significantly different ($p < 0.049$).

DISCUSSION AND IMPLICATIONS FOR CLINICAL PRACTICE

Both studies showed that a brief psychological intervention had the effect of reducing distress amongst the patients attending an A&E department. It also showed that the need for such intervention is considerable, the index depression scores for the Beck Depression Inventory and Beck and Weissman Hopelessness Scale were well into the clinical range. However, the extent of improvement was most seen in patients that attempted suicide and in their individual problems. The results from Study 5 confirmed our

Table 1.6 Number of patients repeatedly attempting suicide, Study 5

Group	Previous frequency of attempts		Repeat suicide attempts six months after allocation to the study	
	Mean	s.d.	Number of patients	Number of attempts per patient
Intervention n=12	2.58	0.9	0 (0%)	0
Control n=8	3.0	0.93	3 (37%)	4

feelings that in the future the CPN will become the most appropriate person to deal with this patient group.

In Study 4 it seems that the intervention may need to be more specifically tailored to the characteristics of this population. The idea behind the study was to apply problem solving in the same way as in parasuicide study. During Study 4 it became evident that the referral was less likely to occur in the acute crisis and in the context of a more medical/somatic pre-occupation. This is sometimes reinforced by the medical services. Future research by CPNs will have to take this into account by using interventions which retain the problem solving approach but de-emphasize crisis management. The research should specifically be targeting physical concerns. Another major factor to emerge from Study 4 was that the five hourly sessions were not going to make a lasting impact on such a chronic and severely psychopathological group. This was reinforced by two patients making suicidal attempts in the course of Study 4.

In Study 5 the intervention outcome results are seen to be more sub-stantial, particularly in reducing the distress experienced by patients at high risk of repeated suicide attempts. Shorter term effectiveness in terms of repeated attempts was also demonstrated. The use of individualized outcome measures is an important advance in this type of study, as it allows the impact of intervention on main problems identified by each patient. This is especially relevant as intervention focused on training in problem solving. A further important factor was that no patients dropped out of the two groups studied. This shows the importance of CPN intervention in the community. However, it is difficult to evaluate an intervention package of this kind, and the contribution of different components of intervention. As intervention was carried out by one CPN we cannot rule out that the response was therapist specific. Also the amount of repeated home assess-ments carried out may have had some impact on the control group. Whilst not conclusive, the present study appears to indicate that a brief problem solving package is effective in reducing distress experienced by a group of repeated suicide attempters and has an impact on the repeated attempts in the short term.

Using patients attendance at A&E departments is a way of identifying at least some of the more distressed patients needing psychiatric intervention. This seems to be practical and acceptable to patients such as those seen in the study. It seems that such patients are highly distressed and have not solved the problems in previous visits when no such service was available to them. Providing psychiatric out-patient care is rarely acceptable to this group of patients. The efficiency of medical emergency facilities would be enhanced if patients with distress leading to consultation that was psycho-logically determined, could be more appropriately treated with the attach-ment of a CPN to A&E departments. This seems to be the most cost-effective strategy in the absence of an acceptable psychiatric emergency service.

ACKNOWLEDGEMENTS

The author is grateful to the staff of the Psychiatric Liaison Team and the Accident and Emergency departments of Leeds General Infirmary for their co-operation. Special thanks go to Paul Salkovskis for his enormous contribution to this study and to A.F. for a new beginning. The study was supported in part by Grant LW 49 from the special trustees of the Leeds General Infirmary.

REFERENCES

Beck, A.T., Kovacs, M. and Weissman, A. (1979) Assessment of suicidal intention: the scale for suicidal ideation. *Journal of Consulting and Clinical Psychology*, **47**, 343–52.

Beck, A.T., Ward, C.H., Mendelsohn, M., Mock, J. and Erbaugh, J. (1961) An inventory for measuring depression. *Archives of General Psychiatry*, **4**, 561–71.

Beck, A.T., Weissman, A., Lester, D. and Trexler, L. (1974) The measurement of pessimism: the hopelessness scale. *Journal of Consulting and Clinical Psychology*, **42**, 861–5.

Buglass, D. and Horton, J. (1974) A scale for predicting subsequent suicidal behaviour. *British Journal of Psychiatry*, **124**, 573–8.

Department of Health and Social Security (1981) *The development of the community psychiatric nursing service*, CNO (81), HMSO, London.

Department of Health and Social Security (1984) *The management of deliberate self harm*, 1HN(84)25, HMSO, London.

Gath, D. and Catalan, J. (1986) The treatment of emotional disorders in general practice: psychological methods *v.* medication. *Journal of Psychosomatic Practice*, **30**, 381–6.

Goldberg, D.P. and Hillier, V.F. (1979) A scaled version of the general health questionnaire. *Psychological Medicine*, **9**, 139–45.

Hawton, K., Bancroft, J., Catalan, J., Kingston, B., Stedeford, A. and Welch, N. (1981) Domiciliary and outpatient treatment of self-poisoning patients by medical and non-medical staff. *Psychological Medicine*, **11**, 169–77.

Hawton, K., Salkovskis, P.M., Kirk, J.W. and Clark, D.M. (1989) *Cognitive Behaviour Therapy for Psychiatric Problems: a practical guide*, Oxford University Press, Oxford.

Linehan, M.M., Camper, P., Chiles, J.A., Strosahl, K. and Shearin, E. (1987) Interpersonal problem solving and parasuicide. *Cognitive Therapy and Research*, **133**, 111–18.

McNair, D.M. and Lorr, M. (1964) An analysis of mood states in neurotics. *Journal of Abnormal and Social Psychology*, **69**, 620–7.

Mulhall, D. (1977) *Personal Questionnaire Rapid Scaling Technique (Manual)*, National Foundation for Educational Research, Windsor.

Schotte, D.E. and Clum, G.A. (1987) Problem solving skills in suicide psychiatric patients. *Journal of Consulting and Clinical Psychology,* **55**, 49–54.

Zigmond, A.S. and Snaith, R.P. (1983) The hospital anxiety and depression scale. *Acta Psychiatrica Scandinavica,* **67**, 361–70.

CHAPTER TWO

A role for the CPN in supporting the carer of clients with dementia

Liz Matthew

SUMMARY

This study is concerned with the carers of people with dementia, and how information is communicated to them, both to increase their understanding of the nature of the illness and to make them aware of services available to help.

A questionnaire was administered to a sample of informal carers on community psychiatric nurses' (CPNs) case-loads ($n=32$) that was followed up by selective secondary interview. The results highlighted the lack of communication on the part of the health care professional in general and the CPN in particular, and a lack of understanding by the carer.

Consequently, the study suggests that the CPNs develop a role of facilitator in helping carers for people with dementia. This includes having a recognizable strategy for the planning, implementation and evaluation of care, the establishment of closer working relationships with other health care professionals and a generally more pro-active role in supporting families that care for a client with dementia at home. Additionally, they should take on a key role in advising as well as counselling and taking account of the social and political issues which relate to their clients.

THE CPN AND THE CARERS OF PEOPLE WITH DEMENTIA – A LITERATURE REVIEW

The role of the carer has begun to figure more highly in the nursing literature over the last five years. There have also been attempts, although not on the same scale, to clarify the role of the 'elderly' CPN, but little has been produced which links both these subjects.

Although it is recognized that work with elderly people is the most common specialism for CPNs (Community Psychiatric Nurses' Association, 1985; Simmons and Brooker, 1987), most research has been descriptive and tackles the CPN's function in a generic way, arguing that the basic philosophies of community nursing are the same whichever client group is being worked with.

Pollock (1988), in her evaluation of the work of CPNs suggests that they are not interested in helping the carer to cope unless this is beneficial to the client or the CPN's management of the client. This she attributes to the CPN's focus on the client rather than the context in which the client lives.

This theme is reiterated by Simmons and Brooker (1987) and elaborated by Adams (1987). Adams suggests that the family should be considered as a system in itself. This would help prevent nurses relying solely on the medical model when dealing with people who have dementia. He also recommends the use of interventions such as family, grief and problem solving therapy as well as assertiveness training. Other potential functions of the CPN have also been reviewed. Clist and Brant (1986) suggest that CPNs take a much more active part in the primary health care team. Georghiou (1986) on the other hand concentrates on education and training. He is specifically concerned with CPNs working with the elderly and their role in supporting care for people with dementia in aged persons' homes. He describes the role of the CPN here as that of a clinical advisor.

The ability of the CPN to deliver an effective service was questioned by Watkins (1985) who studied the Italian experience of treatment in the community. She is concerned that the time needed to provide adequate support to the carer would not be available if caseload numbers remained the same as at present.

A study of general practitioners' (GPs) perceptions of the CPN (Conhye, 1987) was more favourable, most responses being positive and recognizing the potential of the CPN's work. However, some GPs were unaware of the CPN or were unclear of the role and function of the CPN.

One of the strongest advocates of nursing intervention in supporting carers is Robinson (1988). As well as identifying general problems, she highlights particular areas where nurses can help – support with difficult tasks, distributing information or establishing carer support groups. She also makes reference to the economic and political factors affecting support.

Intervention cannot be totally effective unless carers are involved in planning their dependant's care and this has been supported by research undertaken in Surrey (Bloomfield, 1986). These findings support the results of this study concerning the needs of carers and will be discussed more fully later.

The Community Psychiatric Nurses' Association and the Psychiatric

Nurses' Association have produced a paper which reports the results of a working group that had drawn up some recognized problem areas for working with elderly people, both at home and in residential settings (Corea, 1987). They felt that a prime issue for the CPN is a confusion about their role in that in the past, it has been easier to recognize physical problems, nurses have therefore concentrated on support based around a medical model. The paper suggests that nurses redefine their role using highly sophisticated psychological and social nursing approaches in order to support psychiatric services for elderly people outside the context of hospital.

Godin (1987) studied a community psychiatric nursing service, questioning clients on the quality of the service they had received and used similar questions to this survey, for example: Did the CPN understand their problem? Could the CPN help with their problem? Were they satisfied with the service? Generally speaking, clients had few complaints about the service but their expectations were also low.

There is wide ranging evidence in the literature that carers of people suffering from dementia experience stress. Gilhooly (1984) found that the tasks of caring took up a large part of the day and she identified the characteristic behaviours of people with dementia. These included night wanderings, bizarre and dangerous behaviours, mood disturbances and demands for attention. These are problematic behaviours for carers to cope with and have also been described elsewhere (Sanford, 1975; Hirschfeld, 1978).

Other authors have suggested, on the other hand, that it is the dementing client's mental state that causes more stress than coping with physical infirmity *per se* (Grad and Sainsbury, 1965; Gilleard, 1982; Wheatley, 1979).

The alleviation of stress by nursing intervention to meet carers' needs has been considered in more depth lately and the more recent literature deals with practical problem solving issues. Watkins (1988) suggests the use of a dementia stress management model based on information giving and promoting problem solving within the family unit, she also suggests strategies for the nurse to deal with this.

One such strategy is the provision of respite care schemes. Tyler (1987) carried out a national study of respite schemes and not unnaturally found a discrepancy in the quality of schemes provided. One of the key issues was whether the intention of respite was to merely provide a substitute care-taking arrangement or whether it should include any therapeutic intervention. The results showed a desperate need for such services. MacGuire (1987) describes a project in Staffordshire which has provided evidence of an 'unexpressed demand' and the importance of involving the family in planning. Adams (1988) on the other hand, concentrates on the psychological effects on carers and points out that respite, alone, will not alleviate their worries entirely as caring itself has an almost unabated effect on the carers' own mental health status.

The whole problem of stress on carers is provoking discussion within the profession as illustrated by the report of the Royal College of Nursing Association of Care for the Elderly (Mangan, 1988). The subject was considered at some length at the Queen's Nursing Institute Conference in 1987 and is reported by Campbell (1987). The problems appear to be similar in the USA and a summary can be found in Baillie, Norbeck and Barnes, 1988. One study of particular interest focuses on relatives involved in hospital care in New York, here the family provides care whilst the nurse acts as both assessor and educator (Doscher, 1986).

There is now a growing interest in carers and their needs. The findings of three studies completed in 1984 have the greatest relevance to this research. Rogerson (1984) examined 127 carers in Derbyshire and Bonny (1984) looked at 60 carers in Southwark. These studies were essentially a series of questionnaires and brief observations. Both highlighted the role of women and Bonny (1984) was particularly concerned with the amount of care the family provided without help. The third study was a national survey by the Equal Opportunities Commission (EOC, 1984) and followed a previous survey (EOC, 1980) questioning 114 carers. As might be expected it was concerned with the role of women and came to the conclusion that their efforts were undervalued and they were obliged to take on the caring role due to social pressure.

More recently, Lewis and Meredith (1988) completed a study of 41 women caring for their mothers. It suggests that the perceptions of service providers tend to neglect the complexities of caring relationships, and uses a series of biographies rather than closed questions and answers to illustrate its point. Although the majority of findings suggest that women generally take on the burden of caring, a local study (Tameside Metropolitian Borough Council, 1988), has found that men can make up a sizeable minority of carers (40%) and that their needs should not be ignored.

One specific area identified as lacking in support is that of services to black elders. Sharman (1985) refers particularly to neglect of support to black carers of dementia sufferers. Cameron, Badger and Evers (1988) attribute this to a failure to put black patients on the nursing agenda, the prevalance of stereotyping and the lack of information about the role of nurses within the black community.

It is only recently that the importance of the CPN is beginning to be high-lighted in the literature. Even so most discussions are of a general nature. Those which deal with elderly people seem to focus on the medical aspects of care rather than the social or political context. Studies of carers needs however, increasingly recognize the latter viewpoint and the role of the family and family participation are considered paramount in effective support. Consequently this study is timely as little exists in the literature which pinpoints the relationship between the needs of carers and the role of the specialist CPN for the elderly.

METHODOLOGY

Initially the research was intended to examine how effectively CPNs communicated information to carers and how it might relieve the stress of caring. The information covered both the causes and effects of dementia, as well as the support services that were available to the carer. Information in this context was defined as concerning: (a) the causes and effects of dementia; (b) local services and support available.

A combination of both quantitive and qualititive methods were employed and a questionnaire designed with both closed and open questions. The aim of the questionnaire was to identify the channels of communication that existed between carers and health care professionals. It also attempted to ascertain if there was a connection between lack of information about dementia and stress in the carer. The intention was then to examine the completed questionnaires and follow up by a telephone call or personal call where appropriate.

The sample was generated by choosing every fifth record from an index of patients referred to the community psychiatric nursing department. Orginally, it was intended to use a sample of 24 but it proved possible only to interview 16 in depth. This illustrated the difficulty of contacting such a group, for example of the 24 who had originally agreed to be interviewed, one carer had been taken into hospital, two dependants had since died and the time-scale was not suitable for the remainder. The attrition rate, therefore, for the targeted sample was 33% ($n=8$). Interviews were conducted in the homes of the participants, often with the dependant present. As the carers took the opportunity to openly discuss their present dilemma it was difficult to be totally objective. In many cases one question was answered with another. In other cases the carers were emotionally distressed at the time of the interview. As a result, after the interview was formally completed, it proved necessary to offer some form of counselling.

When the initial findings were analysed, it was felt that certain areas required a more detailed investigation and particular respondents were followed up for further interview. Not enough information was available on what carers felt their own needs were. The findings on health care workers were surprising and needed further investigation as did those relating to financial status. Although the interviews were structured informally, a series of general questions were asked to direct the conversation. The length of the interviews varied, but they lasted about an hour on average.

As the discussions were tape-recorded the respondents were allowed to answer in their own time and in their own words.

This first study was conducted in 1987. In the early part of 1989, this was extended to a further 16 carers who were given the same questionnaire. This report therefore concerns a total sample of 32 carers generated from referrals to a community psychiatric nursing department over an 18-month period.

FINDINGS

The questionnaire

a) The carer. The study highlighted three areas: the carers themselves; the type of problems their dependants exhibited; and whether or not caring caused them to suffer from stress.

Personal details were collected to build up a profile of the carer, as far as possible, and to compare it to the findings of other studies to gauge how representative the sample was. The dependant's problems were listed to discover the key areas in which a carer might require support and what made most demands on them, both physically and mentally.

The stress of caring was seen as a key issue with possible implications for the role of the CPN. As has been shown, research has consistently demonstrated the pressures of informal care. In particular, Corbin and Strauss (1988) cite the 'Cocoon syndrome' where the carer and dependant deliberately separate themselves from the outside world, this was tested by questions relating to isolation.

The ages of the carers questioned ranged from 34 to 83, their mean age being 68. The majority were in their seventies and the age distribution is shown in Figure 2.1. Sixty-six per cent of the sample were female, 34% were male; as the number of people with dementia is roughly equal between the sexes, this illustrates the concentration of women as carers. The majority of carers were looking after spouses (63%) and only 3% were not related to the dependant.

The length of time that individuals had been caring varied. The longer periods were usually related to other conditions preceding dementia. The most common length of time was between one and five years.

The study was also intended to test the hypothesis that those who worked suffered less stress than those who did not (EOC, 1980, 1984) however, only 28% ($n=9$) of the sample were under 60 years old and so could be reasonably expected to work. Of those young enough, two worked full-time, four part-time and two did not work at all. All those who worked claimed to enjoy it but, with one exception, they found difficulty in combining the tasks of working and caring.

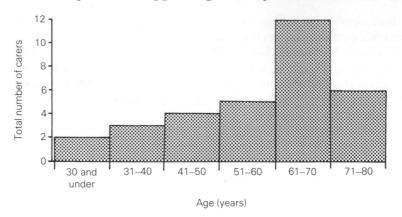

Figure 2.1 The age distribution of carers (mean age = 68 years).

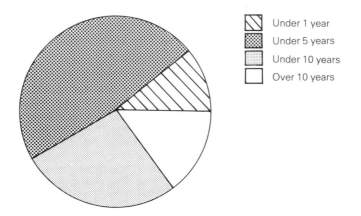

Figure 2.2 Length of caring period (total sample size = 32).

The problems experienced by dependants are listed in Table 2.1 and are typical of those linked to dementia (Hirschfeld, 1978; Machin, 1980). In order to ascertain how affected the carers were by stress they were asked when they had last seen the doctor and why. Fifty-three per cent (n=17) of them had attended a GP's surgery in the last four weeks, the reasons being listed in Table 2.2.

More than one reason for visiting the doctor was often given and the 'stress' category was only used when the carer actually mentioned the word. Although it is difficult to prove that the physical symptoms in the list relate to stress, there was a significant number of instances where the carers

Table 2.1 Difficulties experienced by dependants in rank order

	%	*n*
Remembering things	100	32
Going out alone	97	31
Dressing	88	28
Washing and bathing	88	28
Cooking	84	27
Controlling behaviour	78	25
Going to toilet	69	22
Sleeping	66	21
Walking	59	19
Eating	47	15

Table 2.2 Reasons for visiting GP

Reasons	*Total responses*	*Responses of those visiting in last four weeks*
Heart	8	5
Arthritis	8	4
Stress	5	4
Circulatory	5	2
Gastric	1	—
Back	2	—
Flu	2	1
Menstrual	1	—
Respiratory	2	1

quoted stress as a problem. They were then asked to respond to six state-ments related to stress. These were a mixture of positive and negative statements and were organized so that they did not form a pattern that could be thought to lead the respondent in a certain direction. The responses are given in Table 2.3.

Except for statement (f), all respondents scored highly on stress factors; (f) was included because it had been suggested that lack of money was a common factor amongst carers (EOC,1984). This statement was examined in more detail in the follow-up interview because it seemed incompatible with the other findings.

Table 2.3 Stress statements

Stress statement	Response (%)	n
(a) I usually have an undisturbed night's sleep	66 disagreed	21
(b) Sometimes I don't know where to turn to for help	59 agreed	19
(c) I don't see as much of my friends and relatives as I would like to	81 agreed	26
(d) I never let things get on top of me	84 disagreed	27
(e) Sometimes I feel so frustrated I could cry	88 agreed	28
(f) I often have difficulty making ends meet	81 disagreed	26

b) Initial diagnosis and explanation. One of the primary objectives of the research was to examine the effectiveness of communication between the health care professional and carer and, in particular, the role of the CPN. Gilhooly (1984) had found there was a reluctance for carers to ask for information and a reluctance by some doctors to volunteer it. Saddington (1984) and Muir Gray (1984) had both highlighted the need for the early communication of accurate information and advice and Cloke (1985) highlighted the potential of community health workers in communicating information.

The carers were asked: 'How did you find out about your dependant's illness?', which was intended as an open question. All respondents pointed out that the process was gradual and that there was no particular time when the problem became a crisis. When asked if anyone had explained about their dependant's illness, 22% stated that nobody had (see Figure 2.3). Of those who had, the GP was the most common source of explanation, closely followed by the CPN.

The carers were then asked how long the explanation lasted. As can be seen in Figure 2.4, most explanations were not very long. Interestingly, only one respondent felt that they had been given an in depth explanation and that was as a result of a private consultation.

When asked if there had been any follow-up, either suggesting practical help or by providing further information, 50% (*n*=16) replied positively. Of these, 12 had received written information. These 16 were then asked if they had been referred to anyone. Ten had been referred to a consultant psychogeriatrician. All the other responses were different and included referral to: the CPN, social worker, relative support group, day hospital and meals on wheels.

The sample were asked if they had found out all they wanted to know. The responses were mixed. Forty-one per cent (*n*=13) claimed that they

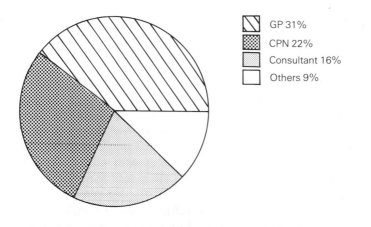

GP 31%
CPN 22%
Consultant 16%
Others 9%

Figure 2.3 Professionals who gave an explanation of the illness. Results relate to the 78% of the sample (*n*=25) that had been given an explanation.

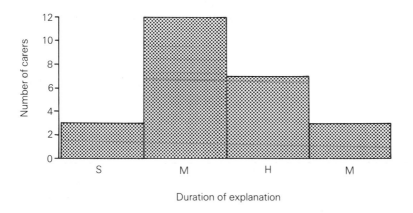

Figure 2.4 Duration of explantion (S, seconds; M, minutes; H, half hour; M, more than half hour).

had found out all that they wanted to know and 37% (*n*=12) had not. When asked if they felt better after receiving the information 37% (*n*=12) felt better, 19% (*n*=6) felt worse and 22% (*n*=7) did not respond. However, only 13% (*n*=4) of the sample felt that they would rather not have known this information.

c) *How formal networks are used.* The study also examined more closely the links between the carer and the health care professionals in order to discover how effective the support offered might be. The role of CPNs was seen as being of particular interest because it was hoped that the study could provide some measure of their effectiveness, as well as comparing them to other workers.

An important point that emerged from the questionnaire interviews was the uncertainty on the part of the carers as to the roles of the various specialists. It also became clear that many had only a vague idea of their exact title. For example a CPN who visited one carer was described as a district nurse. This may partly explain the findings in Table 2.4 when only 53% ($n=7$) of the carers claimed to have contact with CPNs. As the sample was chosen from a file of referrals to CPNs all of them must have had contact at some time or other.

The carers were asked if they had any difficulty in explaining their needs. Seventy-five per cent had experienced no difficulty, but only 44% had been asked what help they needed. The professional cited as being the most helpful was the social worker, followed by the CPN.

d) Information networks. A number of questions were introduced into the questionnaire to test how generally well-informed the carers were. Each respondent was asked whether they had heard of two benefits which may have been relevant to them. These were Invalid Care Allowance and Attendance Allowance. Forty-one per cent ($n=13$) had heard of Invalid Care Allowance and 69% ($n=22$) had heard of Attendance Allowance. From the follow-up interviews it became apparent that although the carers

Table 2.4 Contact with health care professionals/organizations in rank order

	%	*n*
Doctor (GP)	91	29
Social worker	62	20
CPN	53	17
District nurse	47	15
Psychiatrist	47	15
Relative support group	41	13
Home help	31	10
Meals on Wheels	16	5
Geriatrician	13	4
Psychologist	9	3
Health visitor	6	2
Alzheimer's Disease Society	3	1
Age Concern	3	1

may have heard of the allowances most did not understand the conditions for claiming.

Other questions related to services available to give carers a break. Eighty-one per cent (*n*=26) had heard of visits to a day hospital, 59% (*n*=19) had heard of a sitting-in service and 53% (*n*=17) had heard of short breaks in residential homes. Only about half the sample could claim to be informed and awareness of the availability of support did not necessarily mean that it was used, even when appropriate.

The next set of questions were used to elicit to whom carers might turn for help. The results shown in Figures 2.5–2.7 suggest that carers prefer to confide in informal sources rather than the formal health care network.

As a final check they were asked if they felt that any health care professional had not been willing to provide them with information, 13% (*n*=4) felt that this was so.

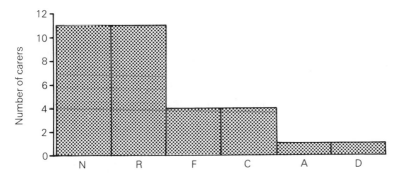

Figure 2.5 Who do you talk your worries over with? (N, nobody; R, relatives; F, friends; C, CPN; A, anybody; D, district nurse).

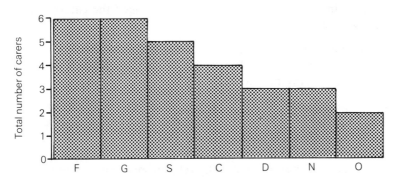

Figure 2.6 If you had a problem who would you contact? (F, family; G, GP; S, social worker; C, CPN; D, district nurse; N, nobody; O, others).

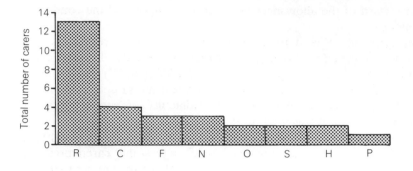

Figure 2.7 Who understands most about your role as a carer? (R, relatives; C, CPN; F, friend; N, nobody; O, other carers; S, social worker; H, hospital; P, consultant psychiatrist).

Follow-up interviews

After the first batch of questionnaires had been completed it became apparent that communicating with health care workers was a significant problem. The questionnaires were examined for examples which highlighted this. Seven participants were identified, but because it was felt that another interview might be personally intrusive for two respondents, only five were interviewed again.

As a result of the answers to the initial questionnaire, it was felt that more data was required on the information that was seen to be important to them, their health care beliefs and their ability to cope financially.

a) Relevant information. One of the objectives of the research was to identify the type of information that carers needed to know. This was done by a general introductory question that encouraged the carers to put forward their own ideas.

> Introductory question: 'Are there any particular areas where you feel you would like to know more. It may be about particular services, or general information. Anything at all?'

It was expected that this would result in a list of priorities but surprisingly, it did not. There were no specific needs identified, their concerns were more general, more basic and more worrying.

One of the carers felt that she needed to be given information regarding her dependant, in circumstances where she relinquished the care to others:

> The day care hospital, examine her and give injections for vitamin supplements and nothing is said unless I discover evidence. I don't like

that. I like to know what the authorities plan for her as I am responsible for her well-being.

More common, however was the assumption that health care workers would decide what care was appropriate, it was therefore irrelevant for them as carers to have information:

I think with the doctor and nurse calling they'll take notice.

Overall there was a feeling of resignation to caring alone, information which offered help was seen to be irrelevant.

b) The role of health care workers. The questionnaire had high-lighted important facts about lack of contact and practical help from health care workers. The follow-up interviews substantiated this.

Introductory question: 'I'd like to know a little about any help you've been offered from the health authority and social work department. Visits from community nurses, social workers for example.'

It seems that health workers do not make contact very often, in some cases not at all.

I never see health workers.
No one comes.

If they do it seems they often appear insensitive and are inept at diagnosing the problem:

They don't realize what you have to put up with. They often mis-interpret your needs. It's luck who you get. Some are OK, others not.
They wouldn't listen to me. They wanted the patient to talk but she couldn't so I had to explain.
I've never been asked what I need. They think you can cope.

It was also clear that most carers had asked for help, but they were usually disillusioned by the response:

I've asked for plenty [of help] but never got it. I feel now it's a waste of time, I'll cope with what I've got.
I don't get the chance to explain what I need. They do their best I suppose. I've asked for help but I haven't got it.

It is often the lack of credibility of the health care workers and their inability to provide support, even of the simplest kind, that causes problems:

When I enquire they say they'll ring you back but they never do.

She came once, said, 'I'll see you in two or three weeks.' That was about six weeks ago and she's not been back since [of the CPN – the carer thought that she was a social worker].

There were other criticisms of the health care network. People could not always differentiate between the specialisms and had little idea of how they were organized. There was also little faith in their ability to work together:

There's a lack of communication. No one sees to know what other professionals are doing.

Not all criticisms were negative, but illustrated some relevant observations:

People who have never coped give sympathy and reassurance but don't know the depth of your experience.

The most common feeling was one of resignation. The majority felt they were on their own and there was little evidence that health care workers did anything significant to alleviate the carers' problems.

They knew I was looking after her. I was entirely on my own. I did everything. I just realized I had to do it.

c) Financial status. It was difficult to ask directly about financial status so carers were invited to take part in a general discussion about money.

Introductory question: It has been suggested that more money should be made available to look after people at home because they cannot go out to work, or are living on a pension. What do you think?

All those interviewed were claiming state pension, and it appeared that this was their major source of income. Although they claimed that money was not a problem, they all gave examples of how difficult it was to manage.

Every time I go shopping it costs more. I have to keep the fire on all the time, he always complains of the cold.
My electrical bills are usually high. My son has offered to help, but he's got a family. I don't like to ask.

There was also evidence that accurate information was lacking on criteria for claiming benefits. Some people had misunderstood what was required:

I get a works pension so I don't see how I could be allowed more money. I didn't bother to claim because I'm not supposed to have it.
I'm not on supplementary benefit so I can't claim things.

Most common however, was the attitude that it was their duty to care without extra financial help, and they appeared to have strong feelings of pride regarding this, often seeing the help offered as being 'charity'.

I can manage with our pension and rate rebate
I make do with what I've got.

d) Health care beliefs. There were no particular questions that related to health care beliefs, but it was noticeable how people viewed dementia and some of their observations illustrated the point that they were not aware in any depth about the causes.

He fell down stairs. I've never said it to anyone else but I think that started it.
I think it started when she had Ménière's disease, she was a confident driver until then.

Summary

The research substantiated the evidence collected by others regarding characteristics of carers. These illustrated the lack of support from statutory services, the predominance of women carers and the stress that caring causes (Rogerson, 1984; Bonny, 1984; Equal Opportunities Commission, 1984).

It was clear that the carers suffered from stress, this was reflected not only in their response to the questions, but also in the attitudes expressed in interviews. For example if the respondent was asked about a service that they had not heard of, they immediately wanted to know more about it.

As a consequence the researcher felt obliged to spend some time counselling and explaining the points she had raised. Gilhooly (1984) had experienced a similar reaction in her Scottish study. As a result the number of clients interviewed had to be limited.

It was apparent that most carers displayed an uncertain attitude to finding out about and accepting help. There was certainly no recognition that it was their right to receive support and in most cases carers thought it was inevitable that they would have to care on their own.

The only exception to this were the younger carers who were also more articulate and assertive in their demands. This difference was particularly highlighted by the fact that the older carers were mainly in their seventies and seemed to adopt a different value system. It would appear from the interviews that the older participants had a higher regard for the authority of doctors and medical staff and tended to be more passive in their accept-ance of care. The younger carers on the other hand, tended to be more assertive and often readily questioned the decisions made by health care workers. The elderly carers had a more developed pride in caring and this included the attitude not to seek help from others. This association was readily established as each questionnaire specified the carer's age and other personal details that could be compared to the responses, especially to the open questions.

The most distressing finding, and one of the most significant, was that health care workers had a minimal effect on helping carers to receive relevant information. Indeed, health workers seemed to often assume that carers possessed knowledge and information; the research demonstrated that this was usually not the case. There seemed to be little evidence of co-operation between workers and a profound lack of planning, and there was evidence of a basic task-oriented service as opposed to one that related to the needs and demands of the client. The result of this was an apathy in the carers and a feeling of no confidence in health workers.

CONCLUSIONS

The results of this survey not only highlight the problems of the carer, but also the problems of the system that can support and advise them. Its intention is not to be negatively critical but rather to identify areas that can be developed. It notes the lack of local policies for helping carers within the health service and the lack of communication between health care workers and carers. Most importantly, it highlights the potential for CPNs. The following suggestions are a direct result of these findings and attempt to address the areas in which CPNs can take a more active part in this support.

CPNs should be clear about their role and communicate this to others

The CPN is just one of many health care professionals working with families of people with dementia. How does the CPN fit into this network, and how does their function differ from that of the others?

There is a general concensus about the role of the CPN in the literature, although how much this is recognized by CPNs themselves may be debatable. As a result there is a need for the CPN to develop research that provides pointers to ways in which the CPN's role with informed carers might be developed. The provision of advice and information is an important function of the CPN. The level of help may vary from written information to supportive discussion. It was apparent from the research that carers are sadly ignorant of many of the services available and it must be remembered that the CPN not only provides information directly but also acts as a gatekeeper to other services. Being well informed also prevents problems. The findings suggest that carers had no forewarning of what to expect from a person with dementia, in fact many of them were totally ignorant of what was happening to their dependant.

Advice can also lead to general support including counselling and listening. The CPN has a great advantage here, being able to use a variety of therapeutic approaches. They can recognize the coping strategies of carers and there is evidence that by using non-judgemental counselling they can reduce stress in the carer (Watkins, 1988).

Despite this the CPN should not attempt to work in isolation, especially when making assessments. Although it is important for a doctor to make a diagnosis, other health care professionals have knowledge and skills which can play a positive part in the overall treatment of the client, many of which can be shared. For example the working methods of social workers with their emphasis on people and family systems may suggest to the nurse a wider view of care.

Skill exchange should work both ways. A vital role for the CPN is training. Being a key specialist in the field of mental health they are invaluable in advising other health workers as well as advising and educating the carers themselves. This skill should not be limited to individuals; there may be value in speaking to carer support groups and staff in elderly persons' homes.

By positive planning of client care the CPN is able to facilitate independence and maintain dignity. This would be their role in hospital and can quite easily be adapted to the community context by supporting the carer. The nurse is a manager of time and resources and has knowledge and skills which can be used to make caring both more efficient and effective, but without taking responsibility from the carer. The carer can then take control of the caring situation and can enhance the choices of care provision. There is an urgent need to develop the participation of carers and their family in decisions about their dependant. Until they have a clearer understanding of the nature of dementia and its effects they will be unable to make these decisions.

If CPNs are to develop their role they will need first to review some of their attitudes to care. Pollock (1988) highlighted the ways in which CPNs often focus on the client without reference to the family. This is of no use to a carer. If CPNs are to offer useful support they will have to widen their experience to family oriented models.

Before discussing role development it may be fruitful to question whether these are legitimate areas for the CPN or whether they would be more properly attributed to other health care professionals. Although the research suggested that there are gaps in supporting carers, what evidence is there that these should be filled by the CPN? From the research the social worker seemed to be the only effective health care professional recognized by the carer, so perhaps the key role is played by the social worker rather than the CPN?

Cloke (1985) suggested that community nurses were ideally suited to help carers, having more time and opportunity to advise them in depth, and having a broadly based but extensive training. CPNs currently may not meet these standards but there is no reason why they should not develop that way. They are in effect specialist care givers and their specialism is their client group, elderly people. They are also able to provide a truly holistic approach that is recognized by other health care professionals. This does not mean that they should work in isolation, or that they should take over the role of a social worker. As one GP suggested to Conhye (1987); 'The CPN helps the patient to cope with the environment, whilst the social worker helps mould the environment to help the patient.' Perhaps the idea of a corporate approach is important, but complementary areas are worth nurturing.

Being clear about one's role is of little value unless it is communicated to others. The survey found very little understanding of what CPNs were and what they did. They were certainly not seen as having a role in providing information. Perhaps this is because a non-specialist will identify roles in a simple way, i.e. doctors, nurses, home helps, etc. Even so, the CPNs should promote their own role much more aggressively both with other health care professionals and with carers.

CPNs should have a recognizable strategy for the planning, implementation and evaluation of care

The research highlighted that CPNs visited carers without any systematic plan of action. Sometimes they failed to keep promises, both in providing help or making further visits. If the CPN has a systematic working method that is carefully monitored, then this problem could be avoided.

Planning is a key issue here. The problem is more often one of poor organization rather than poor service. The support for carers and their dependants should be an important enough issue for the CPN to devote time to planning the provision of high quality support. An important first step here is to recognize the carer's needs and be able to distinguish between *need* and *demand.*

The research clearly highlights that problems are only articulated into demands when the situation is desperate, at the stage of crisis intervention. It also illustrates the multiple problems created by a wide variety of needs and the inability to have these needs recognized. The CPN, along with other health care workers, does not yet have the credibility to be asked for help. The CPN must positively identify these needs and not wait for the carer to articulate them into requests for help when it is too late.

It is possible that the despairing apathy expressed by carers could be partly due to their 'cultural' perception of the role of the health care professional. The concept of a passive receiver may induce a model of helplessness in carers that in itself may be a recipe for learnt helplessness (Seligman, 1974). Involving the carer more can only be an advantage in such a situation, but this does not mean that the CPN can opt out. In reality, the introduction of participative care to a group of people with an average age of 68 years will not stimulate them into taking immediate control of their dependants' care. So the CPN must provide a strong lead and yet ensure that there is adequate opportunity for explanation to the carer.

It would be a very restricted model of care which did not take into account the skills of others. The research has suggested that other health care professionals have skills which are valuable. From the carers' point of view, they were limited and uncoordinated. The key problem was not, as might be expected, a duplication of roles but rather a lack of working together. This is why appropriate joint planning plays such an important part. In some cases close working at all stages of planning may not be possible or desirable but sometimes a clarity of role and function may prove a great help. The GP may be aware of what support a CPN can provide for the newly diagnosed person with dementia, but do they know what support can be provided for the dependant's carer and family?

One dilemma for the CPN may be the delivery of service. On the surface the carer of a person with dementia may seem to make unattainable demands. However, it is essential to differentiate the quality and quantity of service offered. The key to helping the carer is to provide support when required. Although it might appear that carers are in need of constant support a closer consideration will illustrate that they want real help when needed. This can only be achieved by credibility. The research showed an understandably cynical view of health care professionals generated by broken appointments, and a lack of understanding. Before any specific help will be accepted the credibility of the CPN needs establishing. It is the quality of help offered that will solve the problem not the number of visits. The only resources which will be stretched will be the time that should be devoted to appropriate planning.

In summary, the CPN will need to understand the real problem, have a clear idea of what help is available and be able to offer the help that is appropriate. They should provide information readily but recognize that helping is often much more than that. To the health care worker certain knowledge is taken for granted but carers need constant information on how their dependant will be affected and what methods of treatment they will receive and why. The CPN is also in a position to set up and use helping networks and, perhaps most importantly, to ensure that the carer is involved in decision making about their dependant. The CPNs should set up an adequate method of monitoring and use the information they acquire to ensure that an acceptable level of service is being provided to the carer.

This does not preclude the valuable intervention the CPN can make in helping find solutions to pressing practical problems. This will certainly alleviate stress, but the CPN should ensure that it is handled in a way that does not take away the carer's control of the situation.

CPNs should be more aware of the social and political issues relating to the care of elderly people and their dependants

It is essential that CPNs make themselves aware of the wider issues relating to their role. There is a need to realize that the client lives within a context that includes social and political issues as well as physical and psychological ones (Hodges, 1985; Simmons and Brooker, 1987). Traditionally, nurses have not faced these issues and have tended to leave them to others, concentrating on what they would class as practical help – this has invariably meant they have concentrated on a medical model.

When dealing with carers the situation is somewhat different. The issue of caring forces the nurse to widen her conceptual parameters. This may not be pleasant as it can highlight a number of dilemmas. It is also important to remember that a political perception does not necessarily mean a party political perception. Politics is related to all decisions that affect the health service, by whatever political party, on a national level. As the work of the CPN links so closely with the local authority these decisions will also need to be taken into account. The CPN will also need to understand the effect of public attitudes towards mental health, particularly those which relate to elderly people, recognizing, as Sharman (1985) and Cameron, Badger and Evers (1988) have pointed out, that the term 'elderly' is an eclectic one and, for example, black elders may be even more ignored than other groups.

The CPN should furthermore act as a catalyst in encouraging people to take more responsibility for their own health care and encourage them to take up the services to which they are entitled, at the same time persuading them that they will not be belittled in the process.

Finally, the CPN must be aware of the power and control that has traditionally been exercised by the health care professional. It is the transference of this power from the workers to the client, whatever their background, that will need addressing as will its effect on the likely demand for accountability from the CPN that will occur as a result.

REFERENCES

Adams, T. (1987) Dementia is a family affair. *Community Outlook*, February, 7–8.

Adams, T. (1988) A question of caring. *Geriatric Nursing and Home Care*, March, 18–19

Baillie, V., Norbeck, J.S. and Barnes, L.E.A. (1988) Stress, social support, and psychological distress of family caregivers of the elderly. *Nursing Research*, **37** (4), 217–222.

Bonny, S. (1984) *Who Cares in Southwark?* Association of Carers, London.

Cameron, E., Badger, F. and Evers, H. (1988) Old, needy – and black. *Nursing Times*, **84** (32).

Campbell, C. (1987) Helping carers to cope. *Geriatric Nursing and Home Care*, November, 21.

Clist, L. and Brant, S. (1986) A new direction for CPNs. *Nursing Times*, 1 January, 25–27.

Cloke, C. (1985) Who couldn't care less? *Journal of District Nursing*, July.

Community Psychiatric Nurses' Association (1985) *CPN Survey*, CPNA, London.

Conhye, A. (1987) Hidden assets. *Nursing Times*, **83** (35), 49–50.

Corbin, J. and Strauss, A. (1988) Ted and Alice. *Nursing Times*, **83** (14) 32–33.

Corea, S. (1987) Care of the elderly: a joint CPNA/PNA discussion paper. *Community Psychiatric Nursing Journal*, **7** (2), 34–36.

Doscher, P. (1986) When the relative is the nurse ... *Nursing Times*, 28 May.

Equal Opportunities Commission (1980) *The experience of caring for elderly and handicapped dependants*, EOC, London.

Equal Opportunities Commission (1984) *Carers and services: a comparison of men and women caring for elderly and handicapped dependants.* EOC, London.

Georghiou, G. (1986) Home service. *Nursing Times*, 19 March, 57–58.

Gilhooly, M.L.M. (1984) The impact of care giving on care-givers. *British Journal of Medical Psychology*, **57**, 35–44.

Gilleard, C. (1982) Stresses and strains amongst supporters of the elderly infirm day hospital attenders. University of Edinburgh, Edinburgh.

Godin, P. (1987) Keeping the customer satisfied. *Nursing Times*, **83** (38).

Grad, J. and Sainsbury, P. (1963) Mental illness and the family. *The Lancet*, **i**, 544–547.

Grad, J. and Sainsbury, P. (1965) An evaluation of the effects of caring for the aged at home, in *World Psychiatric Associations Symposium – Psychaitric disorders in the aged*, World Psychiatric Association.

Hirschfeld, M.J. (1978) Families living with senile brain disease. University of California, California.

Hodges, B. (1985) The health career model (guide for students). Department of Community Studies, Manchester Polytechnic.

Lewis, J. and Meredith, B. (1988) Daughters caring for mothers: the experience of caring and its implications for professional helpers. *Ageing and Society*, **8**, 1–21.

MacGuire, J. (1987) A welcome break. *Nursing Times*, **83** (32), 48–50.

Machin, E. (1980) A survey of the behaviour of the elderly and their supporters at home. University of Birmingham.

Mangan, P. (1988) Carers – who cares? *Geriatric Nursing and Home Care*, 8 June.

Muir Gray, J.A. (1984) Prevention of family breakdown. *Nursing Mirror*, **158**, 1038–1085.

Pollock, L.C. (1988) The work of community psychiatric nursing. *Journal of Advanced Nursing*, **13**, 537–545.

Robinson, J. (1988) Support systems. *Nursing Times*, **84** (14), 30–31.

Rogerson, B. (1984) Ignore them at your peril. *Nursing Times*, 12 December, 436–439.

Saddington, N. (1984) Courses for carers. *Nursing Times*, 12 December.

Sanford, J.R.A. (1975) Tolerance of debility in elderly dependants by supporters at home: its significance for hospital practice. *British Medical Journal*, **3**, 471–473.

Seligman, N.E.P. (1974) Depression and learned helplessness, in *Friedman, R.J. (ed.) The psychology of depression: contemporary therapy and research,* Winston Wiley, Washington.

Sharman, R.L. (1985) *Ethnic minority groups: a discussion paper,* Bocardo Press.

Simmons, S. and Brooker, C. (1987) Making CPNs part of the team. *Nursing Times*, **83** (19), 49–51.

Tameside Metropolitan Borough Council (1988) The carer surveys. Policy Research Unit, Tameside Metropolitan Borough Council, unpublished report paper.

Tyler, J. (1987) Give us a break. *Nursing Times*, **83** (50).

Watkins, M. (1985) What about the carers? *Nursing Practice*, **1**, 3–6.

Watkins, M. (1988) Lifting the burden. *Geriatric Nursing and Home Care*, October, 18–20.

Wheatley, V. (1979) Supporters of elderly persons with a dementing illness living in the same household. University of Surrey, Guildford.

CHAPTER THREE

Family burden - what does psychiatric illness mean to the carers?

Sue Simmons

SUMMARY

The current trend towards community care for people with psychiatric illness may put an increased burden on the primary care givers, often the family. This has been investigated previously by the use of quantitative measures and structured interview schedules and has frequently been found to be high. However, little work has been done on the *meaning* that family members attribute to their situation. This study employs a guided interview format that covers several themes in tape-recorded interviews with key family members. It was found that interviewees fell into two broad types, those highly involved who were also more closely related, and those living separately who were less involved and less closely related. The experiences of burden were different in the two groups. Other themes also emerged which cross-cut these types, including duty to care and attitudes to the community care movement. Some conclusions concerning the role of the family and the relationship between family and state are drawn, and it is suggested that there are some implications for community psychiatric nursing services.

INTRODUCTION

The past two or three decades have seen major shifts in the pattern of mental health care in this and other countries. Much of the emphasis, particularly more recently, has been on developing forms of treatment in local settings that could be alternatives to hospital care. Closely associated with this movement, community psychiatric nursing has developed rapidly with most health authorities now having some kind of service. There have been various reasons for this. First, the contracting of the large mental hospitals in the early 1960s and the advent of the new tranquillizer drugs enabled psychiatrically disturbed people to live in the community for longer periods of time. Secondly, the disappearance of the local authority mental welfare officer following the implementation in 1972 of the recommendations of the Seebohm Report that social workers take on generic responsibilities, left a gap in the provision of service for psychiatrically ill people (HMSO 1968).

More recently, the trend towards the closure of large mental hospitals and an expansion of community services for mentally ill people has been increasing further. There are proposals to employ large numbers of additional community psychiatric nurses (CPNs) in many districts.

There is, however, very little known about how the community and the families of individuals who would otherwise have been admitted to hospital, experience this change in policy. It is the impression of those working in this area that the families carry a large part of the burden of care, and that the degree to which they are involved with the identified patient may affect the course of his or her illness and need for treatment.

Much work in the field of mental ill health in recent years has looked at the role of the family as a causative factor in the initial breakdown or as a stabilizing influence in continuing illness. For those adopting a psychosocial perspective, the family is seen as a central element in the development of a theory of mental illness.

However, there is another side to this coin. Many studies on the inter-relationship of family and identified patient have concentrated on the experiences of the latter. Relatively few have attempted to gauge the experiences and understandings of the other family members.

The family in our society is the main agent of socialization of new adults and is also the primary care giver in times of ill health (particularly in the case of the women in the family). In the current political climate, this role is being strongly advocated by the government, so that the responsibility of the family to provide care and support may become an even greater burden. Although this governmental move is, I suggest, separate from the ideological moves within the psychiatric services to increase community care, the two developments may have a cumulative impact on the burden of the family.

BACKGROUND

Three main areas of theory and empirical research appear to have relevance to this field. Firstly, various writers have described the philosophy of community care, compared treatment in the community to treatment in hospital, or examined associated developments such as community psychiatric nursing services. Secondly, writings on the role of the family and the relationship between the family and the state provide some of the theoretical background to these developments. Thirdly, work in the specific area of family burden demonstrates that this issue concerns many people in the mental health field.

Community care

In recent years much has been spoken and written about the movement towards community care, both for those who are psychiatrically ill, and for the elderly and mentally handicapped. Some writers have pointed out the ill-defined nature of the concepts of 'community' and 'community care'. For example Walker (1982) suggests that the meaning of community is not shared by all those involved in it. He defines community care as:

> ... help and support given to individuals, including children ... in non-institutional settings. Such care may be provided by informal, quasi-formal or formal helpers or by a combination of all three.

Using this definition he makes it clear that he sees community care, at present, as care in the community, rather than care by the community.

Several factors have been identified as contributing to the community care movement. These include: a greater understanding of psychosocial influences on mental health; a growing belief amongst professionals and the general public that large mental hospitals could be damaging through the effects of institutionalization (Wing, 1981); and advances in tranquillizer drugs, which have enabled some psychiatrically disturbed people to live outside hospital for longer periods of time. Another contributory factor was the Mental Health Act (1959) aimed at the minimization of institutional care, the development of non-institutional care settings and preventive measures against family breakdown and unnecessary admission. However, very little was done to reduce bed numbers in large mental hospitals until many years afterwards. This was despite the fact that the Ministry of Health in 1962 set out plans for the run-down and closure of large hospitals, with care to be provided in smaller units within district general hospitals and in the community (Ministry of Health, 1962). The Mental Health Act (1983) adopts the underlying principle of the 'least restrictive alternative' to hospital admission and thus stresses the need for community facilities (Gostin, 1983). There are now specific plans to close large psychiatric hospitals in many health authorities and a number have already closed.

The establishment of community psychiatric nursing services can be seen as one outcome of these developments. However, the history of the development of community psychiatric nursing services since the first psychiatric nurses worked in the community from Warlingham Park Hospital has been recorded elsewhere (for example, Hunter 1974; Simmons and Brooker, 1986) and will therefore not be repeated here.

The role of the family

Walker refers to the 'informal helpers' in community care. Clearly the most important element in the informal system is the family. This has been recognized by some workers in the field of mental health. Thus Wing (1981) in writing about the 'new long-stay' points out that families carry much of the burden of care, and that services should provide crisis help, holiday relief and a range of residential, occupational and leisure facilities to help them in their task.

In their paper on the role of the family in the rehabilitation of people with schizophrenia, Boyd, McGill and Falloon (1981) stress the importance of families in providing care, but point out the dangers of over-involvement and criticism of the ill member, which may contribute towards relapse. Recent work by psychiatrists and others has described families with a high level of 'expressed emotion' as exacerbating schizophrenic relapse in some people (Brown, Birley and Wing, 1972; Leff and Vaughn, 1985; Tarrier *et al.*, 1988).

Clearly, the role of the family in the field of mental health and ill-health is complex. Not only is the family system central to, and intimately involved in, the mental health 'problem' at a micro-level, both in terms of being a possible contributory factor, and in providing on-going care and support, but it is also involved, albeit unwittingly, at a macro-level in central and local government policies of developing community care.

Walker makes the point that moves towards community care have major implications for the family since at present care for ill, handicapped or elderly people is divided between the state and the family, with the latter taking on most of the burden when the location of care is outside of the institution (Walker, 1982). Recent public expenditure cuts have served to increase the problem of transferring funds to the community. Indeed it appears to be believed by some politicians that greater State help would undermine the family's caring role. For example:

> I think the statutory services can only play their part successfully if we don't expect them to do for us things that we could be doing for ourselves.
>
> (Thatcher, quoted in Walker, 1982)

Walker concludes from this that the State's influence on family life is effected more through non-intervention than by intervention. There is, he says, an assumption that families will do the caring. Little help is provided to facilitate this and the state tends not to intervene until a crisis erupts.

In his study of families caring for an elderly relative or a mentally handicapped child, Moroney (1976) suggests that it is conceivable that some families may be led to question the desirability of community care, and says that the need for services to be provided primarily to those who do not have families means that some families may be penalized for caring, by being deprived of support. By meeting the needs of their members:

> . . . the family, in practice, serves the needs of the State, rather than the more commonly held belief that the State is the servant of its people.
>
> (Moroney, 1976).

Moroney stresses that he does not regard this use of the family as deliberate exploitation, but nevertheless the State clearly benefits from it.

So far this discussion has simplified the relationship between family and State by ignoring the role of the 'formal helpers'. Much of the work in this field has concentrated on social services, but it contains much of relevance to those working in mental health. There is some evidence that these issues are being raised within the mental health professions. Dunham (1974), for example, has raised the question of whose agent are community psychiatrists when they leave the hospital setting. Do they serve the needs of the official agency, or of the community? Walker (1982) describes social service professionals as intermediaries who define the family's needs from the position of the individual requiring care rather than the total family unit. He suggests that social workers and other health professionals are one of the means whereby the State attempts to maintain the traditional caring role of the family.

Both Moroney and Walker conclude that there is a marked need to develop a sharing system of care within the community. Moroney's impression is that there is no evidence at present that families wish to give up their caring function and they should, therefore, be aided in this. Walker argues that we need to know more about the needs of the care-givers and the meaning of community care to them. Services should no longer be simply what professionals think is required or what they wish to provide.

Family burden

Clearly, the growing trend towards caring for those with mental health problems in the community has, as already outlined, major implications for the families of those individuals. How do they experience this development? More specifically, does this change in approach alter the 'burden' that they perceive themselves to be carrying?

Grad and Sainsbury (1963) have described several different effects that they call 'burden' including: disturbances in relatives' health and in social and leisure activities, effects on children, disturbances of domestic routine with less flexibility, and reduction in income. Sladden (1979) suggests that the families of those referred to CPNs are likely to have experienced such stresses and, in some cases, not had access to guidance or support.

The concept of burden can be approached from two different sociological perspectives. Some researchers, treating social facts as 'things', have attempted to develop some 'objective' measure that can be analysed using quantitative methods and compared this with the ratings of other families (for example Hoult *et al.*, 1981; Pai and Kapur, 1982). These researchers have tended to conclude that family burden is not necessarily alleviated by hospital admission. Others have treated the accounts of family members as data that can be analysed using a qualitative approach.

Creer and Wing (1974) examined the problems of people who lived with, or felt responsible for, someone with a diagnosis of schizophrenia. They reported, as have other researchers, that relatives understated their problems, although there were major effects on their lives, and they suggested that the carers had not only become accustomed to their situation, but had also adjusted their own hopes and expectations downwards.

In his study of families with a handicapped child, Wilkin (1979) looked at 'felt needs' and defined these as the help that the families subjectively experience as lacking or inadequate, as opposed to what professionals may assess as the needs. If the felt needs are met there is, he suggested, a greater likelihood that families may be able to keep their child at home. Similarly, I suggest that the felt needs of families with a member who has a major mental health problem may be more pertinent to what happens to that family than are our professional assessments.

Voysey (1975) also interviewed families with a handicapped child and adopted a symbolic interactionist framework to analyse interviews with parents (usually the mother). She argues that parents' accounts can be read as one of several possible accounts, the range of which is limited by cultural constraints that are seen as relevant to the phenomena. The parents' definitions and accounts must compete with those of people in positions of power to determine which is the 'correct' one. Clearly, psychiatrists and other doctors could be in a position to have their accounts accepted as definitive. The longer one such account has been accepted as the definitive explanation for an individual's behaviour or the family situation, the more resistant that explanation is to change. Some features of Voysey's analysis may be extrapolated to an investigation of families with a psychiatrically ill member.

THE RESEARCH

The study attempted some 'illuminative' research (Furler, 1979) into the meanings of some of these issues for those people who find themselves in the position of caring for someone with a mental health problem in the community. My perspective was derived from the school of symbolic interactionism (Blumer, 1969), the most relevant features of which include the premise that the meaning of an object is socially created and hence may be constantly re-defined and re-interpreted through interaction.

Actions are seen to be not simply released responses to stimuli but to be pieced together from many significant elements, including past knowledge and experience, the interpretation of the current situation, and the individual's tendency to act in certain ways. Society's organization and structure provide the framework within which social action takes place, and hence are among the significant things that guide action. However, they do not totally determine it at the level of the individual and the family. In many routine situations previous experience will provide the people involved with a clear understanding of how to act and shared meanings may be easily established. Yet for all of us new situations arise, at times frequently, so that existing rules are inadequate and the interpretative process becomes more complex. Mental ill health may be just such a new situation. Birchwood and Smith (1987), writing on schizophrenia, make a similar point:

> For most families, schizophrenia and its attendant behavioural anomalies will be a novel experience so there will not be an existing repertoire of coping strategies available on which to draw. These will have to be developed afresh . . .

It is, therefore, suggested that within a family the members' understanding of, say, mental illness, help received, and their burden of care may be constructed to take various forms in different situations and at different times, depending on changing meanings and interpretations.

METHODS

The perspective required a method that would neither be too rigid nor limit the scope of the areas to be covered. A guided interview format was therefore used. Melia (1983, 1987) has used this method in her research to discover what student nurses experience in their chosen career. Although she does not describe an interview guide, her reference to a flexible 'agenda' giving the students opportunities to raise different ideas, suggests that she used a similar approach.

The interview guide (see Appendix) covered several issues, including the

Table 3.1 Characteristics of the interviewees

	Relationship to identified patient	Age	Living with identified patient
Mr A	Husband	75	Yes
Mrs B	Mother	59	Yes
Mr C	Husband	80	Yes
Mr D	Brother	53	No
Miss E	Daughter	59	Yes
Mrs F	Mother	45	Yes
Mr G	Father	76	Yes
Mrs H	Sister	70	No
Mrs I	Sister	84	No
Mrs J	Daughter-in-law	52	No

nature of the family problem, the type of help received, perceived burden, felt needs and overall thinking about community care.

The respondents were selected through the community psychiatric nursing team of a central London health district. My decision to use an in-depth interview format limited me to a small number of interviews. However, since my intention was to discover themes rather than to test hypotheses, the principles of random selection in order to generalize from a representative sample did not apply, (Field and Morse, 1985).

Permission for me to interview the respondents was initially sought by the CPN and I would follow this up by letter or telephone call. In all, ten respondents were interviewed, six women and four men. One of the women, Mrs I, was accompanied by her sister who was also involved, but to a lesser extent, with responsibilities for their ill sister. Table 3.1 summarized some of their personal characteristics.

All of the interviews except one were conducted in the interviewees' homes. Assurances of confidentiality were given at my initial contact, and again at the beginning of the interview. In two cases, (those of Mr A and Mrs F) the identified CPN client was present for a brief time at the beginning of the session but left soon after. In the remaining interviews my contact was with the carer only. All of the interviews except one were tape-recorded. All were transcribed in full soon after the interview took place. The interviews varied in length from 40 to 90 minutes.

Within the constraints of an interview guide and certain themes that I wished to explore, I intended to adopt a flexible approach towards the direction of analysis, to allow themes raised by the interviewees to emerge. The early interviews were therefore particularly wide-ranging. Some preliminary analysis was done after conducting approximately half the interviews. This allowed other themes grounded in the data to emerge (Glaser and Strauss, 1967), for example the respondents' understanding of a duty to care for family members. These themes could then be explored in more depth in later interviews. Thus the analysis informed the data collection and vice versa.

FINDINGS

I shall begin by outlining the kinds of problems that family carers describe, and then discuss their accounts of burden and duty to care. This will lead on to an examination of what help the families were receiving and would like to receive. Although the respondents' more general thoughts about community care were addressed in the interviews these will not be discussed here.

Nature of the family problem

I shall deliberately avoid using psychiatric diagnoses in later discussion since I was interested in the families' experiences of living with and/or caring for, not a schizophrenic or depressive, but rather a relative who acts or interacts in certain ways and with whom they have had a lengthy relationship. Nevertheless, it may be useful, at this juncture, to give brief details of the psychiatric diagnoses since they may throw light on some of the types of behaviour and related problems that interviewees described. Table 3.2 summarizes these details.

Table 3.2 Characteristics of identified CPN clients

Interviewee	CPN client	Age of client	Diagnosis	Duration
Mr A	Mrs A	75	Schizophrenia	9 years
Mrs B	Keith B	22	Personality disorder	6 years
Mr C	Mrs C	70	Manic depression	30 years
Mr D	John D	48	Schizophrenia	27 years
Miss E	Mrs E	83	Psychotic illness following bereavement/senile dementia	5 years
Mrs F	Peter F	19	Psychotic illness	6 months
Mr G	James G	51	Schizophrenia	32 years
Mrs H	Mr L	76	Depression	3 years
Mrs I	Miss P	80	Schizophrenia	7 years
Mrs J	Mrs J (senior)	84	Depression/confusion	7 years

In my interviews respondents very rarely made any reference to psychiatric labels when talking about their relative's behaviour. Perhaps not surprisingly in view of what has been said earlier, the problems that were described were almost all rooted in interaction, rather than in intrapsychic phenomena, although the latter are often considered by professionals to be more important. Odd, unpredictable or disruptive behaviour, either in the past or currently, was commonly mentioned, including throwing away clothes or newly-bought food, reversal of sleep pattern, noisy behaviour at night, wandering away from home, going 'haywire' and excessive drinking. The reluctance or inability of individuals to do fairly simple things for themselves, for example cooking, cleaning or shopping, was also described. Several ill relatives* behaved in a withdrawn fashion, perhaps sitting for long periods, smoking heavily or doing nothing. Others behaved with marked impatience or irritability on occasion. These descriptions were seldom presented as complaints but generally accepted as caused by the person's illness, although this was not so often the case amongst the more removed carers.

Mr D described his brother's physical complaints thus:

> There is never a day goes by when there isn't something wrong with him. There are times when you could just go on walking and walking and never ever go back. It gets you to such a pitch, because there is nothing you can do, and you know probably it's the drugs, or withdrawal of drugs.

Mrs B detailed the fits that her son has almost weekly and the injuries he sustains as a result of his excessive drinking.

Several interviewees referred to being unable to allow their relative free access to money, since it would be spent extravagantly and bills left unpaid. They had often learned this the hard way by being confronted with their relative's debts. On the other hand, Mrs H was angered by her brother's refusal to spend money, although he had ample savings.

It was my impression that the most distressing problems, however, were those types of behaviour that conflicted with some norm of social acceptability. For example Mrs I highlighted her sister's shouting 'bad language' at night as a major problem.

> The thing that I can't tolerate is the language. It's terrible. Sex is firmly in her mind. She says everyone accuses her of being a prostitute. She

---

*I refer in this Chapter to the person who is being seen by the CPN as 'ill'. Normally they would be described as the 'client' but this terminology does not seem appropriate when we view the situation from the perspective of the family carers. I do not intend to imply by this acceptance of the medical definitions of psychiatric ill health, but recognize that this debate cannot be entered into here.

suddenly loses her temper and goes to the back gate and bangs it. It shakes things in here, and it's nearly always at night.

Mrs B was greatly distressed by her son's refusal to adhere to her standards of cleanliness.

He will not bath, he will not keep himself clean. He sleeps in his clothes when he's been drinking. He virtually lives here half the week as you would have a down-and-out living with you.

The interviewees were not, on the whole, preoccupied with searching for the reasons for the 'illness'. One possible explanation for this may be that in all but one of the sample the problem had been fairly protracted and the families had therefore come to accept the situation and arrived at some ongoing, fairly stable interpretation. One exception to this was Mrs B whose son had been disturbed for six years. She said that she was still upset by the difficulty in getting through to him.

It's a most peculiar thing to even describe. It's like a brick wall, you can't get through with advice or anything. They all tell me ... that there is no deep mental illness ... but there's something wrong and even I don't know what it is.

Family burden

Hoenig and Hamilton (1966) found in their research that their measure of 'objective' burden on families was generally greater than the families' own 'subjective' rating. One could argue that this discrepancy occurs since family members tend to understate their responsibilities and the impact of these on their lives. I would suggest, in addition, that the difference illustrates the lack of shared meaning or understanding between family and researcher of the concept of burden. Since this shared meaning would arise only through the interactive process and the interaction described was limited to the administration of a questionnaire, the potential for the researcher to get closer to the respondents' understanding was clearly limited.

In my small number of interviews the respondents could be divided into two groups by the degree to which they were involved in the caring of, and were responsible for, their relative. I shall describe them as:

1. highly involved carers, who lived with or had daily contact with their relative;
2. more removed carers, whose contact was less frequent and sometimes irregular.

a) Highly involved family carers. Seven members of my sample fell into this group. In all but one case the carer's relationship with the psychiatrically ill person was that of spouse, parent or child, and apart from the same exception, they all lived with their relative. The exception to this group was Mr D who was very involved in the care of his brother but was married and lived elsewhere. As discussed later, Mr D described himself as 'like a parent' to his brother and had lived with him until his marriage several years earlier. He now visited him at his flat twice a day, six days a week.

All members of this group described themselves as carrying out most of the practical tasks of the household including cooking, cleaning, shopping and handling the finances. Typically, they supplemented the income of their relative (sickness benefit or retirement pension) from their own money, often by a sizeable amount. It was felt that they could not do otherwise since their relative's income was not enough to meet their needs for, say, cigarettes or larger items like clothes. Most were willing to contribute financially, but Mr G pointed out that since he retired it had been much more difficult.

In all cases their caring role had affected other areas of their lives. They tended to describe themselves as being unable or reluctant to leave their relative for long periods of time, and either did not have holidays or, if they did, tended to feel anxious and guilty. Mrs B described herself as having lost her previous routine and having become socially isolated in the six years of her son's illness, saying that nobody now visited their flat.

> I feel I haven't got any normality in my life. I've lost an awful lot of my friends, not only through Keith, but because I can't face people. I mean I haven't got a son that I can talk about in a normal way ... we've both become isolated.

Miss E graphically described the difficulties of living in a one-roomed flat with her elderly mother. For example:

> She'll be sitting there completely absorbed in her book, and then she'll suddenly leap to her feet and start getting her bed ready ... I have to go to bed when she goes to bed, more or less. I have tried sitting up, but she's not too happy, and neither am I, because I'm conscious of the fact that it's keeping her awake. So I either go and sit on the bath to read, or I try to cover my lamp, so that I get the light and she doesn't. Sometimes it works and sometimes it doesn't. Sometimes she says 'Are you going to put that light out?'

Yet despite, or perhaps because of, such problems Miss E was seriously considering taking early retirement from her job to be with her mother during the day.

Members of this group tended to talk about their responsibilities with a mixture of willingness and acceptance. They viewed their relative as ill and therefore attached little or no blame to her or his behaviour. They did, however, describe feelings of sadness and anxiety about the situation. Mr A said of his wife:

> It's been very sad ... I do all the cooking for her. I rather enjoy doing that. But in other words it's not like married life, if you understand that, but I don't mind a bit, as long as I see her moving around.

Frequently comments were made on their worries about the future. For example Mrs B said:

> I did have hope at one stage that things might get better, but I can't see it altering now. I wish I could meet someone in the medical world who would say 'Don't worry, if you're not around, we'll take him under our wing'.

Similarly, Mr A said that his own health had deteriorated recently and caused him added anxiety. This group of involved carers also appeared to live with continual worry that disturbed behaviour might reappear unexpectedly or in some cases that the person might harm themselves. Mrs B said:

> I have this terrible pressure on me at the end of the week, waiting for something to happen, and wondering ... he's had awful injuries in the fits.... It's like living on a precipice, waiting for something awful to happen.

There were no comments suggesting that the respondents feared for their own safety, despite the fact that both Mrs B and Mr G's wife had been threatened with a knife by their relatives during the early stages of their illnesses.

Feelings of fatigue, depression and irritability were generally described. Mr D felt that the strain he was under was not always acknowledged by others.

> I often say it's all right for a doctor to say you should do this, or do that, but you don't live with them twenty-four hours. It's a different thing, like you're just listening to me telling you and you think 'Oh well, I know these things happen', but unless you actually experience it and live with it for a while, and be responsible for it ... it all builds up and builds up until you can quite easily go over the top yourself.

A number of them spontaneously mentioned occasional thoughts that they could be heading for a 'breakdown' themselves and the strain described could at times provoke serious incidents. For example Miss E recounted one such episode.

> I never had much patience. It's doubly a struggle. About two weeks ago she nearly drove me mad, and I picked up a tiny little dish and threw it across the room, and in that instant, just as I threw it, she moved across and it hit her in the eye. She was bleeding and had a real shiner ... I lost about nine pounds weight in a week just worrying my guts out.

Such feelings would at times be dealt with by the carer temporarily removing him or herself from the situation, but did not appear to lead to longer term changes in levels of involvement.

It was my impression that this group of people did initially tend to minimize the burden that they carried but, when given more opportunity to discuss it, they demonstrated, as did Voysey's parents of mentally handicapped children (Voysey, 1975), that they were aware of how different their lives were from those of others, and used this comparison in talking about their situations. Mr G who, with his wife, had cared for a schizophrenic son for more than 20 years since his son's discharge from hospital, now also carried out many tasks for his wife who had become house-bound following a bad fall. Yet he felt able to say:

> Well, I've got rather broad shoulders. You can't go by me. There's some people who could not manage like I do, I can assure you of that ... I don't let things get me down.

Miss E highlighted the apparent discrepancy between the description of her burden and her feelings about it by saying:

> It's not all misery. I love having her there. It has terrible limitations, but if she's not there, I miss her like hell. I can't wait for her to come back.

Members of this group gave moving descriptions of the problems they faced. On the whole they accepted the responsibilities that they saw as having arisen out of their relationship and accounted for their acceptance by referring more to family bonds, affection, and some suggestion that they thought they had little choice, than any concept of 'duty'.

b) More removed family carers. Those carers who had the less frequent or irregular contact (usually around once or twice a week) all lived separately from their ill relative. It was found that their relationship was also more distant, being that of daughter-in-law or sibling. They tended to carry out fewer tasks for their relative but what they did do was generally of a practical nature, including cooking, shopping, collecting the pension, cleaning, and did not include providing company or emotional support. Indeed Mrs J appeared to suggest that she was not prepared to meet her mother-in-law's demands for companionship. She said:

Well, she'll keep on complaining that she's ill, and she's not really ill, she just wants you up there for company. And I'm frightened that one day she'll say 'I'm dying', and she will be dying, and I won't take any notice.

Perhaps because of the geographical distance that separated them from their relative, they tended to suffer less disruption to their routine and consequently less social isolation. However, they did describe feeling anxious about their relatives, and Mrs I felt very depressed that she was unable to help her sister more. These feelings were themselves resented. Like the first group there were comments that the respondents sometimes felt themselves to be close to collapse. However, unlike the first group whose anxiety appeared in the long term to lead them to do more, it seemed that in this group these unwelcome feelings were alleviated by the person becoming less involved. Mrs H said:

When I was closer to him and used to keep going up there, and he was coming up here a bit more often, yes, I did feel bad. He worried me a lot … and I find that through not seeing him so much I feel better. I don't have so much worry.

Gottlieb (1983) has described a similar process. He suggests that if the patient does not reciprocate some of the support given by the carer, the relationship will become increasingly burdensome to the carer and may lead to their withdrawal in order to protect their own well-being. Clearly one consequence of this reduction in contact is that there is even less possibility of the interactants reaching an understanding of each other.

Each of the members of this group spoke fairly critically about their relative, often concerning personal attributes of selfishness or laziness. Mrs H said about her brother:

I used to do quite a lot, but I got a bit fed-up, because sometimes I think he's putting it on a bit. He's always been a lazy man, a person who will not do anything for himself … he used to send all his shirts to the laundry. He won't send them now. If I go up there I bet I find about a dozen dirty shirts.

They were less likely than the first group to make excuses for the person's behaviour. This difference from the highly involved carers suggests that the more removed carers and their relatives had not been able to develop a mutually satisfactory definition of the situation. Members of this group did not interpret their relative's behaviour as caused by illness but by re-calcitrance. They also recounted feeling irritated that their relative had refused the help that had been offered by health and social services. Mrs J said of her mother-in-law:

I don't know that she's had any help really. Your people have offered help, but she won't have any of it. Then she'll ring me up and get me to rush down. That happens quite often, about every ten days. In the meantime we've already been down.

Mrs I suggested that her sister's behaviour reflected on her to some extent.

Permanent worry. It's so humiliating, the things she says and the shouting ... I feel a great sorrow for her, but it is humiliating that people may come here and hear things that you wouldn't want them to hear.... She wore five pairs of socks in winter and no shoes. It's not helpful to meet her in the street as her sister like that.

It was my impression that some of the more negative attitudes to the burden that members of this group felt themselves to be carrying could be accounted for by their relative's not accepting help. The family members would then experience rather uncomfortable, generalized anxiety which could not be effectively utilized (unlike in the more involved group). One possible consequence of this was further withdrawal from the ill person.

Duty

The concept of a duty to care for members of one's family was raised by several interviewees but was most clearly expressed by those people whose relationship to the psychiatrically ill person might, in our society, be expected to be less close, for example, sibling, daughter-in-law, rather than that of spouse, parent or child. Several respondents in the group that I have described as the more removed carers felt able to say that they felt little affection for their relative. Mrs H said:

I haven't got a deep affection for him because he was never a good brother, and he was never a good son ... just now and again I say to myself 'Well, he is my brother, you know, I suppose I better keep an eye on him'.

Similarly, Mrs J commented:

When you said to me why do I look after my mother-in-law, I feel I have to. I'd feel guilty if I didn't. I'm not doing it because I love her, I'm doing it because I feel it's my duty to do it, for as long as I can. As far as I'm concerned she's family.

Mrs H had had little or no contact with her brother for many years, and had only become involved with him since he had started being ill. There had therefore been little opportunity for a gradually developed mutual understanding. In Mrs J's case, although her husband visited his mother every day, she said that it was she who carried out the practical tasks for the old lady. She did not appear to question this but accepted it as a woman's role. She suggested, however, that her willingness to take on the responsibilities of her mother-in-law arose from the continual reinforcement from her husband of their shared interpretation. If he were to hint that he resented the way she related to his mother she would immediately pull out from her commitment and leave it all to him. Hence the meaning of her involvement would have to be reconstructed.

Members of the first group, the more involved family carers, were less likely to resort to the concept of duty to account for their situation. Indeed, the notion of questioning their involvement appeared to be an anathema to them, since their situation was seen to be part-and-parcel of their relationship and as such did not allow for choice. For example, Mrs F said:

> He's my son. I have to do it. I can't just leave him. I don't think any mother would. Well, I know some mothers might have done, but I couldn't do that.

Mr G expressed his position on the alternative for his son if he did not take care of him:

> I don't want to see him walking around the hospital grounds with not a friend in the world and not a fag in the world. But then that's me – I feel that way you see.

There was less frustration in this involved group with the lack of reciprocity in the relationship than in the more removed group. Miss E accounted for her role in caring for her mother by initially referring to emotional bonds but then went on to talk about her mother's former characteristics.

> Oh, because I absolutely love her. She is terrific. She's only a little thing, and my father always protected her so much ... she was always one to give up everything for her family. She devoted herself entirely to the family, and never thought about herself.

Miss E's acceptance of the absence of improvement in her mother's mental state and behaviour appeared to be influenced by her mother's age and the length of her illness. This is not the case for Mrs F who, after explaining her present commitment to her son, went on to say that if the situation was the same in ten years time she might not be too tolerant, unless she could see that he had been trying to change.

When we examine concepts of duty and responsibility, Mr D does not appear to fit the highly involved group as closely as he did previously. When asked if he could explain the origins of his commitment he recounted that he and his brother had been left on their own for much of their childhood, following their mother's death and while their father worked shifts. He had always looked after his brother and now described himself as being like a parent to him. The current relationship between the two had therefore been built up over the years through repeated, similar interactions. A common understanding had developed so that Mr D felt that he was probably the only person for whom his brother had any concern. Mr D was aware that the level of his involvement with his brother was unusually high and pointed out that his wife, who did not view the situation in the same way became distressed by it at times.

Mr D also accounted for his sense of duty by referring to an informal promise that he had made.

> My father was extremely worried about him and said to me; 'I don't know what is going to happen to him when I won't be here'. I said to him, 'Don't be silly, I'll look after him'. And that always comes back, and I feel I should.

Mrs J also expressed a feeling of commitment to another family member (in her case her husband) that brought with it duties towards the ill relative.

> Because she's his mother, as my mother is my mother, and if I couldn't do it I'd expect him to do something for her.

Some of the interviewees in both groups expressed the thought that if they did not carry on their relative would suffer some kind of serious set-back, including relapse, readmission to hospital, becoming a vagrant, self-injury or suicide. This was then used to reinforce their thinking that they had no choice, since there was nobody else who would do what they were doing.

Therefore the concepts of family and reciprocity are central to the ways in which the respondents understood their situation. Reciprocity implies a system in which participants engage in mutual and complementary inter-changes and in which each party has certain rights and obligations. Gouldner (1973) suggests that although the interchanges need not be of equal value at all times, the system will not be maintained if they are markedly unbalanced, unless other compensatory mechanisms exist. There would be exceptions to this however if one party could not be expected to give as much as he or she receives, for example elderly people, children or people who are ill.

Compensatory mechanisms may include culturally shared prescriptions, for example 'generosity'. I would suggest that 'family duty' is such a culturally shared prescription and, as such, is brought in by the more removed carers to justify their continuing role when they are receiving little in return from their relative. The situation is made more complex for the more removed carers by a degree of ambivalence over whether or not their relative should be thought of as ill, and therefore potentially exempt from the obligations inherent in the relationship. Since members of this group appear to be unsure about this, there can be little shared understanding between both parties about what is expected from the other.

Explicit references to duty did not occur among those respondents who had a relationship of spouse, parent or child in which reciprocal interchange could have been a prominent feature in the past, if not in the present. In addition, this group did not appear to doubt that their relative should be somewhat exempt from the usual obligations.

Felt needs

While acknowledging the help currently received by the carers and their relatives, I wished to investigate the interviewees' ideas concerning what was lacking, and what they would choose to help them in their caring role. Wilkin has described the needs expressed by families with a mentally handicapped child as often being overlooked by the service providers (Wilkin, 1979). In a review of relevant literature Birchwood and Smith (1987) found a similar situation in families with a schizophrenic member. They described the carers pleas for help as falling on deaf ears and an atmosphere of suspicion and mistrust existing between families and psychiatric services. I found my interviewees had some difficulty in defining their own needs as opposed to those of their relative. Amongst the more involved carers the felt needs seemed inextricably linked.

Walker (1982) has suggested that professionals tend to define the family's needs in terms of those of the individual requiring care. It would seem that this may also be the case in the more involved families where organization and hence definitions of need revolve around the ill person.

During the course of the interviews, however, a number of different kinds of felt needs were raised, some of a practical nature, others less well defined.

Among those of a practical nature, at one extreme, was the wish that the relative could be removed from their sphere of responsibility completely, by going into some kind of residential facility. This was expressed by Mrs J about her mother-in-law and Mrs H about her brother. Such clear statements expressing the wish for permanent change in the situation only occurred in the more removed group, whereas the occasional need for rather more 'space' in the relationship was articulated by members of the highly involved group, particularly when it seemed that a shared meaning had broken down, for example if a relative became increasingly psychiatrically disturbed or greatly influenced by alcohol. Mrs B described her visits to the homes of relatives which were provoked by her son's drinking bouts and her feelings that she 'couldn't take any more'. Such spontaneous acts of removing oneself led to further anxiety, but it seems that planned breaks were also not without their worries. Mr D observed:

I worry particularly when I'm on holiday. I have to go on holiday because I've got a wife who works all the year, so she's entitled to a holiday. The CPN used to pop in when she was passing just to see that he was OK, which takes a load off my mind.

Another wish for practical help which emerged in several of the interviews was for companionship for the ill relative. It was often said by both groups of carers that the person was isolated and would benefit from someone who might call in for a chat, or take him or her out. Mr A also pointed out that this would alleviate some of his worry.

I'm more contented if I know there's somebody here with her, although she's quite all right on her own.

It seems that Mr A is expressing a need that is as much his as his wife's, since he adds that she is 'quite all right on her own'. Such a felt need could easily be dismissed as being unnecessary by the professional helpers unless we recognize Wilkin's point that by attempting to meet felt needs we may help carers to care more effectively. Wishes for companionship were not always expressed without ambivalence. Mr D certainly felt that it would help his brother but then went on to say that it could be unfair on the helper who may not be able to understand him.

Mr D and others said that they wished they had someone else with whom they could share the day-to-day responsibilities but alongside this wish, there was perhaps a certain ambivalence concerning the effects this would have on their role.

Mrs F differed to some extent from the other respondents who requested companionship, in that she felt her son required the input of someone allocated to co-ordinate his treatment following discharge from hospital, and to encourage him to become involved and interested in different activities.

The third area of practical help related to money. As discussed in the section on burden, money was a recurring theme in many interviews. Mr G expressed his opinion most strongly.

Quite frankly, and you won't like it, do you want the truth? I would like to see old age pensioners like myself and my wife paid a decent pension, even if necessary saving the money on all of these social workers ... it's only money that worries me.

A final practical need that could hardly be ignored by the authorities came from Miss E in her request for more spacious accommodation. Despite the fact that she and her mother were extremely cramped in their current flat, she had not yet been offered anywhere suitable.

Among the less well-defined needs that arose was greater access to information, with several respondents saying that they felt they were not told enough. Sometimes this appeared to reflect the professionals' uncertainty over diagnosis and the future as much as a withholding of available information. At other times it appeared to be a straightforward communication breakdown. It is worth noting that some of the people who had received a great deal of time and been frequently consulted felt that they were told very little. It seems that information may be interpreted in many different ways. The family carers may wish to be told unambiguous, known facts and to have the opportunity to share with professionals an understanding of how the situation is for them. The professionals, however, may feel that in the field of mental health they cannot often deal in certainties. As a result, at times they appear to the families to be avoiding discussion.

Interestingly, among the more removed group, their being given information and being consulted about treatment may not always be entirely welcome. It may be interpreted as recognition by the professionals of their holding a key caring role, which they might prefer not to have. Mrs I and her sister appeared not to have resolved this dilemma concerning their ill sister. Mrs I said:

No, we don't get enough information. We could know more.

Her sister added:

I don't think we should be told everything. It's far too much worry for you. I've seen you terribly upset over it. I think it's wrong.

Only one of the interviewees, Mr C, said that he had no need of any additional help (apart from a wish for more information), although he thought that he and his wife would need more help as they got older. Of the rest, the range of needs was wide, often closely tied up with the ill relative's needs. Perhaps the lack of definition is not surprising considering how seldom family members are asked to express their own needs in relation to their caring role. Gottlieb (1983) has pointed out that people who experience high levels of stress are less likely to develop adverse health consequences if they have the company of, or access to, significant others. While some of the respondents in my study could be said to be providing that kind of support to their relatives (who in most cases otherwise had limited social contacts) it was not always the case that there was someone else providing it for them. Gottlieb suggests that it may be more feasible to increase our support to such primary carers, rather than to attempt significantly to reduce their stressors.

CONCLUSION

As long ago as 1962 Brown and his colleagues reported on a study of the families of people diagnosed as having schizophrenia and wrote:

> Many relatives who lived with disabled patients (probably) subtly adapted their level of expectations so that after a period of years, they no longer reacted according to their earlier hopes and ideals and perhaps had even forgotten them ... Relatives are not in a strong position to complain: they are not experts, they may be ashamed to talk about their problems, and they may have come to the conclusion that no help can be offered which will substantially reduce their difficulties. They must sometimes feel that the doctors and social workers are biased towards taking the patient's point of view. At the same time, a strong feeling of duty and humanity makes many relatives accept the burden of caring for a handicapped patient. It is not necessarily good clinical practice to accept this situation as a justification for 'community care'.
>
> (Brown *et al.*, quoted in Creer and Wing, 1974)

In their report Creer and Wing agreed with these comments. Voysey (1975) also saw family members as relatively powerless and overlooked by professionals. She pointed out that if the explanatory accounts of family members and medical professionals conflicted it was more likely that the accounts of the latter would eventually become accepted by the families as definitive.

It is intuitively plausible that this is more likely to happen if family carers are not asked directly to voice their opinions and describe their experiences, and we know that this is seldom the case. Berger and Luckman (1971) argue that face-to-face conversation enables individuals to gain immediate and continual access to their subjectivity through formulating and hearing their own speech. They suggest that, by this mechanism, language crystallizes and stabilizes people's subjectivity and allows them to know themselves and their opinions more fully. Hence, through being asked to talk about areas that were extremely familiar but possibly not often discussed, the interviewees in this study were able to define and crystallize some of their thoughts.

Certainly, one of the most striking findings in the interviews relates to what has been described by Creer and Wing (1974), Hoenig and Hamilton (1966) and others as the family carers' tendency to understate their degree of burden. This suggests some objective yardstick by which burden can be accurately and reliably measured. I would suggest, however, that burden and the experiences of living with and caring for a psychiatrically ill relative must be individually defined, and that what we are told by interviewees should be treated as an accurate representation of the meaning of their situation.

From this premise we can see that the interviewees did indeed express feelings that they carried a burden, and that the extent to which they thought of this as negative and unwelcome depended on various factors. The respondents fell into two broad groupings, highly involved and more removed carers. By exploring the characteristics of each group it was found that if there was a close kinship tie, a long history to the relationship and if the carer felt that he or she had gained from the relationship either now or in the past, then the responsibilities were seen as less burdensome. Similarly in the case of younger people, when the carer still had hopes and expect- ations of change and improvement the responsibilities might not be shouldered unwillingly. The extent to which carers describe themselves as 'burdened' did not appear to relate directly to the nature of the ill relative's mental health problems.

I think it is possible to draw out some implications for policy and service provision (including that of community psychiatric nursing) from these points. Firstly, there is a pointer in the study to a need for greater access to information relating to health, social services and housing. Birchwood and Smith (1987) also highlighted information as a key need. Similarly, in a study on depression Kuipers (1987) found that a basic requirement of the relatives was information to help them differentiate between 'illness' behaviour and other behaviour. They also sought advice on how to manage difficult situations. Kuipers suggests that carers may assume that the professionals know how to manage such situations and are for some reason withholding this advice. Clearly CPNs could have a key educative role in sharing their knowledge and skills with family carers. Of course this could not be done in isolation from other members of the mental health or primary health care team. Furthermore, not all interviewees in this research were receiving all their entitlements to social security benefits, nor did they know how to go about making the necessary applications. Gottlieb (1983) has made the point that practical help, and especially financial aid, contri- bute to the alleviation of emotional strain. Many CPNs may feel that they do not have the necessary information to fully advise on welfare benefits, however, they may check what benefits carers and clients are receiving and direct them to the appropriate services, if necessary facilitating this contact.

Secondly, the interviews suggest that family members may be somewhat sceptical about the benefits of the transfer of resources from a hospital setting to the community, although the respondents certainly did not dismiss the philosophy outright. There was some confusion over the connection between these moves and much publicized hospital cut-backs. It would therefore seem important that the mental health services explain as fully as possible the thinking behind such policy changes. If CPNs keep themselves fully informed of the plans for community resources in their district they may discuss them with clients and carers and, just as important, act as families' advocates to the planners on the nature of the services that are needed. CPNs may also be able to facilitate a dialogue between planners and client and carer groups.

Thirdly, I think it is important that we pay more attention to what family members tell us and fully recognize that they are often acting as primary carers with the health and social services acting simply as adjuncts. Since in most of the families there was no evidence to suggest that the carers wished to give up their role, the task of the professional services should be to aid the family as far as possible in carrying this out. This is perhaps particularly important where the key carer is receiving little support from other family members, and there is little or no reciprocity in her relationship with the ill relative. In research on the carers of people with senile dementia Gilhooly (1987) found that carers were often reluctant to share problems with other relatives or to ask for help, including help from professionals. From my interviews there is an indication that the people who receive little support are the ones who feel most burdened by their situation and feel that they receive little in return. Gouldner (1973) points out that in such circumstances an unbalanced two-party system may be made more stable by the support of a third party. The support needed may sometimes be emotional and interpersonal, allowing the carer to discuss her feelings openly and honestly. Several of the interviewees expressed some relief in being able to talk to me, although I was able to offer them nothing but a listening ear. More commonly however, carers may need, in addition, more practical help and advice. It is important that their expressions of what help they would like are not quickly dismissed as irrational. Such help as, say, someone to keep their relative company occasionally or relief admissions to allow carers a holiday may be enough to keep them actively involved in caring. Many carers may be helped in their role if CPNs and others were to encourage them to identify and act on their own needs at times, rather than dedicating themselves totally to their ill relative. By not asking the family members what help they would like or, perhaps worse, asking them and then being unable or unwilling to provide it, we reinforce our self-defined role as experts who know what is most important and once again appear to dismiss the family members' central role and knowledge of their relative.

Both Moroney (1976) and Walker (1982) have pointed to the need for a shared system of care. I would suggest that my findings support a similar conclusion. What is needed is a genuine partnership between family members (where they exist and are willing to care) and health and social services in which the latter do not attempt to take over the central role of the family but rather provide a level of support that facilitates the family's continuing involvement.

ACKNOWLEDGEMENTS

I would like to thank Dr Mike Hornsby-Smith of the University of Surrey for his helpful comments on the draft, and the Department of Health and Social Security for the award of a Nursing Research Studentship to undertake the course and this research.

APPENDIX

Interview guide

Nature of the problem

1. Who is the family member who has been referred to psychiatric services?
2. Who are the other members of the family?
3. Who lives with the person who is receiving treatment?
4. How often do you see each other?
5. What sort of things do you do to help your relative?
6. Does anyone else in the family give regular help?
7. How long has your relative had his/her problem?
8. Do you have any particular worries about your relative?
9. What are your main worries?

Structure of help

1. What help have you had in the past?
2. What was the most helpful, to you and your relative?
3. Did you generally receive enough information about what was happening?
4. What help are you receiving now, e.g. from statutory and voluntary agencies, neighbours, etc.?
5. Who do you see as being the main helping person, outside of the family, for your relative?
6. What do you think the job of the CPN is?
7. Do you think the nurse that sees your relative could do more, does too much, or is about right?
8. Does he/she see you regularly?
9. Do you feel you have enough say in what happens to your relative?

Family burden

1. How do your relative's problems affect you, or other members of your family?
2. Have there been any changes in the way you live, e.g. in your routine, contact with friends, your financial situation?

3. Have family relationships been affected?
4. Has there been any effect on your health, either physical or psychological? Or on other family members?
5. What do you see as being the most serious problem facing you at present?
6. Can you say what prompts you to take on these responsibilities?

Alternatives to current situation

1. Do you think other people understand what life is like for you?
2. If you had a totally free choice, what would be the thing that would most help you now?
3. Are you aware of plans to develop more care in the community? What do you think of these plans?
4. What is the most important thing that you would like to say to the people who plan psychiatric services, if you had the chance?

REFERENCES

Berger, P. and Luckman, T. (1971) *The Social Construction of Reality*, Penguin, Harmondsworth.
Birchwood, M. and Smith, J. (1987) Schizophrenia and the family, in Orford, J. (ed.) *Coping with Disorder in the Family*, Croom Helm, London.
Blumer, H. (1969) *Symbolic Interactionism*, Prentice-Hall, New Jersey.
Boyd, J.L. McGill, C.W. and Falloon, I. (1981) Family participation in the community rehabilitation of schizophrenics. *Hospital and Community Psychiatry*, **32**(9), 629–632.
Brown, G.W., Birley, J. and Wing, J. (1972) Influence of family life on the course of schizophrenic disorders: a replication. *British Journal of Psychiatry*, **121**, 241–258.
Creer, C. and Wing, J. (1974) *Schizophrenics at Home*, National Schizophrenia Fellowship, Surbiton.
Dunham, H.W. (1974) Community psychiatry: some neglected realities, in Roman, P. and Trice, H. (eds) *Sociological Perspectives in Community Mental Health*, Davis, Philadelphia.
Field, P. and Morse, J. (1985) *Nursing Research: The application of qualitative approaches*, Croom Helm, London.
Furler, E. (1979) Against hegemony in health care service evaluation. *Community Health Studies*, **3**(1), 32–41.
Gilhooly, M. (1987) Senile dementia and the family, in Orford, J. (ed.) *Coping with Disorder in the Family*, Croom Helm, London.
Glaser, B. and Strauss, A. (1967) *The discovery of grounded theory*, Aldine, Chicago.
Gostin, L. (1983) *A Practical Guide to Mental Health Law*, MIND, London.
Gottlieb, B.H. (1983) *Social Support Strategies*, Sage Publications, London.
Gouldner, A.W. (1973) *For Sociology*, Allen Lane, London.

Grad, J. and Sainsbury, P. (1963) Mental illness and the family. *The Lancet*, **i**, 544–547.

HMSO (1968) *Report of the Committee on Local Authority and Allied Personal Social Services*, (Chairman F. Seebohm) Cmnd 3703, HMSO, London.

Hoenig, J. and Hamilton, M. (1966) The schizophrenic patient in the community and his effect on the household. *International Journal of Social Psychiatry*, **12**(3), 165–176.

Hoult, J. *et al.* (1981) A controlled study of psychiatric hospital versus community treatment – the effect on relatives. *Australia and New Zealand Journal of Psychiatry*, **15**, 323–328.

Hunter, P. (1974) Community psychiatric nursing in Britain: an historical review. *International Journal of Nursing Studies*, **11**(4), 223–233.

Kuipers, L. (1987) Depression and the family, in Orford, J. (ed.) *Coping with Disorder in the Family*, Croom Helm, London.

Leff, J. and Vaughn, C. (1985) *Expressed Emotion in Families*, Guilford Press, London.

Melia, K. (1983) Students' views of nursing. *Nursing Times*, **29**(20), 24–27.

Melia, K. (1987) *Learning and Working*, Tavistock, London.

Ministry of Health (1962) *A Hospital Plan for England and Wales*, Cmnd 1604, HMSO, London.

Moroney, R.M. (1976) *The Family and the State*, Longman, London.

Pai, S. and Kapur, R.L. (1982) Impact of treatment intervention on the relationship between dimensions of clinical psychopathology, social dysfunction and burden on the family of psychiatric patients. *Psychological Medicine*, **12**, 651–658.

Simmons, S. and Brooker, C. (1986) *Community Psychiatric Nursing: A social perspective*, Heinemann, London.

Sladden, S. (1979) *Psychiatric Nursing in the Community: A study of a working situation*, Churchill Livingstone, Edinburgh.

Tarrier, N., Barraclough, C., Vaughn, C. *et al.* (1988) The community management of schizophrenia – a controlled trial of a behavioural intervention with families to reduce relapse. *British Journal of Psychiatry*, **153**, 532–542.

Voysey, M. (1975) *A Constant Burden*, Routledge and Kegan Paul, London.

Walker, A. (ed.) (1982) *Community Care*, Blackwell and Robertson, Oxford.

Wilkin, D. (1979) *Caring for the Mentally Handicapped Child*, Croom Helm, London.

Wing, J.W. (1981) From institutional to community care. *Psychiatric Quarterly*, **53**(2), 139–151.

CHAPTER FOUR

Client satisfaction with community psychiatric nursing

Rachel Munton

SUMMARY

This chapter is a summary of the pilot study of a research project undertaken as part of the English National Board clinical course number 811, Care of the Mentally Ill Person in the Community, at Sheffield City Polytechnic 1988. The research is concerned with inviting evaluative feedback from clients discharged from a period of community psychiatric nurse (CPN) intervention. It aims to discover what aspects of that intervention the client found satisfactory.

The location of care for people with mental health difficulties continues to shift from the institutional setting into the community. With this shift comes a need to review and evaluate the philosophy and framework of care provision, so that it develops in a way that meets the client identified need. The theoretical recognition of this need has resulted in frequent references in mental health literature to consumerism, the devolution of power and a partnership between the providers and recipients of care (O'Neill, 1983; MIND, 1983; Brandon and Brandon, 1987). However, as MIND's Chairperson, Juliet Bingley, writes in her introduction to MIND's proposals for a new mental health service (MIND, 1983): 'The gap between rhetoric and action is nowhere as marked as in the development of mental health services.'

The jargon of 'consumers as colleagues' is seldom translated into reality, in a culture where those with mental health problems remain marginalized (Brandon, 1981). It is a desire to act on the current rhetoric of consumerism that underpins this study. Client satisfaction with community psychiatric nursing services is seen as an important evaluation tool and a critical outcome variable.

In this study, informal, unstructured interviews with Nottingham based mental health consumer groups provided an insight into consumer concerns about community psychiatric nursing practice, and these areas of concern were then incorporated into the research questionnaire. This postal questionnaire for anonymous, retrospective completion was sent to 20 adult clients discharged from a period of CPN intervention over the previous year. Open questions predominated to allow respondents freedom to express attitudes and feelings in their own words with as little constraint as possible. Over a three-week period a 55% response rate was achieved. The resultant rich, subjective data highlighted elements of both client satisfaction and dissatisfaction with CPN intervention.

Central issues related to client satisfaction were the CPNs' willingness and ability to listen, and a genuine understanding of the client. Several other issues of importance to the client were identified, for example explicit invitation by CPNs to be contacted outside visits, needs for increased access to CPNs and preference for domiciliary visits.

It seems that clients value an opportunity to comment on their experience of CPN contact, and are both able and willing to report unsatisfactory as well as satisfactory experiences, and to generate ideas for service improvement. The study of client satisfaction with community psychiatric nursing services is in accordance with MIND's (1983) recommendations for a meaningful community mental health service, in seeking to treat the client as a full citizen with rights and responsibilities, who is entitled to be consulted and to have an active opportunity to shape and influence relevant services, no matter how severe his or her disability.

Community psychiatric nursing, as a relatively young profession, can be innovative in its development and through research into client satisfaction may realize:

> ... a great potential for the views of patients in receipt of community psychiatric nursing care to make a contribution to the planning of services and, by providing valuable information about their preferences, to influence the mode of service operation.

> (Mangen and Griffith, 1982)

With this in mind, the chapter concludes with some thoughts on the methodology and implications of the main study.

AIMS OF THE STUDY

By focusing on client feedback this study aims to:

1. provide a formal opportunity to learn what clients have found helpful and unhelpful in the CPN intervention, and to use this to
2. provide the knowledge base to underpin changes in service provision in order to meet client-identified wants, wishes and desires, and thus

3. reduce the distance between the 'doers' and 'done to' in community
    psychiatric nursing practice.

The need to reduce the disparity of power between users and providers
of the health service is seen as the key factor in attempts to develop
meaningful consumerism.

(Winkler, 1987)

FORMULATION OF THE RESEARCH QUESTION

What aspects of CPN intervention does the client find satisfactory? This
question outlines the study's aim to discover what clients found satisfactory
within the context of CPN intervention so that an assessment of the extent
to which that intervention gratified the wants, wishes and desires of the
client can be made.

Although this is, in part, an evaluative exercise carried out by the CPN's
client, the study neither seeks to appraise individual CPN performance, nor
to uncover the client's particular difficulties which led to that CPN involvement.

The study focuses exclusively on client-reported satisfaction as an
outcome variable. It does not study objective measures of therapeutic
outcome, i.e. the extent to which the CPN's involvement has helped to
solve or ameliorate the problems identified at referral or subsequently.
Although these two areas are not always mutually exclusive, satisfaction
and objective outcome measures are regarded as discrete entities in this
study.

The focus of this study is on the quality of the encounter between CPN
and client, as perceived by the client, because:

> People live in a subjective world as well as an objective one, and there-
> fore one important part of agency effectiveness is clients' subjective
> reactions to their contact.

(Gutek, 1978)

As client satisfaction can be seen to provide only one element of evaluative data, this study cannot be a multi-faceted evaluation of community
psychiatric nursing practice. However, the issue of client satisfaction is
highly relevant to community psychiatric nursing practice. Professionals
often assume a knowledge of what is important to the client without
consultation. The pursuit of the consumer viewpoint is readily justifiable in
a service which strives to be client centred, it is *non*-consultation which
demands justification.

LITERATURE REVIEW

The availability of literature relating directly to client satisfaction with community psychiatric nursing is very small. Four relevant studies will be considered here: Mangen and Griffith (1982), Marks (1985) Hunter (1978) and Pollock (1986b). Literature concerning consumerism in mental health care, and quality assurance initiatives, will also be considered, as will satisfaction studies from disciplines other than community psychiatric nursing.

Most directly relevant to this study is Mangen and Griffiths' (1982) comparative study of satisfaction over an 18-month period with CPN as opposed to consultant psychiatrist out-patient follow-up. As part of a larger study by Mangen *et al.* (1983), three main areas of CPN and standard out-patient department follow-up were considered:

1. efficacy in terms of symptom alleviation, social role performance, expressed consumer satisfaction, and patients' families degree of burden;
2. actual pattern of treatment received;
3. the comparative costs of both modes of follow-up.

Clinical and social outcomes were found to be comparable in both follow-up groups; community psychiatric nursing care was more expensive initially but subsequently and over the whole study period it was cheaper. Using an interviewer-rated questionnaire and self-report schedule at the end of the study, satisfaction with CPN and out-patient treatment was compared in a sample of 71 neurotic patients. Significantly greater consumer satisfaction was expressed by the CPN patient group. Whilst Mangen and Griffith (1982) acknowledge that rated satisfaction with health care is usually high, compared with the out-patient follow-up group:

> Nurses were regarded as more easy to talk to, kinder, more caring, displaying more interest, pleasanter, putting patients at ease and better at their jobs.
>
> (Mangen and Griffith, 1982)

At the conclusion of the study, 100% satisfaction was reported with CPN follow-up.

However, whilst domiciliary care was favoured as it enabled the clients to form more confiding relationships with the CPNs, due to the increased duration of visits and informality, clients in the study: '... in both groups considered themselves only partly informed about the nature of their disorders and likely prognosis.' (Mangen and Griffith, 1982). Mangen and Griffith therefore recommend that more energy should be expended in giving information to clients, particularly that which will assist in the development of coping strategies to overcome the effects of long-term illness.

Mangen and Griffiths' study looked at client satisfaction as one of many outcome variables. It was a comparative study and concerned a specific client group by diagnosis. This makes translation to other client groups questionable. However, it does provide an insight into the values of the CPN as perceived by the client.

Marks' (1985) study also evaluates the clinical outcome for neurotic patients of nurse behaviour therapists in a primary care setting, in comparison to treatment by the general practitioner (GP). Marks found that patients allocated to a nurse behaviour therapist showed greater improvements than the GP group at both 6- and 12-month follow-up. Particularly relevant to this study is the finding that patients preferred the primary care treatment setting (home or GP's surgery) as it was more familiar and felt to reduce stigma.

Marks (1985) also makes reference to the unmeasured results of the survey: that brief (one session) behavioural counselling was of benefit to clients; and that the GP sought wider advice from the nurse therapist than was expected, resulting in an extended role which Marks likens to that of a CPN.

Hunter's (1978) research concerned a patient group with the diagnostic label of schizophrenia. His study was undertaken over a five-year period and examined the viewpoints of patients, carers, and the practice of CPNs. It sought to reveal what influence, if any, CPN involvement had on the lives of the people concerned. The group of patients supported by a CPN were compared retrospectively with a group without this intervention. During the study, the patients in the CPN group were admitted to hospital more frequently, and spent longer periods there once admitted. The study did not seek to explain reasons for this in detail, but postulated that it may be due to a recognition by the CPN of behaviours which warrant further treatment, behaviours that may have gone unobserved in the control (no CPN) group. However, over the five-year study period, the CPN group reported relatively few problems, compared with the control group.

Hunter (1978) found that 23 out of 30 carers described the CPN involvement as helpful, with 16 of these respondents giving strong positive indications of the value of the CPN visits. The seven carers who described the CPN's visits as of no help were those who continued to be distressed by the patients' behaviour, or felt that continuity of care was not provided. The results of this study provide valuable insights into the CPN's value to the carer and patient, with valuable verbatim reports illuminating their perspectives. The study concludes that the CPN's value as expressed by those concerned can be summarized as follows:

1. the CPN's provision of a special feeling of security through expertise in mental illness (for example, discerning difficulties, not being fooled by the patient);
2. the long-term support and security this brought for the carer in particular (for example, taking time to talk and being friendly, reliable, etc.);
3. the function of the nurse as an agent of the service, particularly their association with a psychiatrist and the authority this conveyed.

Hunter (1978) was also able to make recommendations for beneficial changes in CPN intervention. These include a change in focus from exclusively patient-centered care to an approach which views the carer and social situation as a whole. Linked with this is the adoption by the CPN of a more active, therapeutic approach, with an explicit discussion of its nature with all concerned. This would move towards a recognition of the central importance of the care giver.

Most frequently commented upon in Hunter's (1978) study were the personality and attitudes of the CPN: 'High on the list of the nurses' positive attributes in this study were friendship and understanding'.

Within a specific diagnostic group, CPN intervention was assessed in a multidimensional analysis of outcome, including carers' and clients' perspectives, which are reported verbatim to provide a genuine insight into their individual perspective, and is in this respect directly comparable to this study.

Pollock (1986b) contributed to CPN outcome research in a study that aimed to describe and compare two community psychiatric nursing services, elicit family and patients' views of these services, and through comparison, identify CPN activity which the family and patient find useful. This research is described more fully in Chapter 6. Arguing that her use of the Personal Questionnaire Rapid Scaling Technique (Pollock, 1986a) lends reliability and objectivity, she specifically focuses on the extent to which carers' experiences of problems were relieved by CPN intervention.

Pollock (1986b) explains:

The patients' views of community psychiatric nursing were also obtained because I considered it unethical to approach relatives without the permission of the psychiatric patients in the study.

Therefore, clients' own evaluation is elicited as an adjunct to carers' opinion, rather than as a primary focus.

Pollock's (1986b) study shows that carers found CPNs did not help with the: 'daily drudgery of caring' but responses to the questions eliciting carers' opinions of CPN activities were uniformly positive. The CPN was perceived as helpful in a specialist crisis capacity; the carer finding that this availability offered security. However, not all CPNs made themselves available in this capacity.

Carers found CPNs to be patient-oriented, and helpful to the carer in understanding their relatives' illness. Sixty per cent of carers did not see the CPN as an outsider; Pollock (1986b) suggests that this means that the CPN is seen as a friend or family member. This may be an assumption as there is a wide middle ground between outsider and family member, into which the CPN might fall. Carers reported their relationship with the CPN to be trusting and caring, facilitating problem sharing.

Pollock (1986b) looked specifically at CPNs' frequency of visits, case-load size, and carers' reported perceptions of the skill of individual CPNs; this resulted in three significant findings:

1. Busy CPNs were seen as less helpful than quiet ones when respondents replied affirmatively to the statement: 'I have to take care not to upset the patient'.
2. Female carers found CPNs less helpful than male carers in response to the statement; 'I don't know if I do the right things'.
3. All but one CPN was considered to be significantly helpful in response to the statement; 'The nurse is easy to talk to'.

Pollock (1987) also reports the emphasis placed by CPNs on developing relationships, which demonstrates a shift from the medical models' use found in previous studies (see Sladden, 1979). Pollock concludes that there is a need for explicit aims and goals in CPN service provision, and local evaluation and monitoring of performance.

Sladden's (1979) research, a comprehensive process study, aimed to analyse and describe the functions and skills of CPNs in clinic and domiciliary settings. She chose a descriptive rather than evaluative study, arguing that evaluation is meaningful only when it follows the identification, reproduction, recognition and replication of the activities to be evaluated. At the time of her study, these activities had not been examined.

Sladden's (1979) work did not set out to evaluate efficiency or effectiveness of the CPN; nonetheless, some pertinent observations about the CPN's role are made which are relevant to the study of client satisfaction. Frequent reference is made throughout the study to the importance of the emotional component of the treatment relationship. This was enhanced in the domiciliary CPN group, who adopted a more psychosocial frame of reference than their clinic-based counterparts, demonstrated through lengthier contact, involvement of the client's family, and greater continuity of care.

Sladden (1979) notes that the most outstanding features of nurse–patient contact were sheer persistence, durability and a practically indissoluble commitment to care. However, CPNs' work was found to be largely conservative and non-dynamic in nature, and Sladden describes CPNs as the mobile arm of the parent hospital, facilitators of hospital care rather than substitutes for it.

The current relevance of some of Sladden's findings are limited by virtue of a number of changes that have taken place within community psychiatric nursing practice since her study. These include a wider, more open referral policy, with closer links with primary care health workers. This has resulted in a more diverse client group, with whom CPNs work in a primary and secondary preventive framework, thus broadening the spectrum from the more traditional tertiary prevention (Caplan, 1961). These issues cannot be discussed at length here, but can be argued to challenge the direct translation of Sladden's (1979) findings to current community psychiatric nursing practice.

The small number of CPN–client outcome studies, particularly where client satisfaction is the primary focus, justified the exploration of studies from related disciplines in this literature search. There is a vast amount of such material, recurrent themes of which are outlined below.

Hill (1969), in an American study of women psychotherapy clients, found two broad client satisfaction clusters. The first cluster is expressed as:

> Satisfaction of having had a person to person relationship with the Therapist and having gained greater insight, self-understanding and self awareness as a consequence of therapy.

The second and less commonly reported cluster was the symptom relief cluster, for example achieving greater mood control.

Hill (1969) also draws attention to the therapists' de-emphasis on giving advice and guidance, and the low level of reported client satisfaction with this. Hill notes that working towards a specific goal increased client satisfaction.

The studies of both Kline *et al.* (1974) and Hill (1969) suggest that focused, goal-oriented work, where the therapist is prepared to be directive and advisory, increase satisfaction, and Hill (1969) shows that the interpersonal relationship afforded to the client is the most satisfactory element of therapy.

> While the patients' satisfaction with ongoing therapy is hardly a criterion of ultimate success, it does represent a partial fulfilment of those personal needs which lead a person to seek therapy, and undoubtedly influences the maintenance of the therapeutic relationship.

Kline *et al.* (1974), in an American study of clients evaluating psychiatric out-patient services found that three therapist behaviours caused client dissatisfaction as expressed through termination of contact:

1. feeling the therapist was not interested in them;
2. finding the therapist too insensitive or working in a way inappropriate to their needs;
3. feeling that the therapist was incompetent or insufficiently trained.

Clients reported most dissatisfaction about receiving insufficient specific advice and direction. The studies of both Kline *et al.* (1974) and Hill (1969) suggest that focused, goal-oriented work, where the therapist is prepared to be directive and advisory, increase satisfaction and Hill (1969) shows that the interpersonal relationship afforded to the client is the most satisfactory element of therapy.

Loff *et al.* (1987) surveyed client satisfaction with mental health treatment in a group of adolescents, their parents, and the parents of child clients under the age of 13. The authors make reference to the very few studies which have focused on satisfaction specifically, as opposed to those which consider it as a small part of total outcome evaluation. Using a client/patient satisfaction rating scale, the respondents showed good to moderate levels of satisfaction (124 out of 377 questionnaires were returned). Of particular interest is that 45% of adolescents, and 37% of parents found individual therapy, as opposed to family or group therapy, most satisfactory.

The study of Loff *et al.* (1987) is directly comparable to this study in that it focuses exclusively on satisfaction as an outcome measure. However, Loff *et al.* (1987) acknowledge that their study falls foul of some of the formidable methodological problems of such research (for example poor response rate) which will be discussed later in this chapter.

Within social work, particularly mental health social work, the area of client satisfaction studies has been described by Fisher (in Booth, 1983) as 'burgeoning'. The pioneering work *The Client Speaks* (Mayer and Timms, 1970) marked the beginning of this new era in social work research. Fisher (in Booth, 1983) suggests this was underpinned by two main theories. Firstly, that the degree of client satisfaction would be the barometer of a healthy service, and that dissatisfaction would pinpoint areas for improvement; and secondly that social workers have a value to their clients beyond narrow outcome measures.

Mayer and Timms (1970), in a retrospective study, found that clients who were satisfied in seeking help with interpersonal problems had four common traits:

1. they had been able to unburden themselves of their problem;
2. they were given emotional support;
3. they were enlightened about their situation, with regard to both internal and external factors;
4. they had found that the social workers did not hesitate to give direct guidance through suggestion, advice and recommendation.

The study makes the analogy that offering psychosocial or other support to an individual whose material and/or financial needs remain unmet, is like offering a set of clothes to a drowning man.

Fisher (in Booth, 1983) links the interest in client studies in social work with the adoption of a consumer model of service delivery, where consumer preference becomes a critical influence. This shift in emphasis is currently mirrored within mental health care provision and is broadly termed consumerism. This concept has attracted much attention recently and published material on consumerism in mental health provision is plentiful. The main arguments are summarized here.

Winkler (1987) identifies the emergence of the supermarket analogy of consumerism from the Griffiths' Enquiry report (1983). She regards this as a retailer model of customer relations, with its focus on cutting down queues and exchanging goods. Winkler defines this as the 'harmless version' of consumerism, requiring very little serious change, but much public visibility. 'It does not extend, even at Marks and Spencer, to inviting the customers onto the board.' (Winkler, 1987)

This service model relationship is criticized by Fisher (in Booth, 1983) as inappropriate in mental health services. He argues that clients are *not* like consumers, in that their preference to a particular type of service ought directly to lead to an increased provision of that service. Fisher (in Booth, 1983) argues that social work clients are not free agents in a service market; and that this captivity of the client, his or her limited knowledge of other sources of help, and his or her possible acceptance of low standards of care, all threaten the usefulness of satisfaction studies within a mental health care context.

Although the last two criticisms may be true of the CPN's client, the CPN, unlike the social worker, has no statutory powers or responsibilities. This makes the issue of 'captivity' less relevant in the CPN's work, as the client must, to some extent, wish to be involved in their interaction for it to continue.

In a mental health care context, the service model relationship of consumerism is also challenged as simplistic:

> For hoovers and toasters, this may be a relevant assumption, but for the disturbed relationships which characterise the lives of Social Work clients, such an approach is naive.
>
> (Fisher, in Booth, 1983)

Mangen and Griffith (1982) also criticize the attribution of a consumer status to clients, which may suggest a supply and demand interpretation to what is, in fact, a complex negotiation between therapeutic agent and patient.

Consumer research within this commercial definition and framework is analogous to commercial market research, often finding out what the researcher wants, not the client, and providing hard data, through a structured format, on which policy decisions may be based (Fisher in Booth, 1983). For these reasons, consumerism within this framework is fraught with difficulties in the translation to mental health care provision (Winkler, 1987).

Chambers (1987) offers a definition that is more appropriate to the mental health forum:

> A more sophisticated definition should perhaps encapsulate the idea of developing an awareness and a sensitivity to the needs and expectations of the consumer in the planning and running of services.

This can be seen to be a slightly wider expression that takes into account the substantial interaction between services and users, and acknowledges that attention should be paid to users' views (Chambers, 1987). Fisher (in Booth, 1983) argues that small-scale, qualitative research methods are the most useful in eliciting those views.

It is this concept of consumerism that underpins this study, and is in line with many recommendations for consumer participation in mental health care. To dismiss consumerism as inapplicable because of its usual connotations of market choice, or supply and demand, may be used as an excuse to avoid taking up elements of this philosophy to provide a more client-centered service. One way in which this can be achieved is through the study of client satisfaction.

It can be seen that client evaluation of services, and satisfaction as an element of that evaluation, is supported by clients, authors on consumerism, current mental health care philosophy and quality assurance initiatives alike. However, the recurrent theme throughout the discussion of client satisfaction studies is the methodological minefield which must be negotiated.

Methodological difficulties in the study of client satisfaction

In the face of much evidence which shows that uniformly high levels of satisfaction are reported, even in areas in which satisfaction is known to be low by 'common knowledge' (for example assembly line work, marriage ending in divorce) the fundamental validity of clients' reports of satisfaction is often questioned (Gutek, 1978). Because of this, it is argued that satisfaction data should be viewed with some suspicion as *objective* behavioural indicators of satisfaction (for example absenteeism from work, non-attendance at planned appointments) are frequently incongruous with *subjective* reports of satisfaction.

Lebow (1982) suggests that mental health service satisfaction data derived using unobtrusive, objective measures such as monitoring utilization of services may infer that if a client attends or participates in treatment, this in itself indicates satisfaction with that treatment. However, participation *per se* is equally likely to be influenced by the very same factors that threaten to invalidate satisfaction data, for example social desirability, or lack of alternative forums for help.

Gutek (1978) also reports discrepancies between an individual's evaluation of his or her own experience, the experience he or she imagines others have had, and the service as a whole. Fisher (in Booth, 1983) also notes that respondents may differentiate between the *way* a service is provided and the adequacy of that provision. This issue of dimensionality is raised by Lebow (1982) in a discussion of methods which may enhance the specificity of client and treatment variables in relation to satisfaction.

Satisfaction with an interaction/relationship may also be unrelated to levels of therapeutic improvement and it is on this count that Fisher (in Booth, 1983), in line with relative deprivation theorists, questions the pertinence of client satisfaction studies. Can the client who is *less* lonely, or *less* likely to take an overdose, really describe him or herself, or be described, as satisfied?

Gutek (1978) also discusses the influence of the contrast effect, where positive elements are found in an experience about which negative attitudes prevailed. Such contrasts may inflate levels of reported satisfaction.

Mangen and Griffith (1982) also acknowledge that a client's responses may be influenced by what he or she knows of the therapist's role, indicating a naivety about treatment rather than an informed decision process reflecting the adequacy of that treatment (Lebow, 1982). Clients may also differentiate professional roles:

> It is apparent that patients have different expectations of care provided by psychiatrists and nurses; whilst patients may attach great value to the inter-personal relationship with the nurse, they may regard the technical aspects of that treatment as being more firmly within the reins of the doctor.
>
> (Mangen and Griffith, 1982)

Validity in client satisfaction studies is challenged in many ways; the problems of acquiescence, reactivity, social desirability, mood and halo effects may result in responses more favourable than the clients' reality; respondents may not be able to recall negative experiences, or may not be able to articulate their views (Gutek, 1978; Mangen and Griffith, 1982; Lebow, 1982).

For the specific client group of his study, Hunter (1978) argues:

Psychiatric patients and their relatives can be in a particularly difficult position concerning the open expression of their views. Many recognise their continuing dependence on the service, and expect this to continue indefinitely.

Although Hunter speaks of a diagnostic group (schizophrenics) for whom long-term involvement may be particularly likely, the specific issues raised in this quotation of dependency, vulnerability, and their influence on honest client response, must be considered in the context of this study as the sample is drawn from those who have, or have had, mental health difficulties.

Further threats to validity are caused by the poor response rates characteristic of mental health client surveys. This is due in part to a high geographic mobility in this client group and other motivational issues (Lebow, 1982). Potential distortions may also occur through selective attrition, and some studies suggest that respondents differ from non-respondents in ways which are likely to affect the reporting of satisfaction, i.e. those who are dissatisfied may be those who do not respond (Loff *et al.*, 1987; Lebow, 1982; Hawkes, 1987).

As satisfaction is a multi-faceted and divisible function, the most critical issue in satisfaction studies is what does satisfaction actually *mean*. Lebow (1982) argues that it may be best considered as conceptually separate from other outcome measures in order to discover its meaning to the respondent. Mangen and Griffith (1982) argue that because satisfaction as a concept is rarely defined, often only a small segment of that concept can be tapped in client satisfaction studies. The need to move beyond superficiality in such studies is emphasized by Gutek (1978) in order to develop a fuller understanding of what respondents actually mean in their answers to satisfaction questions. Focusing must be sharp and measures improved, answers checked for reliability through questions being repeated in alternative forms to encounter check responses (Gutek, 1978).

There is, within this methodological minefield, one way to avoid these various and complex issues, as Gutek (1978) suggests: 'The most drastic approach to the apparent problem of subjective satisfaction involves abandoning the attempt entirely.' However tempting, this would deny clients the right to offer their feedback, and would omit a central element in the evaluation and monitoring of the CPN–client interaction. Satisfaction studies are one element of this evaluation and whilst they cannot be regarded as the sole criterion of success, must be taken into account in the review and planning of client centred services. 'The client has a unique view of the treatment process, and an important conception of the quality of service.' (Lebow, 1982).

THE PILOT STUDY

Design and conduct

The design and conduct of the pilot study aimed to offset many of the potential methodological problems of client satisfaction previously outlined. Through this the reliability and validity of the data is enhanced. In this pilot study, two main research tools were used: informal unstructured interviews, and a retrospective self-report postal questionnaire.

Retrospective evaluation was chosen as discharged clients may be less fearful of reprisals from their participation in such an evaluative study and, as a result, more willing to answer questions honestly. Clients in current contact with services may be particularly fearful of effects on their treatment as a consequence of their responses (Lebow, 1982).

Anonymity was considered critical in the pilot study to enhance honest, reliable responses, truly indicative of client satisfaction. The retrospective nature of the study assists in furthering anonymity, by creating a distance between the respondent and service being evaluated. Lebow (1982) summarizes some of the potential influences on a client's response:

> Consumers may alter their responses as they consider who will read these surveys, how the surveyors will regard them, and how the surveys will affect their future requests for service, and the careers of the practitioners who offered them treatment.

Introduction to the Nottingham mental health and community psychiatric nursing services

Nottingham and its immediate environs are divided into six mental health sectors, each served by a multidisciplinary team. The pilot study was conducted in one of these sectors, the North Nottingham and Hucknall Sector Team. The population served by this team is approximately 90 000 (1981 census).

The community is essentially an urban part of the Nottingham conurbation. Within the sector, there are two areas which are demographically disparate. Hucknall itself has many features of a self-contained small town. Here, the majority of dwellings are owner occupied. In October 1986, Hucknall colliery closed down, and only 540 of the 1300 made redundant were re-employed in other collieries. This had a significant effect on the unemployment profile of Hucknall. The sector also includes large areas of accommodation owned by the local authority, in both old established estates and city overspill estates. Two of these estates were described in the Social Services' County Deprived Area Study as 'areas of extreme disadvantage' (Pearson, 1987). This may be a contributory factor in the high level of psychiatric morbidity recorded in the sector, which in 1987 received the second largest number of referrals of all six sectors, the largest being the inner city sector.

Potential clients are referred to the Sector Team as a unit by a GP. Very occasionally, referrals can be accepted from other health workers or community groups. All referrals are dealt with at a weekly multidisciplinary team meeting, and an assessor is decided. The assessor feeds back his or her initial contact with the client and a key worker is identified. The assessor and key worker may be a member of any discipline. An emergency rota is established to provide an immediate response for clients whose needs dictate.

Unstructured interviews with consumer groups

Whilst constructing the pilot study questionnaire, the researcher sought opinions from various consumer groups in order to provide an insight into the consumers' perspectives of CPN work. The use of a non-structured interview to achieve this allowed spontaneous questions and free responses, most likely to be truly indicative of consumer concerns. The aim was to include in the pilot questionnaire items linked with these concerns. Lebow (1982) warns that the:

> Evaluator must not assume that clients attach the same degree of importance to various aspects of service provision as do the professionals.

The following Nottingham branches of consumer groups contributed to the pilot study:

- The Manic Depressive Fellowship
- Incest Survivors Group
- Anorexic Aid
- The National Schizophrenia Fellowship
- The Patients' Council.

The following groups in contact with potential clients were also notified of the study and invited to comment, but have not reported feedback to date:

- Nottingham MIND; Women at MIND
- Nottingham Community Health Council
- Nottingham Health Strategy Group.

The consumer group feedback showed several common themes that were taken up in the pilot study questionnaire.

1. Access to CPNs should be made easier, without the client needing to

be referred through a GP or consultant psychiatrist.
2. CPNs' working hours should be extended to include evenings, weekends and out-of-hours emergency work.
3. CPNs should work in a relative-centred as well as client-centred framework.
4. CPNs should work within a clearly defined appointment system, and make explicit invitations to clients to contact them outside appointment times as needed.
5. Any new development within the CPN service should be effectively and immediately communicated to consumer groups.
6. Clients should be able to choose the sex of their CPN.

Consumer group feedback frequently mentioned the value clients place on the 'friendly' relationship they enjoy with the CPN.

Definition of terms used in the research question

Question: 'What aspects of CPN intervention does the client find satisfactory?'
A CPN, for the purpose of this pilot study, is:

1. a registered mental nurse (RMN), male or female, working in the North Nottingham and Hucknall Sector Team;
2. a charge nurse/sister II grade staff member, with a minimum of 6 months in post as a CPN.

Intervention
Not as in its common usage, but as defined by Heron (1975) in terms of interaction processes, i.e. the client–therapist encounter, where:

1. there is some formal differentiation of roles between the one who is practising the intervention and his or her client, so that: 'The diffentiation is such that the practitioner is offering some kind of enabling service and skill to the client.' (Heron, 1975);
2. there is a clear and explicit voluntary contract between practitioner and client, so that they both agree to be freely involved in the interaction.

Client
A man or woman, aged 18–65, who has been discharged within the last 12 months from a period of CPN contact, irrespective of length. The client must not have been seen by a CPN prior to this period of contact. Someone who, fulfilling the above criteria, was not seen by any other discipline within the team apart from the CPN.
Satisfactory
The expressed gratification of the wants, wishes and desires of the client in

respect of his or her CPN intervention. The *Shorter Oxford English Dictionary* definition of 'to satisfy' is: 'To meet or fulfil the wish or desire or expectation of; to be accepted as all that could be reasonably desired; to content.'

The pilot study sample

Three CPNs (two male, one female) provided a list of 23 client names. No groups of clients were excluded by diagnosis or demographic factors. CPNs put forward all clients' names who met the criteria outlined above.

Clients who saw another multidisciplinary team member were excluded to avoid role confusion in evaluation. Similarly, clients who had had a previous episode of CPN contact were excluded to provide a specific evaluation exercise of current services; it was for this reason also that discharge within a 12-month period was considered the maximum acceptable. From the 23 names, 20 names were picked at random, 10 of the sample were male, 10 female.

The research tool

These 20 individuals were each sent:

1. an introductory letter;
2. a questionnaire;
3. a stamped addressed envelope to the researcher.

a) The introductory letter. The introductory letter aimed to add a personal dimension to the request for questionnaire completion, by using a handwritten personal name and signature. For ethical reasons, the researcher gave in this letter a full explanation of the purpose of the study, and the use to which replies would be put, to enable clients to make an informed choice about their participation. The anonymity of the study was emphasized, and how the individuals' name and address had been obtained was explained. An assurance was given that the CPN would not be identified or penalized through feedback received. An accurate estimation of the time required to complete the questionnaire was included (tested through completion by a client known to the researcher but not in the pilot sample). Clear instructions regarding return procedure and deadline were also included.

b) The questionnaire. A questionnaire was chosen as the research tool as it would enable clients, through anonymous completion and postal return, to consider their responses at length and openly express their views (Mangen and Griffith, 1982). To further this end, the self-report questionnaire consisted mainly of open questions, their purpose being to allow respondents freedom to express attitudes and feelings in their own words, with as little constraint as possible. The resulting rich, subjective data gives the most accurate client view of CPN intervention derived from the clients' own ideas and thoughts.

Questionnaires such as the one used in this study have the advantage of being free from interviewer bias (in a well-constructed tool) and thus more indicative of clients' views rather than the researchers' agenda. Offset against this advantage are the disadvantages of poor compliance, superficial or incomplete responses and comprehension difficulties. In designing the questionnaire, the following general principles were used to offset these problems:

1. Questions were short and concise (less than 20 words in length) and dealt with only one topic at a time. The total number of questions was limited to encourage completion (13 in all).
2. Wording of questions was straightforward, unambiguous, free from bias and built-in clues.
3. The amount of space allocated was metered in order to influence response length, maximized to facilitate comprehensive responses.
4. Questions progressed from simple to more complex topics, from the general to the specific.
5. Items to be answered in a similar way were grouped together, simple instructions were built into the questionnaire items.
6. Back door and indirect questions were used to check clients' responses to similar items. Questions were re-phrased to achieve repetition, and items included for the expression of dissatisfaction amongst those general elements with which respondents were satisfied.

A reminder letter was mailed, to be received by all respondents/non-respondents, two weeks after the original questionnaire, one week before the deadline for return. The timing of this was chosen to enable non-respondents to complete and return the questionnaire before the re-stated deadline. The reminder letter shared the same aims and style of the introductory letter sent with the questionnaire.

Therefore, because of the well-documented problem of poor response rate in client satisfaction and mental health consumer studies, the researcher attempted to enhance the response rate by the inclusion of a full explanatory letter (followed by a reminder letter) a straightforward questionnaire with a realistic deadline for completion, and by both ensuring and demonstrating anonymity of the client and CPN. However, this anonymity prevented the differentiation of respondents from non-respondents, and therefore any specific prompts for the latter group. A 55% response rate was achieved (11 questionnaires), which compares favourably with other client satisfaction studies (Lebow, 1982).

Analysis of findings

The pilot questionnaire's aims have been discussed earlier in this chapter: the data from the respondents is rich, qualitative and subjective in many instances, by virtue of the study's aim and design. Although trends and statistics can be derived from some of this data, in general the use of verbatim quotes and subjective interpretation predominates in this analysis.

The pilot study results will be considered within three main areas: elements of the CPN intervention that clients found satisfactory; elements of the CPN intervention that clients found unsatisfactory; and other incidental findings concerning the CPN–client intervention.

Three questions were posed to elicit the satisfactory elements of the CPN–client intervention.

1. What sort of person would you like a CPN to be?
2. If you need to talk over a problem with someone, what do you look for in that person?
3. Please write down what you found most helpful about the CPN.

It appears that clients would like CPNs to have a core cluster of characteristics:

- a willingness to listen
- an ability to listen
- empathy and understanding
- a non-judgemental acceptance
- genuineness
- an ability to air their own views
- an ability/willingness to give constructive help or advice.

These findings are best substantiated through clients' verbatim quotes:

He sat and listened to me which people need.

He understood the way I was feeling and he explained to me why I was feeling that way.
She got me through a difficult time when I just needed someone on my side.

His obvious sincerity and willingness to listen to the problem without being too cloying.

Questions that aimed to elicit areas with which clients were dissatisfied or could offer suggestions for improvement were:

1.   Please write down what you found most unhelpful about the CPN.
2.   In your opinion, how could the CPN service be improved?

Once again, a core set of criticisms emerged in response to the questions:

- a feeling of loss and dissatisfaction when the client–CPN intervention ended;
- feeling CPNs were inaccessible;
- suggestions that the hours that CPNs work are too limited;
- complaints about the lack of information given to the client about his or her situation;
- a desire to see more publicity and promotion of the role of CPNs.

Once again, these findings are best substantiated through client's verbatim quotes.

> Give the patient more information about what's happening with his or her case.
> To follow through without leaving the patient with a sense of loss.
> I would like to see more advertising as I think prevention could be a great asset rather than at present it appears they call after the event.
> It was difficult to arrange meeting times [due to having to take time from work].

In the face of much literature claiming that mental health clients are reluctant and/or unable to offer criticisms of the service they received, it is encouraging to find that even in this small pilot study,

1.   73% of the respondents reported unhelpful factors about the CPN;
2.   87% of respondents reported ways in which the service could be improved;
3.   37% of clients distinguished between the *way* the service is provided and the adequacy of that provision, for example: 'I think they do their best: it can't be easy for them, there are so many people who need help.'

This demonstrates the value of providing a formal feedback opportunity to clients.

In addition to these main areas of satisfaction and dissatisfaction, a number of incidental findings emerged:

1.   91% of clients were seen in their own home, often making strongly positive comments about this, for example: 'Very good because you really feel relaxed and able to express your feelings better.'
2.   No connection was found between visit frequency and satisfaction, but

clients expressed a desire to negotiate this with the CPN.

3. 45% of clients received visits of one-hour duration. All of these clients reported satisfaction with this length of time.

4. 73% of clients were invited to contact the CPN outside arranged visits: all these felt this was good. However, it was clear from one client's response that this should be made as an explicit invitation. 'It was said as they were leaving and not said with feeling!'

5. Two female clients suggested that CPNs of the same sex would have been preferred: 'I felt if I had spoken to someone of the same sex, it would have made things a little easier.'

Conclusion and discussion

This chapter has examined the design, conduct and findings of a small-scale research project concerning client satisfaction with CPN intervention.

The subjective data resulting from the pilot study can provide a base from which to move towards a more objective format in the main study without sacrificing the richness of individual perception. The inclusion of such perceptions, and the resultant qualitative data can be argued to be an inevitable feature in the study of nursing, which in itself is:

> Complex, multi-dimensional, difficult to define and understand, and may not be amenable to rigid experimental design which requires identification and control of intervening variables.
>
> (Cormack, 1984)

The pilot study has shown that clients *do* value an opportunity to disclose their opinions about their experience of CPN contact, and are well able to recall unsatisfactory as well as satisfactory experiences and to generate ideas for service improvement. This alone provides sufficient grounds for continuing with the main study, and to persevere with the theme of client satisfaction as the primary focus.

However, it has become clear that the study has not exclusively focused on the outcome of intervention, as many comments on the process of community psychiatric nursing have been made. This client view of the CPN intervention process has raised specific issues that can become foci in the main study.

Although firm conclusions cannot be drawn from this small pilot study, it appears that clients place a special value on the interpersonal relationship with the CPN. This finding is congruous with those of Hunter (1978), Pollock (1986b) and Mangen and Griffith (1982).

In terms of the aims of this research, as outlined earlier in the chapter, the pilot study has offered a formal opportunity to learn what clients find helpful and unhelpful in CPN intervention and has begun to provide the knowledge base on which service changes can occur.

The third aim, to reduce distance between the 'doers' and the 'done to', can only result from a continued and varied investment in client centred activities.

Eliciting clients' views can only be one part of that investment, but the pilot study allows for optimism: client satisfaction data *is* available on request, despite methodological problems. The main study will seek to further tap this critical form of evaluative material, a small beginning in the reduction of professional power and influence, and a corresponding increase in that of the client.

What becomes of them and of us will depend largely on the dismantling of barriers. Old attitudes survive new buildings and new systems.

(Brandon, 1981)

ACKNOWLEDGEMENTS

Thank you to those clients, friends and colleagues who have helped and encouraged me, to Margaret Grainger for her word processing, but above all to Ross, for everything.

REFERENCES

Booth, T. (ed.) (1983) *Social Services Monographics Research in Practice*, University of Sheffield, Sheffield.

Brandon, A. and Brandon, D. (1987) *Consumers as Colleagues*, MIND, London.

Brandon, D. (1981) *Voices of Experience: Consumer perspectives of psychiatric treatment*, MIND, London.

Caplan, G. (1961) *An Approach to Community Mental Health*, Tavistock, London.

Chambers, N. (1987) Developing a consumer strategy in the NHS or getting things right. *Hospital and Health Service Review*, **83**, 12–14.

Cormack, D.E.F. (ed.) (1984) *The Research Process of Nursing*, Blackwell Scientific, Oxford.

Gutek, B.A. (1978) Strategies for studying client satisfaction. *Journal of Social Issues*, **34** (4), 44–56.

Hawkes, J. (1987) *Patient/Client Satisfaction Surveys and their Methodology*, Quality Assurance Department, Wessex RHA.

Heron, J. (1975) *Six Category Intervention Analysis*, Human Potential Research Project, Guildford.

Hill, J.A. (1969) Therapists' goals, patients' aims and patient satisfaction in psychotherapy. *Journal of Clinical Psychology*, **25**, 455–9.

Hunter, P. (1978) *Schizophrenia and Community Psychiatric Nursing*, National Schizophrenia Fellowship, Surrey.

Kline, F., Adrian, A. and Spevak, M. (1974) Patients evaluate therapists, *Archives of General Psychiatry*, **31**, (11), 113–16.

Lebow, J. (1982) Consumer Satisfaction with Mental Health Treatment. *Psychological Bulletin*, **91** (2), 244–59.

Loff, C.D. Trigg, L.J. and Cassels, C. (1987) An evaluation of consumer satisfaction in a child psychiatric service: viewpoints of patients and parents. *American Journal of Orthopsychiatry*, **57**, 132–4.

Mangen, S.P. and Griffith, J.H. (1982) Patient satisfaction with community psychiatric nursing: a prospective controlled study. *Journal of Advanced Nursing*, **7**, 477–82.

Mangen, S.P., Paykel, E.S., Griffith, J.H., Burchell, A. and Mancini, P. (1983) Cost effectiveness of community psychiatric care of neurotic patients. *Psychological Medicine*, **13**, 407–16.

Marks, I. (1985) Controlled trial of psychiatric nurse therapists in primary care. *British Medical Journal*, **290**, 1181–4.

Mayer, J.E. and Timms, N. (1970) *The Client Speaks: Working Class Impressions of Case Work*, Routledge and Kegan Paul, London.

MIND Publications (1983) *Common Concern: MINDS' Manifesto for New Mental Health Service*, MIND, London.

O'Neill, P. (1983) *Health Crisis 1000*, Heinemann, London.

Pearson, A. (ed.) (1987) *Nursing Quality Measurement: Quality Assurance Methods for Peer Review*, Wiley & Sons, Chichester.

Pearson, D. (1987) *North Nottingham and Hucknall Mental Health Team*, Annual Report Nottingham Social Services, March 1987.

Pollock, L. (1986a) An Introduction to the Use of Repertory Grid Technique as a Research Method and Clinical Tool for Psychiatric Nurses. *Journal of Advanced Nursing*, **11**, 439–45.

Pollock, L. (1986b) An Evaluation Research Study of Community Psychiatric Nursing Employing the Pesonal Questionnaire Rapid Scaling Technique. *Community Psychiatric Nurses Journal*, May/June, 11–21.

Pollock, L.J. (1987) *Community Psychiatric Nursing Explained: An Analysis of the Views of Carers, Patients and Nurses*, Phd Thesis, Edinburgh University.

Sladden, S. (1979) *Psychiatric Nursing in the Community: A Study of a Working Situation*, Churchill Livingstone, Edinburgh.

Winkler, F. (1987) Consumerism in Health Care: Beyond the Supermarket Model. *Policy and Politics*, **15** (1), 1–8.

CHAPTER FIVE

Information for practice through computerized records

Maura Hunt and John Mangan

INTRODUCTION

The need for a common core regional information system for the Community Psychiatric Nursing (CPN) Services is discussed. The development of such a computerized system is presented in relation to the planning of its content, the technological aspects and its organizational and location requirements. The participation by the users of the system in creating its content is stressed so that the values, methods of working and expected outcomes of the service are made explicit. The design of the system to meet clinical information needs, as well as managerial requirements, is described together with the processes undertaken in piloting the system. The potential uses of the system for research, quality assurance and auditing are explored. The need for CPNs to develop more questioning and critical approaches to their practice is proposed so that the information available is exploited and comparisons can be made between the working methods outcome of individual CPNs.

> ...being able to provide useful information depends on having the right data and an effective way to process them   (Rippington, 1985)

Community nurses, such as health visitors and district nurses, traditionally have maintained records on services provided to individual patients and clients. In addition they have presented weekly or monthly accounts of their activities to managers. Despite this accumulation of data community nurses have been reported as viewing information derived from their returns as giving limited, if not distorted, pictures of their work. Dawtrey (1978) has reported that weekly returns among health visitors were known as 'the weekly liar' and because the forms used were open to such a variety of interpretations 'no reliable data could be derived'. As a relatively new community nursing service, community psychiatric nurses (CPNs) have assumed similar recording systems. The deficiencies of the systems being developed were revealed in 1983 in the responses to the Department of Health and Social Security Chief Nurse's request for information on the community psychiatric nursing services.

When the inadequacies of available information were recognized in the South East Thames Regional Health Authority (SETRHA) an attempt was made by the Regional Nursing Research Officer to carry out a survey of the community psychiatric nursing services. It was identified that CPNs in all district health authorities, (DHAs) had developed idiosyncratic recording systems and, as the services were changing rapidly, it was recognized that a one-off survey would produce merely historical data. McKendrick (1981) found a similar situation in a national survey of CPNs' recording systems concluding that: 'There is thus a need for widespread review of forms to determine the critical information content'. At that time the Körner Working Groups were reviewing the National Health Service information systems and the chairman of the Working Group D, on Community Health Services (Department of Health and Social Security 1983) commented:

> The present statistical returns, based on staff groups, obscure rather than illuminate the nature of community services. They add little to our understanding of how resources devoted to these services contribute to the overall effort of the Districts: nor do they assist operational and strategic decisions on priorities between hospital and community services or among the latter.

THE DEVELOPMENT OF AN INFORMATION SYSTEM

In view of the situation outlined in SETRHA it was agreed that a working group of CPN representatives from all the region's DHAs should be established, coordinated by the Regional Nursing Research Officer. The aims of the group were:

1. to review the existing CPN recording methods in each DHA for differences and similarities in information collected;
2. to identify common core information considered essential by CPNs for clinical practice and to meet management requirements;
3. to devise standardized methods of collecting the agreed information appropriate for computerization.

To achieve these aims it was considered that there should be full communication between the producers and users of the information. Historically nurses seemed to view individual patient/client records as *aide-mémoires* for practice and the aggregated information submitted to managers as of no use or interest to practitioners. Since there was limited feedback from managers on how data was used it is not surprising that the collection and submission of information was regarded often by practitioners as a useless chore. To overcome these difficulties it has been proposed that the planning of an information system should involve dialogue between producers, users of the system and technical specialists involved in the following stages (Härö, 1980):

1. planning of the information content;
2. planning of technical and methodological aspects;
3. planning of the organizational structure, location etc. of the health information system.

The planning of the information content

Reaching agreement among CPNs in the Working Group as to the core information content of the proposed system required lengthy and often heated discussions. Härö (1980) has suggested that it is a misconception to believe that:

> ... it is relatively simple to know what information is needed and how it should be used. In most cases decision-makers are not aware of their information needs and much effort is needed to discover what should be known.

In addition the CPNs, still in the process of developing an identity, were forced to examine collectively what their work values, skills and objectives were and how their performances might be judged. This process was often upsetting and demanding but promoted a critical and creative climate. It was agreed that the information requirements of the CPN records should be client centred. The decision was reached to regard the recipients of their services as 'clients' rather than 'patients' with its passive, dependent connotations. This value was reflected also in not giving prominence to psychiatrists' diagnoses but rather focusing on the 'problems' the clients' conditions generated for them. 'Problems' expected to be associated with the CPN clients' and their family situations were generated from the CPNs experience, reviews of records and Brooker's (1984) problem categorization. This led to the production of a structured 'Menu' list of potential 'problems' from which CPNs and their clients/families could select those that were most appropriate for them. Through testing and re-testing in practice the 'problem' lists were repeatedly modified and refined until the CPNs were satisfied that they were realistic and usable.

It was intended that the clients/families should collaborate in the identification of what constituted 'problems' for them, with the establishment of priorities for interventions and their outcomes. This process was made explicit in the records constituting an acceptance that: 'the record is not just a passive receiver of information but can play an active part in influencing the collection of that data' (Rees, 1981). The record format conformed to the requirements of the individualized care, 'nursing process' model that included assessments, plan of care and resulting outcomes (Walton, 1986). Efforts were made to consider carefully the purpose of collecting the information that was considered necessary, how it might be used and the extent to which it was justifiable to probe into all aspects of the lives of clients and their families. The nursing process movement seems to have been uncritical of its requirements to collect unlimited social and biographical information about clients and patients in the interests of achieving individualized and 'whole person' services. Armstrong (1982) has pointed out that traditional aspects of medical practice, which was concerned mainly with the diagnosis and treatment of illness, was explicit about its boundaries and only focused on circumscribed aspects of the patient. In contrast the 'whole-person' approach:

> in processing the whole person, offers the potential of total surveillance. Social control becomes truly individualised.

It has also been proposed that power is promoted as much through encouraging speech as through inhibiting it (Foucault, 1979). This supports the old adage that 'knowledge is power'.

Most of the Working Group's efforts concentrated on CPNs' method of practice and clinical requirements and commonly used key terms were explicitly defined to reduce interpretative errors. For example definitions were produced of 'case-load', 'referral' and 'discharge'. The managerial requirements in the form of monthly returns of CPNs' activities were dictated by the Körner recommendations that became mandatory.

When the first draft of the records was completed each representative on the Working Group undertook not only to acquire comments from all CPN colleagues, but also to obtain volunteers willing to test the new records in practice. When the records were tested in the majority of DHAs they were changed and modified in accordance with the CPNs' responses. A number of further tests and adjustments were carried out until no further changes were suggested and the records became more structured and streamlined.

The planning of technical and methodological aspects

When the records were completed CPNs in a number of DHAs commenced their day-to-day usage manually. It was recognized that without computerization the information generated from the records could not be exploited, so plans were made to achieve this aim. A small, volunteer sub-group of the larger Working Group was formed to deal with this stage. A member of the Regional Computer Centre was invited to join the sub-group. It has been erroneously assumed in the past that information system development can be left to the technical expert but as Härö (1980) points out:

> Such an expert cannot advise on *what* should be known but the role of the technical expert is fundamental when decisions are made about *how* data should be collected, processed and presented.

In collaboration with technical experts a functional specification and the appropriate software were developed. The software was designed to be menu-driven and operate on PICK operative systems. This was chosen because it was appropriate for use with the hardware available in most health authorities in SETRHA. In addition, it was considered that the PICK system had the following advantages.

1. Its relational database prevents the storage of items more than once and is flexible and easy to use for interactive data processing and information management.
2. Its variable length of data storage maximizes the use of disk space.
3. Its data dictionaries enable easier access to data without requiring costly programming.
4. Special access routines allow the users to design their own reports with very little training, check their accuracy and give warning if there is a problem.
5. Security and validation routines are designed to conform to the Data Protection Act (1984) and prevent sensitive data being seen by unauthorized personnel.
6. It has the ability to share the data between the community psychiatric nursing system and other proprietary software.

The planning of the organizational structure

It was planned that the CPNs would have direct, daily access to the computer system. Terminals or microcomputers had to be made available in all the CPNs' work locations of which there were several in most DHAs. Fears were expressed by CPNs that if they were responsible for accessing and removing all the data it would be time-consuming and reduce their contacts with clients. Recommendations were made that some secretarial support should be made available to CPNs to undertake the standardized and routine tasks. The issue of time expended would be determined during the pilot study. Technical experts who produced the software and staff of the Regional Computer Centre advised on the appropriate hardware required and the installation of the software. They also undertook to act as consultants during the pilot study and to deal with any problems that might arise.

THE PILOT STUDY

To test the efficiency of the software in practice it was planned to establish pilot studies in two health authorities. Because of staff changes and problems in obtaining appropriate hardware in one of the health authorities a pilot study was carried out in one authority only. During the pilot study the authority had from 16 to 25 in-post CPNs dealing with general psychiatric and elderly mentally ill patients, sited in two locations. During the pilot study an addiction centre was set up serviced by CPNs who participated in using the computerized system.

The objectives of the pilot study were:

1. to ensure that the software met the requirements of the functional specifications;
2. to identify and rectify any problems or deficiencies;
3. to promote the proficiency of the CPNs and the secretaries in using the system;
4. to find out the extent to which CPNs used the data and reports produced for clinical and managerial purposes;
5. to develop the CPNs' abilities to identify information needs about their clients and to provide practice for auditing and quality assurance purposes.

To prevent breaches of confidentiality dummy data was generated and used in the early stages of the pilot study. This data used fictitious biographical details of clients and, though real information was drawn on from clients' case-notes to preserve authenticity, the data was disguised so that nobody could be identified. The dummy data was used to produce both standard and Körner Reports so that by the CPN's interrogation of the system its potential was tested and any problems and need for improvements were identified. After the appropriate adjustments had been made by the technical expert it was agreed that 'live' data would be put on the system so that a trial could be done and it be used 'for real'. The Regional Data Protection Officer had been co-opted as a member of the Working Sub-group to develop a strategy for ensuring confidentiality. Those authorized to have access to the system were identified and issued with access passwords which were changed every three months.

Secretaries of the CPN teams undertook to load on to the system all the

CPNs' current 'live' case-loads. It was estimated that each client record took six minutes to load on to the computer. This process highlighted the previous lack of explicit definition of what constituted 'live' case-loads since no systematic methods of formally discharging clients existed. Such a review raised the issue of the need for more accurate case-load profile information as a basis for allocating equitable case-loads and defining priorities which have manpower and financial implications (this will be discussed further later). The identification of live case-loads highlighted the inaccuracies of previous estimates since it was found that they included a number of clients who were receiving no services from CPNs, thus falsely inflating their case-loads. The introduction of the formal discharge system promoted more explicit decision-making and accountability. In addition, the introduction of a review of clients on CPNs' case-loads for three months or longer promoted questioning of the need for, and purposes served by, indefinite CPN involvement with clients.

Data produced

The system was designed not to replace entirely the use of manual records but to synthesize critical information that could be retrieved in the form of reports considered necessary for clinical and management purposes. It also provided opportunities for CPNs to interrogate the system so that correlations between variables could be made in relation to defined clients, and to compare the clinical practices of CPNs, working both individually and in teams, with their clients' outcomes.

The data in the system that can be drawn on emanate from:

1. biographical, social and health histories of clients;
2. referral information;
3. assessments of problems generated for clients or their families;
4. interventions or therapies planned and given;
5. outcomes achieved;
6. work-load and daily activities of CPNs.

Assessment and therapy processes

In contrast to most nursing process records the assessments of clients' requirements on the CPN records were structured, explicit and confined to the critical information needed and the defined problems that are commonly presented to CPNs (as discussed previously). In relation to nursing process documentation the suggestion often made is that un-structured assessment forms, or even blank sheets of paper, would result in every assessment made by nurses being non-standardized – each tailored to suit the individual patient. This assumption is questionable, since in a review of nursing process records, in hospitals where assessment forms were unstructured, it was clear that all patients/clients were asked standardized questions despite the fact that nurses did not see each other carrying out the assessments (Hunt, 1987a, 1989). This supports the findings of studies of professional practice in which a close similarity was found in the interviewing processes among individuals of the same occupation. Rees (1981) describes this process in the interviewing of house doctors in hospital as did Sudnow (1965) among American public defenders dealing with criminal offences. In relation to social workers' assessments of clients Smith (1973) has observed:

> The social worker selects some materials for specific attention while paying less attention to those facts of the case for which no categories are readily available. The interview resembles a moulding process in which the client and his situation are reconstructed to render them manageable within existing agency routines.

The lack of making explicit the critical information required by nurses from all patients by the structuring and standardization of assessment forms appears to lead to unnecessary questioning of all patients and clients and the recording of narrative data that is often vague and open to numerous interpretations. In addition, when no information on an issue was recorded, it was not clear if the appropriate information was sought or just found not to be of sufficient importance to record (Hunt, 1987a). If clients' and patients' records are to serve, not merely as *aide-mémoires* for individual nurses, but as a means of communication between them and as a basis for planning care, ambiguities in the method of questioning and in the responses recorded need to be reduced. Making explicit the critical information required from all clients can lead to clarification as to how the information might be used realistically by nurses. It could also make explicit the nurses' accountability for taking action on the basis of the collected information which, it is suggested, sometimes has appeared unclear to clients (Walton, 1986). Delineating the critical information required need not lead to assessments that are not individualized. The first screening assessment done could identify clients from whom further information may be required, tailored to their needs and the nurses' abilities to meet them, thus providing a better rationale for questioning than the not uncommon one given by nurses: 'it's just for the records' (Hunt, 1989).

Problem identification

The potential problems listed on the CPN assessment form were categorized and sub-categorized in the following way:

Mood related	Depressed
	Elated
	Other
Thought disorder	Delusional
	Incongruent
	Other
Drug/substance problems	Alcohol
	Drug controlled
	Solvents
Relationships	Family
	Marital
	Friends
	Work
	Others
Social	Financial
	Employment
	Housing
	Isolation
	Other
Behavioural	General anxiety
	Phobic/obsessional
	Habit
	Sexual
	Eating
	Sleeping
	Other
Loss	Bereavement
	Divorce/separation
	Physical
	Other
Self-injury	Overdose
	Lacerations
	Other
Confusional states	Dementia
	Toxic
	Cause unknown
	Other

Other (specify)

A study was undertaken to determine the extent to which there was agreement among CPNs in their interpretations and selection of the problems. A range of descriptive data on client assessments, derived from

CPN records prior to the computerization project, were selected. These were given to all CPNs in SETRHA to translate into problem identifications selected from the menu of standardized categories as given above. The results indicated that over 80% of CPNs ranked the same three problems as priorities. This suggests an acceptable level of interpretative congruity. Descriptive data explaining and amplifying the identified problems can be accommodated on the records. The problems identified by the referrer, the client/family, and the CPN are recorded and compared before plans are made for intervention and therapy. The client's physical health is also assessed. The sharing of the problems identified by the referrer and the CPN with the client/family clearly illustrates the partnership approach that is currently being advocated by professionals. If differences become apparent between the referrer's, the CPN's and the client's/family's perceptions of the priority problems, then discussions have to be engaged in and agreement reached before intervention can be planned.

The therapies or interventions planned are categorized in the CPN system as:

- Drug supervision
- Drug administration
- Support/practical help
- Individual counselling/psychotherapy
- Marital counselling/psychotherapy
- Family counselling/psychotherapy
- Group counselling/psychotherapy
- Re-referral to other agencies
- Discharge
- Other.

Again, descriptive data giving details of the therapy planned can be recorded and comparisons made between the recommendations made by the referrer and the CPN and the wishes of the client/family.

Evaluation of outcomes

A summary of the clients' progress and treatment outcomes can be completed at intervals and whenever discharge or re-referrals of patients are planned. The treatment outcomes and discharges have to be agreed between the CPNs and the clients with the latter recording their responses. The definition of discharge that was agreed on was: 'clients no longer being offered, or given services by CPNs'. Identified reasons for discharge are:

- Completion of treatment
- Failure to keep appointments

- No indicator for continued CPN involvement
- Death
- Other (specify).

The treatment outcomes are related to the extent to which the clients' problems have been ameliorated or assessed by the clients/families and CPNs as having improved. The assessments are based on the following scale.

Significantly	Client not distressed, able to cope with presenting problems and find own solutions.
Moderately	Problems not causing high degree of distress. Client can cope with support (specify).
Little or no significant change	Requires different help (specify).
Condition deteriorated	Requires different help (specify).
Not known	
Other (specify)	

Narrative can be recorded to expand on treatment outcomes and reasons for discharge.

Daily activities

CPNs, or their secretaries, enter daily records into the system that include details of clients referred and seen, where they were seen, the personnel that were present and the purposes of the contacts and the interventions/treatments given. This data provides the information required for the Körner Reports and other standard reports requested by CPNs.

USES OF INFORMATION

It has been suggested that:

> . . . information of itself has little value. It is a tool to be used to aid decision-making and to monitor and perhaps improve performance of tasks. It provides the basis for accountability in an organisation and, as such, is enmeshed in its functioning and management.
>
> (Klein and Scrivers, 1987)

An important objective of the pilot study was to find out how the information provided by the system could be exploited and used for clinical and management purposes. In addition to the standardized Körner reports, the data generated monthly standard reports that were made available to provide case-load information for individual CPNs and teams in the general, elderly and addiction services. These case-load profiles include new referrals and all clients that are being given services, their biographical details, the length of time they have been on case-loads, their treatment outcomes and discharges.

During the pilot study CPNs, working both separately and in teams, found this regular up-dating of case-load information very useful in planning their work. Acquiring such information on a regular basis before the computerized system was established had been time-consuming and the information had often been found to be inaccurate or not up to date. Further developments of the case-load profiles are possible as Hunt (1982) has suggested in relation to health visiting.

In the current climate of setting priorities, making the best use of resources and monitoring the quality of services provided (Department of Health and Social Security, 1989) case-load information is necessary (this will be discussed further later). Discussing physiotherapy, Williams (1989) presents a system of 'case weighting' which was being developed to determine work priorities and work load concluding that:

> ... a simple system of monitoring caseloads and weighting cases was necessary for good management and that, together with the development of clinical-outcome measures was an urgent and important next step in relation to the data, work load, manpower and costing systems currently being developed.

'Case weighting' is a method of grouping clients into categories representing 'light' or 'heavy' in their demands on the service with four to six weighting bands that are similar to the patients' dependency levels. From experience and data derived from their computerized system CPNs could develop criteria representing the 'weight' of defined categories of patients in terms of the time required and the demands made on the CPNs, for example clients requiring occasional supervision and medication will be at one end with those needing frequent and lengthy contacts at the other. The comparison of CPN case-loads thus 'weighted' could contribute to equitable distribution of referrals and work-loads and, over time, help to identify changes in referral patterns with potential manpower needs and training requirements.

ACCUMULATING CLINICAL INFORMATION

Community nurses at work are invisible to each other and many have few opportunities to acquire skills and knowledge from each other. Dingwall (1977) has observed, in relation to health visiting:

> Unlike work in many bureaucratic organisations, health visiting work is virtually invisible to monitoring by supervisors ... the only public area of

a health visitor's performance is her record keeping. Thus for a field health visitor to demonstrate satisfactory work it is crucially important that she should keep satisfactory records which can be called upon to demonstrate that she has operated in an organisationally correct manner.

Clark (1981) supported this view when she wrote that health visitor's records: 'provide the ongoing information which alone can document changes over time'. CPNs are in a similar situation to health visitors and, despite the accumulated data in their records, little information has been derived from them about their practice.

In the past because of the narrative nature of their records it has been prohibitative to extract and analyse data manually to provide information about CPN practice. With the computerized system it is possible to overcome these difficulties. The system can be interrogated to produce information about particular categories of clients with specific 'problems', how long they are on CPNs' case-loads, what therapies and interventions were made and their outcomes. Examples of such processes could be (a) the requesting of data from all CPNs' files about women over 40 years of age with depression as their primary problem correlated with their lengths of time on case-loads, the therapies and interventions made and their outcomes or (b) similar information obtained for men under 40 years of age with alcohol addiction 'problems'. From the 130 items of information in the system about clients further data could be acquired for specified clients such as their social and family circumstances, physical health, civil status, duration of their problems etc. With this data CPNs can compare each other's methods of practising and their outcomes and identify examples of effective therapies and build up a repertoire of standards and auditing indicators.

A survey by three researchers of district nursing (Badger, Cameron and Evers, 1989) produced information that can now be obtained about CPNs' case-loads by interrogating the computer system. For example: 'In relation to the distinctive and differing characteristics, if any, of recently referred and long-stay patients'. Badger, Cameron and Evers concluded that:

Although covering similar areas of the health authority, nursing teams varied in the proportions of recently referred and long-stay patients, suggesting that individual nurses' caseload management is a crucial determinant of length of time on the books ... Current pressures on all community services mean that practitioners must give more detailed attention to evaluating patient outcomes and caseload review ... In order for caseload monitoring to be facilitated, practitioners need relevant local and patient based data in order to make inter-team comparisons.

One-off studies to acquire such information are expensive and because of the time needed to collect the research information the reports produced can be out of date. The CPN system overcomes this difficulty by allowing repeated reviews and comparisons to be made concurrently and retrospectively.

QUALITY ASSURANCE

In recent years increasing emphasis has been placed on the institution of quality assurance programmes in the National Health Service. This involves the setting of agreed standards to be attained and the development of methods to ensure that they are reached in practice. Currently, the development of standards for community psychiatric nursing practice is difficult. They rarely are derived from research-based knowledge of what CPNs do, how they practice and with what results. Simpson (1989) in a review of available CPN research concluded that:

> There appears to be no research at all indicating whether community psychiatric nursing interventions are in fact, systematic and rooted in sound theoretical and research based practice. Aspects of community psychiatric nursing activity which could be based on research include clinical practice, service organization, local consumer needs and cost effectiveness among others.

Schön (1983) suggests an alternative to the traditional reliance on the creation of a body of knowledge by theorists and researchers in higher education who pass it on 'like a package' to be used by practitioners. He argues that inquiries that create epistemologies of professional practice are lacking because universities, which influence research approaches, are committed 'to a view of knowledge that fosters selective inattention to practical competence and professional artistry'. Schön's suggested alternative approach involves practitioners' engagement in 'Reflective research' which is triggered by situations occurring in practice. These situations can be generated from the community psychiatric nursing computer system as already pointed out and can provide a means by which CPNs, who work in isolation from colleagues, can communicate to each other private insights and problems and test them against the experiences and views of their peers. The values, theories and knowledge underpinning what seems to be good practices can then be made explicit and reflected upon. This process could raise questions about the development of theories and models of practice that nurses have been creating from an academic stance, with the expectation that nurse practitioners will implement them. Without testing and validation in practice such theories and research recommendations may be inappropriate for the contexts in which the nurses are working, may be difficult to implement and create stresses for practitioners unless necessary organizational and resource changes are made (Hunt, 1987b; Procter, 1989; Fielding and Llewlyn, 1987).

NURSING AUDIT

The auditing of records requires that they are structured and that criteria constituting of good practice are defined so that interventions and outcomes can be appraised. Phaneuf (1976) describes the process as:

> The nursing audit is a method for evaluating quality of care through appraisal of the nursing process as it is reflected in the patient care records for discharged patients ... Evaluation is part of professional accountability ... The audit is one way through which nurses can help to satisfy the accountability that is inherent in professional practice.

Structured computerized records makes it easier for CPNs to carry out auditing and for managers to engage in more focused supervision with indicators of good practice generated from how the service is actually provided. Schröeder and Maibusch (1984) demonstrate the value of nurse practitioners being actively involved in generating standards for auditing and quality assurance and in the monitoring of their practice through peer reviews, thus creating a climate of innovation and concern for the quality of services provided.

THE PROCESS OF CHANGE

The implementation of the community psychiatric nursing computer system was not merely a different form of recording but necessitated considerable changes for practitioners and managers as noted during the pilot study. Most CPNs had no previous experience or knowledge of using computers and expressed concern about their abilities to use the technology or had unrealistic expectations of what might be achieved by the system. Though the system is user-friendly it took some time for CPNs to become comfortable with it as part of their daily working methods. Even towards the end of the pilot study not all CPNs had achieved this ease and familiarity. Because the means have not been available in the past to produce information and make comparisons between CPN practice and outcome, the techniques of raising questions about these issues and problem-setting have not been learned by practitioners and managers. There can be an understandable reluctance by practitioners to expose their method of working and its results to the scrutiny of their peers and managers. Time is needed to break down the mystique CPNs have tended to create about their work that, whilst serving as a protective mechanism, can prevent the provision of information to justify its worth. To effect the necessary change towards more open and critical approaches requires time for, as Marris (1974) points out:

> Whenever people are confronted with change they need the opportunity to react, to articulate their ambivalent feelings and work their own sense of it.

The availability of more defined information about their method of practice also creates changes in practising CPNs' interactions with their managers. Supervision can become more focused and accountability for planning and manpower service development more soundly based.

CONCLUSIONS

Currently, the information that the community psychiatric nursing computer system can produce has not been fully exploited and continuing efforts will need to be made to promote CPNs' abilities to question it. If this aim is fully achieved it is likely that demands will be made in the future for a more sophisticated system and its integration with other relevant systems. In the meantime the CPN system provides a means for practitioners to become computer literate and to make explicit their roles, practice standards and means of evaluating it. The Department of Health's (1989) *Strategy for Nursing* makes it clear that in the future the development of nursing information systems will be vital, it states:

> The nursing professions will increasingly use clinical technology with their direct delivery of health care in every setting, and it will be necessary to ensure that they are appropriately prepared for this.... In all aspects of health care delivery, computer information systems will play a vital role. Tomorrow's health practitioners will need to use the computer with the same confidence that they today use the telephone. Whether in hospital or in the community, it will be the primary source of information and competence.

Computer education for nurses will be greatly enhanced if future students have available in practice computer systems which are being used by practitioners in their everyday work.

The involvement of nurse practitioners and managers in the development of discrete computer programmes tailored to meeting their needs is worthwhile, not only for the outcomes achieved, but for the processes engaged in. The developmental processes involve making explicit the practitioners' methods of working, their values, aspirations, skills and differences from other allied professionals. This contributes to the clarification of identity and the development of more effective interdisciplinary working relationships where unique and different skills are recognized and used. Having practice-based information easily accessible to justify their services can give nurses professional confidence in negotiating with other disciplines for, as Marris (1974) suggests:

> To negotiate a common platform, the constituent parts must first be confident that no resolution will overwhelm their right to be themselves. If the groups are intrinsically insecure, still unsure of their integrity and purpose, any alliance may seen threatening.

ACKNOWLEDGEMENTS

To all the SETRHA CPNs who participated, in particular, the members of the Working Sub-group, David Dumbrell and the Medway CPNs who undertook the pilot study. The pilot study was sustained by the CPNs' secretary Thelma Sheriff whose efficiency, interest and hard-work were invaluable. The contributions of Peter Brocklesby and the Regional Computer Centre Staff were appreciated as was the financial help acquired from the SETRHA Endowment's Trust Fund.

REFERENCES

Armstrong, D. (1982) *Medical knowledge and the modalities of social control,* Mimeo, Sociology Unit, Guy's Hospital Medical School, London.
Badger, F., Cameron, E., Evers, H. (1989) District nurses' patients – isues of caseload management. *Journal of Advanced Nursing,* **14,** 518–527.
Brooker, C. (1984) Some problems associated with the measurement of community psychiatry nurse intervention. *Journal of Advanced Nursing,* **9,** 165–174.
Clark, J. (1981) *What do health visitors do? a review of the research 1960–1980,* Royal College of Nursing, London.
Dawtrey, E. (1978) *The health visitor in primary care,* MSc Thesis, Medical Architecture Research Unit, North London Polytechnic, London.
Department of Health (1989) *A Strategy for Nursing,* HMSO, London.
Department of Health and Social Security (1983) Working Group D (Community Health Services), January, Körner Steering Group on Health Services Information Reports, HMSO, London.
Department of Health and Social Security (1989) *Working for Patients,* White Paper, HMSO, London.
Dingwall, R. (1977) *The Social Organization of Health Visitor Training,* Croom Helm, London.
Fielding, R.G. and Llewlyn, S.P. (1987) Communication training in nursing may damage your health and enthusiasm: some warnings. *Journal of Advanced Nursing,* **12** (3), 281–290.
Foucault, M. (1979) *The history of sexuality, Volume 1,* Allen Lane, London.
Härö, S.A. (1980) Information systems for health services at the national level, in

McLachlan, C. (ed.) *Information Systems for Health Services.* World Health Organization, Regional office for Europe, Copenhagen.

Hunt, M. (1982) Caseload profiles – an alternative to the neighbourhood study. *Health Visitor*, **55**, 521–525, 606–607, 662–665.

Hunt, M. (1987a) *Review of 'nursing process' assessment records in hospitals.* South East Thames Regional Health Authority.

Hunt, M. (1987b) The process of translating research findings into nursing practice, *Journal of Advanced Nursing*, **12** (1), 101–110.

Hunt, M. (1989) *Dying at home: its basic ordinariness displayed in patients' relatives' and nurses' conversations*, PhD thesis, Dept of Sociology, Goldsmiths College, University of London.

Klein, R. and Scrivers, E. (1987) The politics of information, in Mason, A. and Morrison, V. (eds). *Walk, don't run*, King Edward's Hospital Fund, London.

Marris, P. (1974) *Loss and change*, Routledge and Kegan Paul, London.

McKendrick, D. (1981) Statistical returns in community psychiatric nursing, *Nursing Times*, 16 and 23 September, 108, 101–104.

Medical Audit (1989) *Working for Patients: Working Paper 6*, HMSO, London.

Phaneuf, M.C. (1976) *The nursing audit: self-regulation in nursing practice*, Appelton – Century-Crofts, New York.

Procter, S. (1989) The functioning of nursing routines in the management of a transient workforce. *Journal of Advanced Nursing*, **14** (3), 180–189.

Rees, C. (1981) Records and hospital routine, in Atkinson, P. and Heath, C. (eds) *Medical work – realities and routines*, Gower, Farnborough.

Rippington, J. (1985) Financial information, in Mason, A. and Morrison, V. (eds), *Walk, don't run*, King Edward's Hospital Fund, London.

Schön, D. (1983) *The reflective practitioner: how professionals think in action*, Basic Books, New York.

Schröeder, P.S. and Maibusch, R.M. (1984) (eds) *Nursing Quality Assurance: A unit based approach*, Aspen, Rockville, Maryland.

Simpson, K. (1989) Community psychiatric nursing – a research based profession? *Journal of Advanced Nursing*, **14**, 274–280.

Smith, G. (1973) *Ideologies, beliefs and patterns of administration in the organisation of social work practice*, PhD Thesis, University of Aberdeen, Aberdeen.

Sudnow, D. (1965) Normal crimes: sociological features of the Penal Code in a Public Defender Office. *Social Problems*, **12**, 255–276.

Walton, I. (1986) *The nursing process in perspective: a literature review*, Department of Social Policy and Social Work, University of York, York.

Williams, J. (1989) Weighing up your workload. *Health Service Options*, November 16–17, 116–117.

CHAPTER SIX

The goals and objectives of community psychiatric nursing

Linda Pollock

SUMMARY

It is not clear from the literature what goals community psychiatric nurses (CPNs) are aiming for. The goals for community psychiatric nursing activity tend to have been stated in imprecise, broad terms, and the available quantitative measures tell us little about their attainment. Some goals of community psychiatric nursing activity can, of course, be measured in quantitative terms, but many others, for example improving patients' social skills or their capacity to cope with stress, are less amenable to quantitative measures. The research presented below aimed to provide a broad analysis of community psychiatric nursing practice and to examine the values and assumptions underpinning the work of the CPNs. The work of community psychiatric nursing specifically with carers was also explored.

INTRODUCTION

In reviewing the current policy documents on provision of psychiatric care, it was found that there is a lack of elaboration of strategy towards defined goals. The author explored whether or not this was also the case for community psychiatric nursing. The goals and objectives of community psychiatric nursing as detailed in the literature, are elaborated below.

Strategy and community psychiatric nursing

The lack of elaboration of strategy towards defined goals, evident in policy documents, raised questions about whether this is also the case for community psychiatric nursing. Use of the word strategy suggests a plan or method (the term has military derivations which include 'the art of

113

manoeuvring an army effectively' and 'a large-scale plan for winning a war'). By implication, plans have objectives and goals.

A review of the community psychiatric nursing literature provides evidence that authors are searching for 'explanations' of service development rather than citing evidence of planning towards achievable goals. Publications which present details of strategic aims of community psychiatric nursing services are scarce (Simmons and Brooker, 1986). Many of the descriptions provided do not mention any theoretical framework surrounding community psychiatric nursing service development, and much of the information presented is anecdotal (Brennan, 1981; Ainsworth and Jolley, 1978; Sencicle, 1981).

Reasons for development of community psychiatric nursing

Reasons for service development seem to be stated in preference to highlighting goals. The 'reasons' given for developing local community psychiatric nursing services include various expressed purposes or intentions, recommended/prescribed tasks and perceived advantages. These illustrate the ambiguity of the word 'reason' but yield information about implicit goals, objectives and 'process' criteria.

The reasons for the development of community psychiatric nursing reflect two different levels of argument: one, arguing for the development of community psychiatric nursing and the other, arguing at the level of why specific services have developed. Often rationales are not separated clearly. Thus the confusion that surrounds definitions of 'community care' at the conceptual level is mirrored here (see Pollock, 1989).

An examination of accounts of service development reveals a number of different types of rationale, some having quite complex ramifications, variations and structures. A typology of the rationales behind community psychiatric nursing service development is listed numerically below. It shows that the stimulus for community psychiatric nursing development has come from: a desire to improve (a) the organization of services to patients – hence improving patient care (see rationales numbered 1–4, 6 and 8 below), (b) the family's coping capacity (see rationales numbered 7 and 8 below), (c) inter-professional relationships (see rationale number 5), (d) psychiatric nursing itself (see rationales numbered 10, 11 and 12 below); and for economic reasons (see rationale number 9 below). There are diverse motivations spurring the development of community psychiatric nursing: local factors, presence or absence of professionals and willingness of other professionals with whom to collaborate, combined with theoretical discussion of the preference of community care to institutional care, have given an impetus to community psychiatric nursing in specific areas.

The rationales.

1. Institutional care leads to secondary handicap which is considered undesirable and it is therefore argued that patients should not be admitted to hospital but preferably nursed at home (Roberts, 1976).
2. In accordance with government policy (and current professional practice), there is a desire to reduce the numbers of in-patients and length of hospital stay (MacDonald, 1972). Pressure on hospital beds requires early discharge to vacate beds (MacDonald, 1972; Sharpe, 1975). There is evidence in the literature that discharge can result in 'the revolving door syndrome' where a pattern of short-term treatment and early discharge becomes repetitive. Nurses were therefore commissioned to undertake a supervisory and after-care service (Nickerson, 1972; Willey, 1969; Kirkpatrick, 1967; Marais, 1976; Sharpe, 1975) to try and avoid this relapse pattern. Psychiatric nurses were considered the ideal group to assume this role by providing 'continuity' from hospital care and by using the developing relationship to effect change (Kirkpatrick, 1967; Warren, 1971).
3. Nursing of the patient outside the hospital is preferred to institutional care as patients can avoid being labelled (Shires, 1977; Cohen, 1978; Jeevendrampillai, 1982). Stobie and Hopkins (1972a,b) talk of avoiding the crisis of admission and Harker, Leopoldt and Robinson (1976) comment that contact with CPNs avoids stigma. It is argued that care outside hospital can allow patients to maintain their social role for as long as possible (Stobie and Hopkins, 1972a,b) and responsibility can be maintained within the social group of the family (Pullen and Gilbert, 1979a,b; Ritson, 1977).
4. The availability of drugs, particularly the long acting preparations of phenothiazines, is considered effective in preventing relapse of patients, particularly schizophrenic patients whose frequent readmissions were (assumed to be) related to failure to comply with drug regimes (Warren, 1971). CPNs were considered the most appropriate professionals to administer these drugs in the home situation (Nickerson, 1972; Warren, 1971; Leopoldt, 1974).
5. Implicit in the literature is the suggestion that community psychiatric nurses can influence and change the attitudes of professionals and the public (Higgins, 1984; Stobie and Hopkins, 1972a,b; MacDonald, 1972; Sharpe, 1980). Psychiatric nurses possess particular skills (Kirkpatrick, 1967; Haque, 1973) that are transferable and useful in the community setting. Roberts (1976) has commented that CPNs can act in a consultative capacity to non-psychiatric nurses who may have problems dealing with people showing symptoms of mental disorder. Clarke (1980) uses research evidence on psychiatric morbidity to argue that CPN and health visitor liaison is needed. Anderson (1972) has

commented on the need for CPNs to educate other professionals in psychiatric knowledge.

6. Assessment at home by the CPN enables contact with relatives and, accordingly, can give greater insight into a patient's behaviour (Hunter, 1978; Stobie and Hopkins, 1972a; Henderson, Levin and Cheyne, 1973) and provide supplementary information on social history and living situations (Weeks and Greene, 1966; May, 1965a,b).

7. Home assessment also enables CPNs to offer support to the family and carers of the patient (Barker and Black, 1971; Roberts, 1976).

8. CPNs can implement treatment quickly and early help can be given which helps patients and carers (MacDonald, 1972; Leopoldt, 1979a,6).

9. CPNs can relieve medical staff out-patient clinics (Leopoldt, 1973; Sharpe, 1975) and can see patients previously dealt with by a psychiatrist (Leopoldt, 1975) or compensate for a shortage of psychiatric social workers (Sharpe, 1975).

Three other reasons have been given to justify the continued development of community psychiatric nursing:

10. The work of the CPN is considered rewarding and interesting and may involve learning new skills (Henderson, Levin and Cheyne, 1973), increased job satisfaction (Maisey, 1975), and reduction in wastage of psychiatric nurses (MacDonald, 1972).

11. Experience provided by community psychiatric nursing teams was considered beneficial to students and trained nurses whose training was considered to be too institutionally oriented (Sharpe, 1975).

12. CPNs were considered to fulfil a useful function as disseminators of information on family and social aspects to the team and institution (Maisey, 1975).

As can be seen from this list, most of the writing about reasons for development took place in the 1970s. This seems to have coincided with a marked growth in the speciality of community psychiatric nursing; documentation of 'reasons' for development may be linked to the need for the speciality to gain recognition. Since the 1970s, community psychiatric nursing has gained acceptance within the field and the literature of the 1980s has moved on from general comments about the reasons why CPNs are needed, to looking more systematically at the factors influencing the growth of community psychiatric nursing services (Brooker, 1987), and to focusing on specific issues like education and training, details about practice and evaluation of the effectiveness of services (Simmons and Brooker, 1986; Richards, Butterworth and Shrubb, 1988; Pollock, 1989).

Goal setting and community psychiatric nursing

Therefore, community psychiatric nursing services, according to the literature, do not seem to set goals for their corporate activities; note however, that individual services may indeed have aims which are unpublished and hence unavailable for open scrutiny. If the published literature represents practice in the field, individual nurses seem to be increasingly using a systematic approach to care; more recent papers, for instance, suggest that goal setting is a feature of CPNs' work with individual patients (Persaud, 1985; Ditton, 1984): this is related to increased use of the 'nursing process' and assessment approaches taken by some CPNs (Williamson, 1982; Jones, 1988). Goal setting otherwise, does not appear to be a feature of the work of CPNs. Goals can be inferred from the reasons given but authors do not elaborate on these or find out if specific aims are met.

Statistical data, although not entirely satisfactory as a means of evaluating services, may be utilized to ascertain goal attainment. Inasmuch as one can make general comments based on the literature, descriptive statistics on community psychiatric nursing services appear to be collected routinely, analysed retrospectively and used to justify changes in patterns of community psychiatric nursing care rather than for forward planning (Sharpe, 1980; Maisey, 1975; Leopoldt, 1979a,b). Only three articles provide evidence of statistics being used for forward planning: those of Sharpe (1982), Holloway (1984) and Brooker and Simmons (1985). Sharpe (1982) conducted a survey of general practitioners (GPs) in the Croydon area, in order to plan a future community psychiatric nursing service. He found that 84% of the GPs wanted an attached CPN and was able to gain a clear idea of these GPs' expectations of the CPN. Holloway (1984) carried out a project that demonstrated the value of a proposed mental health centre and resulted in improvement and changes in future service provision. Brooker and Simmons (1985) examined two models of community psychiatric nursing care delivery – day hospital – and primary health centre-based CPNs; they analysed the routine statistics collected by the nurses and used the findings to argue that future developments (in the services studied) be towards primary health care-based CPNs. Of course, these three papers could be the tip of a large hidden iceberg, but the lack of statistics at national level (see Pollock, 1989) would give some support to the conclusion that statistics are not used for planning services. The present study looked at the goals set by two community psychiatric nursing services and investigated the work of community psychiatric nursing to examine the values and assumptions underpinning the work at local level.

THE STUDY

Research studies can be categorized into studies that focus on 'structure' (the study of factors of the system, for example equipment, staffing levels, etc.), 'process' (the examination of what is being done, this includes not only visible behaviour but also invisible behaviour such as decision making), and 'outcome' (the results of care are explored in terms of change in the recipient of care) – see Donabedian, 1966. My study focused on the 'process' and 'outcome' of community psychiatric nursing – aspects of community psychiatric nursing work that had been little studied previously. The work formed the substance of a PhD thesis (Pollock, 1987). I studied and compared the work of CPNs in two hospital-based services situated in rural settings surrounded by small pockets of urban population. The study combined qualitative and quantitative methods (see Pollock, 1989) and produced a wealth of information for analysis. Data were obtained about the CPNs' own views of their work and the goals they were working towards. A second body of data was also accrued on the families'/carers' views of the CPNs. Each data set was examined in its own right but cross-comparisons were also made that enabled comment to be made about the links between 'process' and 'outcome'. Information about one of the methods used in the study and the findings about the 'goals' of community psychiatric nursing work are presented below.

RESEARCH TOOLS

The repertory grid method

A step by step guide to the method of repertory grid technique, was published in the *Journal of Advanced Nursing* (Pollock, 1986). Repertory grid technique was developed as a methodological component of a theory of personality (Personal Construct Theory) proposed by a psychologist, George Kelly (Kelly, 1955 and 1963). Kelly believed that humans develop predictive hypotheses which are tested, modified or discarded in order to survive; he considered this an active process which influences and conditions how individuals see the world, and he believed that individuals build up a network of hypotheses (based on unique experiences) which is called a 'construct system'. Repertory grid technique offers the opportunity for an individual's 'construct system' to be elicited.

'Constructs' are treated as if they are bipolar dimensions of judgement, a description that always has an opposite, for example, light is nonsense without a sense of its opposite – that could be heavy or dark; this opposite may not always be the dictionary opposite but the semantic opposite which conveys individual meaning and understanding.

The repertory grid technique. The technique has been described as a type of structured interview, the format of which enables the collection of individuals' descriptions ('constructs'); this elicitation of constructs is triggered by a sorting procedure (triadic elicitation), where the topics of interest ('elements') are written on cards. The technique involves three distinct stages: element choice, construct elicitation and grid construction.

The laddering procedure

This is a procedure, described by Hinkle (1965), for eliciting increasingly superordinate constructs, that is, constructs of a higher order of abstraction than those initially elicited. It is a conversational technique developed from repertory grid, and is aimed at systematically obtaining information from an individual to explore the meaning of one given construct. McCall and Simmons (1969) have stated:

> In exploring for possible factors affecting some given variable, or for chains of causes and effects constituting a 'process' there appear to be two basic techniques ... the second is to ask people themselves to explain what happened and to give their reasons for acting as they did. The basic question is always why?

In the laddering procedure the interviewer repeatedly asks the question: 'why?' Wright (1970), demonstrated the clinical use of the technique by using it to explore the meaning of psychological symptoms necessary, he argued, for behavioural change. The laddering procedure has had limited use in research application: Allsop (1980) and Hazelden (1981) used the procedure with teachers to explore the reasons for reading difficulties and truancy respectively.

According to Landfied (1971) the 'laddering' procedure provides a tool for documenting the conversation. This was used by Allsop (1980) and Slater (1976). Hinkle's procedure has been called 'laddering up' from a construct. The laddering procedure is explained clearly and at length by Judkins (1976), Fransella and Bannister (1977), Stewart and Stewart (1981), and Wright (1970). Constructs can also be explored by 'laddering down', where the respondent is asked 'how' one side of the construct differs from the other (see Figure 6.1 for an example of the procedure 'laddering up' – as used in the present study). All the laddered conversations were taped, to allow for qualitative analysis of the interview data (see Pollock, 1989).

LP   What we are going to do today is talk through some of the things you told me about last time and really it will be getting you to state the very obvious about your work. I want you to tell me in your own words about your work, what you do and why. I've taken the descriptions you gave last time and we'll go through them.

LP   Family support – not
       Tell me how someone with family support differs from somebody who doesn't have it, to give me an idea of what you are talking about.

F   If someone has family support you are getting a more objective picture of what is going on and you are getting somebody other than the patient's views. If someone has family support you'll find out quickly if there is anything going wrong, if there is adverse change in the situation. You may find the family tend to overreact and you are called to crises that are not really, in the crisis situation you are more likely to be able to keep them out if they have family support.

LP   OK, let's take these separately. Why do you like to get a more objective picture?

F   To get a broader picture. Most of the information you get is subjective. You get a broader view if you speak to the family – of what is going on and what you are dealing with.

LP   Why do you want to do that?

F   Because we are not treating an illness, we are treating an individual and the only way to get to know them as a complete person is to get to know them.

LP   You want to get to know them as a complete person – why?

F   To provide a better standard of care, of comprehensive care.

LP   Why do you want to do that?

F   To give a good service. An illness and symptoms cannot be just treated, they have got to be looked at as an individual in his or her entirety.

LP   Why would you want to hear if there was something going on?

F   Sometimes you do and sometimes you don't. We can maybe take action to prevent further crisis and prevent an admission or any further trauma to the patient.

LP   Why do that?

F   That is difficult; The nurses' job is not just treating people, we owe it to our patients to give as good a service as we can, part of this is preventive medicine, primary care.

LP   Why is it useful for you to know if someone doesn't have support?

F   The CPN's information gathering processes would be more difficult. We would have to look for other sources of information, like neighbours which would have ethical implications. Or we may have to visit relatives who live a distance away.

LP   Why do that?

F   To get more information . . .

Figure 6.1 Excerpt from the laddering procedure.

THE CONCEPTUAL FRAMEWORK OF THE STUDY

The research question formulated for examination at the outset of this research study was: 'Is community psychiatric nursing effective?' With this in mind, the next paragraphs present some of the literature in the area of health care evaluation and how this influenced the present study.

Two major influences on the present study can be identified; these are Suchman's model of the intellectual process of evaluation (Suchman, 1967) and Donabedian's model of the foci or mind's eye objects of evaluation (see previous elaboration of structure, process, outcome). The relevance of the former to the exploration and analysis of the 'goals' of community psychiatric nursing work, is presented below.

Initial reading indicated that the word 'effective' focused on the ability of a programme to be carried out successfully. Other words 'effects' and 'efficiency' continually emerged in the literature in relation to 'evaluation': 'the effects' of a programme are defined as the ultimate influence of a programme on a target and 'efficiency' is defined as how well and at what cost this is achieved relative to other ways of producing similar effects (Wright, 1955; Cochrane, 1971).

The mere mention of some of the phrases and words – 'ultimate influence', 'successfully', 'relative to other ways,' suggested that the task ahead would not be easy! 'Ultimate influence' suggested that activities may have grades of influence; who judges whether an action is successful or not?; the same activity may be judged both unsuccessful and successful by different assessors. Suchman (1967) defined 'evaluation' as:

> ...the determination (*whether based on opinions, records, subjective or objective data*) of the results (*whether desirable or undesirable, transient or permanent, immediate or delayed*) attained by some activity (*whether a program, or part of a program, a drug or a therapy, an ongoing or one-shot approach*) designed to accomplish some valued goal or objective (*whether ultimate, intermediate, or immediate, effort or performance, long or short range*). This definition contains four key dimensions: (1) process – the 'determination'; (2) criteria – the 'results'; (3) stimulus – the 'activity'; and (4) value – the 'objective'. The scientific method ... provides the most promising means for 'determining' the relationship of the 'stimulus' to the 'objective' in terms of measurable 'criteria'.
> (Suchman, 1967) [my italics]

This definition, although helpful overall, tends to confound values with objectives. Suchman continues:

> The value-laden nature of one's objectives constitutes a major distinction between evaluative research and basic research aimed at hypothesis testing. A precondition to an evaluation study is the presence of some activity whose objectives are assumed to have value.

Values generally are seen at a higher level of abstraction than the goals derived from them. According to King (1962): 'Values are the principles by which we establish priorities and hierarchies of importance among needs, demands, and goals'. In terms of King's definition, values underlie or determine our goals and are thus of a prior and separate order from either goals or objectives. 'Values' of course, are very closely tied to the setting up of goals – one does not ask if something is of value without asking: 'value for what?' This is recognized by Suchman (1967) who argues that the evaluation process itself stems from and returns to the formation of values.

Figure 6.2 shows Suchman's final visualization of the evaluation process. To take an example from community psychiatric nursing, the value could be that the dignity of individuals should be preserved or that all adults have a right to participate in community life; arising from this, the goal set could be: admission to psychiatric hospital should be avoided or the number of admissions to psychiatric hospital reduced. In order to measure whether or not this goal is achieved, statistics on admissions could be obtained and the 'goal attaining activities' could then be identified, for example: early sufferers detected; support services developed in the community for patients and families; domicilary visiting organized. These activities would then be put into operation: liaison with GPs, health visitors and social workers would be organized on a regular basis; premises secured for day centres, social clubs or self-help groups which would be advertised locally and *via* professionals; practical arrangements made about who would run and organize the group. These goal-directed operations would be assessed

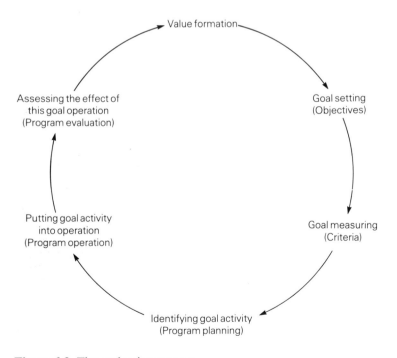

Figure 6.2 The evaluation process.
Source: Suchman (1967).

to see if the stated predetermined objectives were achieved. Finally the initial value is reassessed. This scheme suggests that it is possible to isolate dimensions to be measured. The present study attempted to examine the values, assumptions and goal activities of the CPNs and see if these were identifiable and separable.

Separation of the assumptions and goal activities of CPNs may not be possible.

> The many difficulties suggested – the breadth of the thing subsumed under a particular objective, the multiple objectives encompassed by many programs, the ambiguity inherent in any or all of the objectives as stated, and the disagreement as to the objectives – are characteristic of many programs and are enough to stagger the imagination of the evaluator.
>
> (Hyman, Wright and Hopkins, 1962)

Despite the fact that health care programmes have multiple objectives, three types of 'goals' have been described: immediate, intermediate and ultimate goals.

> Practically, there can be very little argument about this requirement that immediate and intermediate goals constitute valid steps toward the attainment of some ultimate goal. Otherwise activity becomes substituted for effect and the goals that lead to the adoption of certain means tend to be forgotten as the means become ends in and of themselves. However knowledge is never complete and there must always be gaps in the 'cause/effect' sequence which can only be filled by making assumptions concerning the validity of the intermediate steps ... such linkages are often if not usually taken for granted but upon challenge they must be reproducible.
>
> (Suchman, 1967)

This study used this framework and examined the goals of community psychiatric nursing as described by CPNs.

THE FINDINGS

The immediate, intermediate and ultimate goals of the nurses

The constructs elicited by the triadic sorting procedure (see above for an explanation of these terms), could be described as 'immediate goals'. This can be justified on the grounds of the theoretical discussion (Pollock, 1989) that focused on the importance of the nursing process in community psychiatric nursing work. Based on the literature it was hypothesized that the CPNs would use the nursing process, the first stage of which is assessment and information gathering. The interview data confirmed that these activities featured in the nurses' work.

Strictly speaking, the initial goal of this part of the nurses' work is to obtain baseline information. Elicitation of 'constructs' reveals headings for the nursing assessment and details the sort of information which the nurses used to plan care. As such the constructs can be taken to be 'immediate goals' of community psychiatric nursing work. The laddering procedure (see above) was then used to explore the thinking underpinning the relevance of each 'immediate goal'; from this exploration it was possible to examine the nurses' accounts of the work and identify the intermediate and ultimate goals of the nurses.

Each CPN was able, when led, to give a version of goals relevant to his or her work, and the findings suggest that there is a disparate list of values underpinning the work of each CPN. The elaboration of the goals into a triadic hierarchy is not as clear as the theory above suggests: this probably reflects the difficulty of being explicit about the complicated life scenarios with which the CPNs have to deal. Often there was not just one 'intermediate' goal, but several, see Figure 6.3, an example of a 'laddered construct' using data from the present study.

The decision to describe a goal as 'intermediate' was based on the researcher's interpretation of whether or not this appeared to be a 'step' aimed in the direction of achieving an 'ultimate goal'. Regardless of how the goals were described, this analysis showed that the nurses, contrary to the expectations of the literature, were able to discuss clearly the goals in their practice. Table 6.1 provides a summary of the values, intermediate and ultimate goals described by the CPNs in this study.

Examination of the immediate goals

With the help of a content analysis (see Pollock, 1989 for a fuller discussion of this method of data handling) the 'immediate goals' were examined to ascertain the CPNs orientations and to see whether the constructs showed evidence of concern for the carers on the part of the nurses. The headings for the content analysis were chosen with this purpose in mind. The final headings used in the content analysis arose partly out of comparison of previous construct categorizations reported in the literature (detailed below) and were chosen because the descriptions fitted the data. An attempt to further check the validity and reliability of the content analysis (by sending it to experts in the field) failed. The choice of headings however, was sufficient to show the predominant focus of the CPNs' work.

Bearing in mind the advice of Berelson (1952), definitions of the details of the headings used for the content analysis are described below and

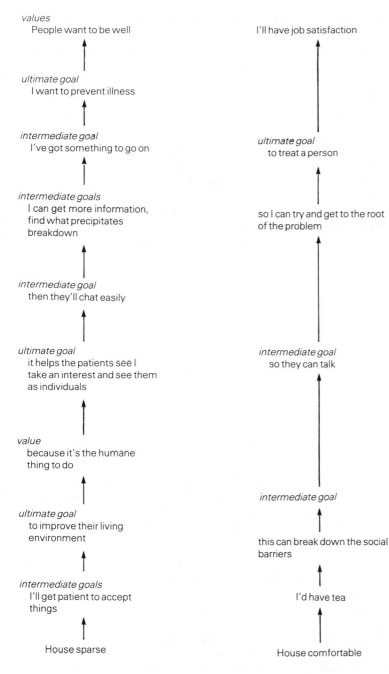

values
People want to be well

ultimate goal
I want to prevent illness

intermediate goal
I've got something to go on

intermediate goals
I can get more information,
find what precipitates
breakdown

intermediate goal
then they'll chat easily

ultimate goal
it helps the patients see I
take an interest and see them
as individuals

value
because it's the humane
thing to do

ultimate goal
to improve their living
environment

intermediate goals
I'll get patient to accept
things

House sparse

I'll have job satisfaction

ultimate goal
to treat a person

so I can try and get to the root
of the problem

intermediate goal
so they can talk

intermediate goal

this can break down the social
barriers

I'd have tea

House comfortable

Figure 6.3 Details of a laddered construct with superimposed interpretation of goals and values written alongside.

Table 6.1 A summary of the values, intermediate and ultimate goals described by the CPNs

	Patient-centred goals	
Intermediate goals	*Ultimate goals*	*Values*
Improve patient coping capacities	Help patient cope	Autonomy
Help individual change	Help patient manage	
Develop relationships	Increase confidence	
Help individual achieve	Increase confidence	
Get person to talk	Able to offer self	
Give opportunity to improve	Promote independence	
Encourage patient to do things	Better to help self	
Discourage the sick role	Promote self-sufficiency	
Focus on precipitants	Avoid hospitalization	Community
Help person solve problems	Avoid relapse	care is good
Set realistic targets	Avoid relapse	
Aim to work through feelings	Avoid escape to hosp.	
Help person deal with stress	Avoid escape to hosp.	
Help person cope with stress	Prevent illness	
Look for early warning signs	Prevent illness	
Get person to ventilate	Prevent illness	
Provide company and stimulation	Prevent illness	
Avoid uprooting person/family	To reduce stress	
Keep people in families	Maintains roles	
Keep person in community	Won't learn sick role	
Want to get to know a person	Provide individual programmes	Respect for
Get information to work on	Provide individual care	individual
Show that I care	Interested in person	
Be a friend to patient	Individual feels valued	
Get person to accept gifts	Improve environment	Quality of
Reduce myths about mental illness	Educate the public	life
Put support services in	Avoid risks	
Make self available	To prevent crises	
Help give person a role	Increase self-esteem	
Help individual mix socially	Feedback from others	
Help person to go out	See life is worthwhile	
Maintain daily living skills	Enable person to survive	
Help person self-medicate	Opportunity to socialize	

Family-centred goals

To develop respite services	To relieve the family	Family care is
Make carer's life easier	To reduce the burden	good
Give carer practical help	Improve coping capacity	
Help family understand	Improve communication	
Improve home relationships	Patient stays at home	
Keep relatives informed	Family continue caring	
Give carer support	Family continue caring	
Allow carer to ventilate	Family continue caring	
Prevent crisis	CPN and carer cooperate	

Nurse-centred goals

I would lower my expectations	Avoid getting frustrated	Job is
Collect maximum possible information	Provide efficient service	satisfying
Get to know patient well	Use time well	
Avoid hospital admission	Prevent blocked beds	
Reduce myths about illness	Make job easier	
Educate the public	Others' expectations fit	
I want to use my skills	To use my training	

shown in Figure 6.4. (All the constructs produced by each nurse, sorted into the headings used in the content analysis are available for scrutiny in Pollock, 1989). I tried to sort the constructs consistently under a particular heading. The headings are not mutually exclusive and it is acknowledged that some constructs could have equally well been sorted under another heading. For instance, constructs that mentioned 'family' in relation to 'self-sufficiency' were put in the latter category, although they could have been inserted into the home situation grouping. For this reason the choice of headings is not entirely satisfactory.

The content analysis showed that the majority of constructs were patient focused and that the nurses seemed little concerned with the families' needs; additionally, many of the constructs showed that the nurses were concerned with medical problems. The findings may be partly due to the choice of patients as elements for the repertory grid technique (see Pollock, 1989). However, the results of the qualitative analysis that explored the usefulness of the constructs with the nurses, did not reveal a marked change in this focus of concern.

The content analysis also revealed that each nurse produced a varied number of constructs, and placed different emphasis on the production of some types of constructs rather than others (see Figure 6.5). The concern

1. Home situation
   Any description where home situation is described.
2. Illness
   Any description where illness label is used.
3. Treatment
   (a) Patient response
       Any description where patient response to treatment is mentioned.
   (b) Description
       Where treatment offered is detailed.
   (c) Medication
       Any description where medication is mentioned.
   (d) Time orientation
       Any description denoting future orientation or expectancy or past orientation or expectancy of patient contact with community psychiatric nursing services.
4. Social interaction
   (a) Any statement in which face-to-face, ongoing interaction is indicated or lack of face-to-face, ongoing interaction is indicated.
   (b) Interpersonal statements that might curtail interaction with others or encourage it.
5. Work – finances
   Any descriptions where work or finances are mentioned.
6. Self-sufficiency
   (a) Any statement denoting interdependence, initiative, confidence and ability to solve one's own problems or the opposite.
   (b) The ability to attend to aspects of daily living (hygiene, washing, dressing, nutrition) or inability to attend to aspects of daily living.
7. Factual description
   A characteristic so described that most observers would agree that this is factual and not open to question.
8. Self-references
   Any statement where the nurse refers directly to himself or herself.
9. Value judgement
   Any description which is subjective and suggests moral evaluation.
10. Problems identified
    Any statement where problems are focused on.

Figure 6.4 Content analysis: headings and definitions used.

of this analysis was not to explore details of the working practices of individual CPNs. The purpose of exploring individual's descriptions was to draw conclusions about community psychiatric nursing work generally and specifically in relation to care of the carers.

The content analysis. Few category systems have been developed for construct analysis. Existing category systems were reviewed to see if they could be used in the present study. Systems of categorization have emerged from previous researchers' data: Davis (1984) used Duck's (1973) classification of constructs. Duck classified constructs into 'psychological', 'role' and 'other' categories which, he claimed, allowed his constructs (on friendship) to be placed into exclusive and exhaustible categories. These categories seemed too broad to classify the constructs used by the CPNs.

Philip and McCulloch (1968) using repertory grid, identified two clusters of constructs used by social workers to describe patients. These groups concerned the degree to which a patient functions and copes socially and the feelings of the social worker towards the patients. These groupings were relevant for classification of the constructs produced by the CPNs but were limited in that they did not enable description of the range of constructs produced by the nurses.

Lifshitz (1974) studied the perceptions of trained and untrained social workers and developed seven categories:

1. task orientation;
2. a description of concrete situations;
3. abstract intrapsychic characteristics;
4. abstract inter-personal or interpsychic characteristics;
5. abstract social values;
6. intellectual characteristics;
7. affective – egocentric approach.

The categories developed by Landfield (1971) proved to be the most helpful in guiding the construct categorization used in this study. Landfield (1971), developed a manual that provides 22 categories into which constructs can be placed. Some of these descriptions were borrowed: social interaction, self-sufficiency, factual description, self-reference. Combined with these headings, I developed six other categories. The definitions used with the headings are described in Figure 6.4. The findings of this analysis, the quantitative data base for the extraction of goals, are presented in Pollack (1989).

Examination of values, intermediate and ultimate goals

The laddering procedure revealed that different CPNs produced varied lists of values, intermediate and ultimate goals which, it can be assumed, influence practice. These findings are worthy of future study.

The results of other parts of the study in effect provided feedback of whether or not attainment of the goals was achieved (see Pollock, 1989). In the following pages, the values, intermediate and ultimate goals referred to by the CPNs are presented and discussed in relation to what the patients and carers said about the 'process' of community psychiatric nursing.

The phrases presented in the Table 6.1 present information about what the nurses said about goals. All the phrases used are not listed, those chosen, give a flavour of the range of descriptions of goals given by the CPNs (for example the list shows that 'to maintain the daily living skills of patients' and 'to help people be independent', are intermediate and ultimate goals; another nurse mentioned 'to increase the social skills of individuals' and 'to help the person take a more adult position in life', these were judged by the researcher to be similar). Different CPNs used different phrases and the chart here represents a summary of the goals aimed for by the CPNs.

The list of values, intermediate and ultimate goals, can be read vertically as lists in their own right. Alternatively, the list can be read horizontally, as the information is presented using the links between intermediate, ultimate goals and values, that were provided by the CPNs. Some of the intermediate goals could be linked to a number of the ultimate goals, for example the intermediate goal 'to maintain daily living skills' could be linked to the ultimate goal of either 'to increase independence' or to improve quality of life'. Similarly, some of the intermediate goals could be ultimate goals, for example 'keeping an individual in the community' is presented as an intermediate goal, with 'to stop the individual adopting the illness role' but it could have been presented the other way around, and was by some of the CPNs. The classification of the goals, therefore, is somewhat arbitrary.

In assessing professional function one can operate at the level of aims (the terms used here to discuss aims are 'intermediate and ultimate goals') and take values for granted. This study has focused on what the nurses did (the qualitative analysis showed that the nurses use the resources they have got to make the 'system' work), what they were aiming to achieve (the expressed goals) and an analysis of the outcome (the carers' and patients' view of the service, which gives an objective measure of goal attainment).

It is only when one starts to ask 'was it worth doing anyway?' that one gets into a political level of discourse where an examination of values is indispensable. At this level of debate, there are no purely objective criteria. In this sense detailing 'values' is less appropriate for the level of functional analysis, the concern of this study. The 'values' of the CPNs are detailed however, as they provide information about the value base of the CPNs' work that influences the way in which the CPNs rank the goal setting aspect of their work.

The CPNs could be described as working from a basis that embraces values to do with autonomy and self-sufficiency; preservation of a dignity and quality of life; respect for the individual and beliefs about care in the community (i.e. it is better to avoid hospitalization and institutional neuroses and promote care in the family situation). As Downie and Telfer (1980) have commented, values are essentially comparative in nature and this was borne out by the manner in which the CPNs referred to values (the CPNs commented, for example that 'autonomy is better' implying a negative comparison). The description of 'values' is related to the content of the 'ultimate goals'. In Table 6.1 these values are displayed alongside the goals with which they were most often linked. As mentioned for the goals, this presentation is somewhat contrived and is not intended to be expounded as a rigid prototype, but rather a rough guide to the framework of values referred to by the CPNs in this study.

Broadly speaking the CPNs' goals could be described as either patient centred, job centred or family centred in nature, although these were linked. If asked to clarify the goals to do with 'family', the CPNs talked about helping the family cope in order to improve the patient's quality of life. When asked to explore the importance of 'patient autonomy' they referred to the importance of running an economic service or getting job satisfaction from seeing patients manage on their own.

Patient and carer feedback about goals

The limitations of space here means that it is impossible to give lengthy detail about the process of community psychiatric nursing (see Pollock, 1988a and 1989). The statements made by patients and carers provided comment about how the goals, as expressed by the CPNs were perceived and experienced by the consumers.

For the purpose of presentation, the statements made by patients and carers (that were used in the 'outcome' measure, Personal Questionnaire Rapid Scaling Technique (PQRST), used in the study) were reclassified into the goals and value groupings used in Table 6.1. 'Values' are included in this presentation for illustrative reasons only. (The intention of this section of the analysis is not to fit the consumers' views into the same set of values as the CPNs. This would be unreasonable: job satisfaction, a value of the CPNs, could not be expected to figure highly in the patients' and carers' scale of values). The point at issue in this analysis is not to compare the nurses' and consumers' value systems, but rather, the level of comparison is that of goals.

(a) The patients' view of goals. Analysis of the comments of patients at the day centres suggest that many perceive the intermediate goals of the CPNs (see Table 6.2 that reclassifies the contents of the day care PQRST in relation to the goals and value groupings discussed above). The ultimate goals were less accurately perceived by the patients; the most obvious omission is that the patients did not explicitly focus on the work of the CPNs as being aimed at 'avoiding hospital admission', 'preventing illness' or 'keeping individuals with families'. Neither did the patients see the CPNs as educating them about mental illness, although this could be implied by reference to seeing 'other people at the day centre being different'. A further point of note is that the patients also commented on

the work of the CPNs in terms of their activities: these descriptions could be likened to the task centred definitions, of community psychiatric nursing, referred to earlier.

A similar interpretation can be used to comment on the perception of the patients who were visited at home (see Table 6.3 for a reclassification of the contents of the home visiting PQRST into the goals and value groupings detailed earlier). The patients visited at home discerned the intermediate goals described by the CPNs and the patients also focused on the task centred nature of the work. Analysis further showed that the goals emphasizing 'individualized care' are experienced most keenly. The goals grouped under 'autonomy' and 'community care is good' were compara- tively little used. The 'home visited' patients referred especially to the 'manner' or way in which the nurses worked. These comments could be converted into the intermediate goal expressed by the CPNs of 'showing they care' or 'befriending'.

(b) The carers' view of goals. Feedback from the carers about community nursing work was restricted to comment about the CPNs rather than to problem relief or stress (see Pollock, 1989). For this reason Table 6.4 presents a breakdown of the PQRST, the 'nurse aspects' section only. One fifth of the statements in this section of the PQRST refer to the patients (and are classified under the patient centred goals); the carers therefore considered some of the CPNs' patient centred goals to have been realized. The carers especially commented on the 'talking' behaviour of the nurses. The carers were much less specific and less varied in their range of descriptions of intermediate and ultimate goals than were the CPNs. The CPNs were considered to work with patients 'to prevent hospital admis- sion' and 'to prevent relapse of illness' (goals not perceived by the patients). The format of the visiting situation was commented on, suggesting that the carers endorsed some of the CPNs' comments about community care; again what the CPN actually does, i.e. the activities of the CPNs, were mentioned by the carers.

The remaining statements in the nurse aspects section of PQRST suggest that almost all of the intermediate goals expressed by CPNs and included in the family centred goals list (see Table 6.4) were endorsed by the carers. The exception to this was the goal of 'improving of relationships within the family'. Few of the ultimate goals were elaborated on by the carers.

The outcome information suggests that objectively the CPNs did not help very much with a high proportion of the carers' problems. Neverthe- less some goals were attained, because *some* carers experienced relief of problems and help with the feelings associated with looking after a mentally ill relative at home (see Pollock, 1989). Many of the patient centred goals identified by the carers, were also attained – as evidenced by

Table 6.2 Statements from the day care PQRST, grouped in relation to the goals and values expressed by the CPNs

---

Autonomy:
    I made friends at the day centre
    the day centre is like a family
    people there are worse off than me
    I meet others with similar troubles
    the nurses talk to me
    the nurses have time for discussion
    I talk to nurses about things I couldn't discuss elsewhere
    the nurses let me see things differently
    the day centre builds up my confidence
    the nurses tell me not to get dependent
    I make my own way to the day centre
    the nurses delve into my past

Quality of life:
    the day centre is a place to go
    the centre has a nice atmosphere
    I can phone the nurses any time
    the nurses give me support
    I feel I am helping others
    I am kept busy at the day centre
    I get a meal at the day centre

Respect for the individual:
    the nurses take an interest in me
    the nurses make me feel important
    the nurses care
    the nurses say things that comfort me
    the nurses don't treat me badly
    the nurses listen to me
    the nurses ask how you are feeling

Community care is good:
    I can get things off my chest
    I have company at the day centre
    others at the day centre are different

Task orientated definitions of the work:
    I attend a group
    we play games
    the nurses give me my medication
    the nurses arrange for me to see a psychiatrist

Unsorted statements:
    the nurses are cheery
    the nurses have special qualifications

Table 6.3 Statements from the home visiting PQRST grouped in relation to the goals and values expressed by the nurses

---

Autonomy:
>   a relationship has developed

Quality of life:
>   you get to know the nurse
>   I know the nurse's circumstances
>   I can talk to the nurse confidentially
>   the nurse brings things I need
>   the nurse talks to me

Respect for the individual:
>   home visit promotes better idea of me
>   the nurse takes an interest
>   I know I am not forgotten
>   the nurse cares
>   the nurse asks how I am keeping
>   I can trust the nurse
>   the nurse visits informally

Community care is good:
>   same nurse visits all the time
>   there is no waiting at the house
>   it is convenient at the house

Task orientated definitions:
>   the nurse has a cup of tea
>   the nurse has a look around
>   the nurse takes blood
>   the nurse gives medication
>   the nurse visits regularly

Unsorted statements:
>   the nurse has other qualifications
>   the nurse cracks jokes
>   the nurse is patient
>   the nurse is attentive
>   the nurse is cheerful

---

the high evaluations of scores given to the items in the nurse aspects section of the questionnaire.

Before concluding this section it is worth commenting that there is limited information about the CPNs' goals that were not commented on by carers or patients. It could be concluded that lack of reference to a goal means that the CPNs were not working towards an expressed goal. This conclusion is not entirely accurate. Some aspects of the CPNs' goal-seeking behaviour may, by virtue of the nurse–patient relationship, be mis-interpreted by the recipients of care. Further, the goal, as defined by the CPNs, for example work aimed at 'promoting independence' such as encouraging someone to go to the day centre, may be experienced as something totally different by patients and carers, such as the nurse showing care and interest. It would be unreasonable for all the expressed goals of the CPNs to be interpreted in the experiences of the carers or patients. It should also be said that the findings may demonstrate that the goals are not mutually negotiated by nurse and patient/carer, and that the goals are never made explicit by the CPNs to either the patients or the carers.

Suchman's statement (1967) that goals (aimed for by practitioners in a service) should be attainable has already been referred to. This analysis has shown that the CPNs in the two services studied were able to do this: the CPNs clearly detailed 'goals' which they aimed for. This is contrary to the information previously documented in the literature.

This analysis has also shown that there is a good deal of congruence between what the CPNs sought to achieve and what the clients ex-perienced.

IMPLICATIONS FOR CLINICAL PRACTICE: SOME LIMITATIONS OF THE STUDY

Before elaborating on some of the implications for clinical practice that arise out of this research study, it is worth devoting some paragraphs to comment on the limitations of the work, and the wider application of the findings. This study examined the process and outcome of community psychiatric nursing. The nature of community psychiatric nursing itself constitutes a whole spectrum of activities ranging from the one-off pro-vision of information and physical help to a complex amalgam of practical and/or emotional support, counselling and collaboration with various agencies and professionals. The task of attempting to link change in patient behaviour with community psychiaric intervention may always be an almost impossible endeavour. In these circumstances, the 'natural' course of the condition being treated is unknown, and the question of whether any care is better than none will always remain unanswered. This study did not have

Table 6.4 Statements from the family PQRST, grouped in relation to the goals and values expressed by the nurses

---

Family centred goals:

 carer can see nurse when patient visited
 carer feels can approach nurse if worried
 carer feels can talk to the nurse about anything
 carer finds nurse easy to talk to

 carer can call the nurse
 nurse will visit if something is wrong

 helps the carer understand illness
 gives the carer backing
 nurse tells the carer they are doing OK
 makes the carer feel less alone

Patient centred goals:

Respect for the individual:
 patient needs to talk to the nurse
 nurse comes to see the patient
 the nurse assesses the patient
 carer leaves patient alone with the nurse
 nurse can talk to patient and say things carer can't
 the patient's presence inhibits the carer
 carer dislikes talk behind patient's back

Community care is good:
 the nurse staves off recurrence
 the nurse prevents hospitalization

Quality of life and autonomy:
 nil

Task orientated definitions of the work:
 nurse stops carer seeing a psychiatrist
 nurse arranges day care
 nurse arranges admission

Unsorted statements:
 meeting on my territory is best
 the nurses are freer
 the nurse is an outsider
 nurse arrives unannounced

---

any of the conditions sufficient to establish whether the outcome measures can in fact be linked to the community psychiatric nursing intervention, for example random assignment of the population to an experimental and a control or comparison group, different interventions offered to each of these groups, clear specification of the types of intervention being used (with separation of the effect of the method used from the influence of the person giving the help). Bearing these factors in mind the findings presented above must be viewed with caution.

Any attempt at evaluation is a matter of assessing the value or worth of an activity; if this is accepted, it follows that evaluations are essentially subjective judgements, varying with the viewpoints and the roles of the evaluators. The criteria used in this study to explore value were viewed from the vantage point of the families of patients visited by CPNs. The carers' view is only one, though important, element in the constellation of factors that need to be taken into account in judging effectiveness. A fuller picture of effectiveness may have emerged if other kinds of data had also been acquired which could have supported these measures. Further, it should be noted that follow-up data are of little use unless comparison can be made with the state of affairs at the start of the intervention. For this a prospective study would be required. As with any piece of research, the endeavour raises more questions than it answers; the findings provide merely pointers to areas of future study, and indicate possibilities and options for service developments.

Other reservations about the design of the study include the fact that the number of carer respondents was small; this must limit the applicability of the findings. Another factor worthy of note is that, as only a small number of CPNs were involved in the research, it is unclear whether the findings are applicable to community psychiatric nursing as a whole. The findings do have a certain amount of face validity in that they appear reasonable to the author as a clinician and to community psychiatric nursing audiences (including the nurses who were involved in the study) to whom the results have been presented. The fact that the findings in the second site confirmed the qualitative analysis in the first area also gave a certain amount of validity to the conclusions.

The major finding of the analysis of the goal seeking activities of the CPNs is that some criteria for assessing the nurses' success in meeting their own aims have been fulfilled and that there is a good deal of congruence between what the CPNs sought to achieve and what the clients experienced. An issue that should be mentioned here is that of using the same data about CPNs' goals to both define them and assess how far they have been addressed. To examine a body of data in two different ways, although not intrinsically wrong, does introduce a circularity into the argument. In reality it is unknown whether the CPNs in the practice situation, did actually attempt to attain the goals that they talked about in the interviews, and details about how these goals were actually achieved are also lacking.

PRACTICAL IMPLICATIONS

The methods

I have already argued that repertory grid is a useful method for clinicians (Pollock, 1986). My study has demonstrated that the method can be used (and enjoyed) by CPNs. I would maintain further that the method could be of practical use in supervision sessions. Here managers (or whoever) are in the business of case-load management and helping the CPN to explore practice issues. The repertory grid is an ideal method to help in this task.

Using repertory grid technique, constructs and elements are traditionally integrated into a grid format, with each element rated in terms of the construct; this allows the primary data to be clearly presented for discussion. The ability of the technique to provide quantitative information that can then be analysed using statistical packages is a factor that recommends its use (Fransella and Bannister, 1977). The computer analysis undertaken by the author proved to be less helpful than expected and did not provide additional information to that gained from the 'laddering' interviews. Interpretations of the computer print-outs go beyond the bounds of the data and should, according to the seminal work on repertory grid technique, be negotiated with the respondents. I would, however, promote the method as a useful, structured conversational technique which could have a variety of valuable uses for CPNs (see Stewart and Stewart, 1981). The laddering procedure, little used previously in research, provided a useful means of exploring the initial constructs. Laddering has some of the problems of normal conversation but has the advantage of being much more focused.

The challenge to future practice must be for managers and clinicians to document their work and argue that community psychiatric nursing is a worthwhile and valuable exercise to all concerned (practitioners, other professionals and consumers). This task requires evaluation and systematic examination of practice to ensure quality provision and will be a requirement of future practice. This, if anything, must be one of the strong messages arising out of the National Health Service review paper (1989 white paper) – messages which must be heard by CPNs, clinicians and managers alike. Perhaps the framework used for goal analysis may be helpful in this respect.

The results

Elaboration of the findings detailed in Table 6.1 providing information about individual CPN's work/assessments was irrelevant to the purpose of the above study. For a supervisor of clinical practice or a manager of a community psychiatric nursing service, however, this finding should be examined closely, and in particular how the values actually influence practice in the individual nurse–patient situations and how each nurse establishes priorities within the goals they set, need to be identified. This remit is the clinical supervisor's. The content analysis (see Figure 6.4) could be a useful tool for managers or supervisors, and help make comparisons between the individual CPNs in any one service. Thus it could be ascertained whether the differences in constructs produced represent differences in the way the CPNs used models or reflect varied theoretical orientations of the CPNs; the differences may result from the varied contexts in which the CPNs work or be related to differences in the patients.

As detailed above, the findings may demonstrate that the goals of community psychiatric nursing practice were not made explicit nor mutually negotiated by the CPNs. Negotiated contracts with patients are a feature of particular model use (Peplau, 1988) and learning contracts are increasingly used to support change and plan ways to meet mutual goals (Luther and Wolfe, 1980; Jarvis, 1986; Keyser, 1986). This is an area that is worthy of discussion if not future action at practice level.

CONCLUSION

This chapter has explored and analysed the goals and objectives being aimed for by community psychiatric nurses. These findings were based on the examination of the work of two community psychiatric nursing services and formed part of a larger study which focused on the 'process' and 'outcome' of community psychiatric nursing (Pollock, 1989). The literature has been reviewed and the reasons for community psychiatric nursing service development have been presented. This has been set against the reality of close scrutiny of the assumptions and goal activities of a selected group of community psychiatric nurses. Analysis showed that the framework of immediate, intermediate and ultimate goals can be used usefully to explain the rationales underpinning community psychiatric nursing practice, and that these were either patient, job or family centred in nature. The further finding was, using comparative outcome data, that a considerable number of the expressed goals of the nurses were achieved. The methods used in the study and the results detailed have implications for practice and as such this research should be used as a springboard to improve and build on the work of present day community psychiatric nursing.

REFERENCES

Ainsworth, D. and Jolley, D. (1978) The community nurse in a developing psycho-geriatric service. *Nursing Times*, **74** (21), 873–874.

Allsop, N. (1980) *An exploration of infant teachers' explanations of reading difficulty.* MSc Thesis, Educational Psychology, Edinburgh University, Edinburgh.

Anderson, D. (1972) Working with the family doctor – a programme for mental health. *British Medical Journal*, **4**, 781–784.

Barker, A. and Black, S. (1971) An experiment in integrated psychogeriatric care. *Nursing Times*, **67** (45), 1395–1399.

Berelson, B. (1952) *Content analysis*, Free Press, Illinois.

Brennan, P.J. (1981) A family close to crisis. *Nursing Times*, **77** (32), 1390–1392.

Brooker, C.G.D. (1987) An investigation into the factors influencing variation in the growth of community psychiatric nursing services. *Journal of Advanced Nursing*, **12**, 367–375.

Brooker, C.G.D. and Simmons, S.S. (1985) A study to compare two models of community psychiatric nursing care delivery. *Journal of Advanced Nursing*, **10**, 217–223.

Clarke, M.G. (1980) Psychiatric liaison with the health visitor. *Health Trends*, **12** (4), 98–100.

Cochrane, A.L. (1971) *Effectiveness and efficiency: random reflections on Health services*, Nuffield Provincial Hospital Trust, London.

Cohen, D. (1978) Psychiatry at home. *New Society*, 2 March, 486–487.

Davis, B.D. (1984) *A repertory grid study of formal and informal aspects of student nurse training.* PhD Thesis, London University, London.

Ditton, L. (1984) *Student nurse placement within the community psychiatric nursing team.* Hampstead District Health Authority, unpublished paper.

Donabedian, A. (1966) Evaluating the quality of medical care. The Millbank Memorial Fund Quarterly, **44** (3), 166–206.

Downie, R.S. and Telfer, E. (1980) *Caring and curing. A philosophy of medicine and social work*, Methuen, London.

Duck, S. (1973) *Personal relationships and personal constructs*, John Wiley, Chichester.

Fransella, F. and Bannister, D. (1977) *A manual for repertory grid technique*, Academic Press, London.

Haque, G. (1973) Psychosocial nursing in the community. *Nursing Times* **69** (2), 51–53.

Harker, P., Leopoldt, H. and Robinson, J.R. (1976) Attaching community psychiatric nurses in general practice. *Journal of Royal College of General Practitioners*, **26**, 666–671.

Hazelden, J. (1981) *Exploring the views of four guidance teachers and five truants in a Scottish secondary school.* MSc Thesis, Educational Psychology, Edinburgh University, Edinburgh.

Henderson, J., Levin, B. and Cheyne, E. (1973) Role of a psychiatric nurse in a domiciliary treatment service. *Nursing Times*, **69** (41), 1334–1335.

Higgins, P. (1984) Mental Health Education. *Nursing Mirror*, **159** (19), 28–29.

References   141

Hinkle, D. (1965) The change of personal constructs from the viewpoint of a theory of construct implications. PhD Thesis, Ohio State University, Ohio.
Holloway, R. (1984) One step beyond. *Nursing Times*, **80** (8), 44–49.
Hunter, P. (1978) *Schizophrenia and community psychiatric nursing*, National Schizophrenia Fellowship, Surbiton.
Hyman, H., Wright, C.R. and Hopkins, T. (1962) *Applications of methods of evaluation: four studies of the encampment for citizenship*, University of California Press, Berkeley.
Jarvis, P. (1986) Contract learning. *Journal of District Nursing*, November, 13–14.
Jeevendrampillai, V. (1982) Coming out of long stay. *Nursing Times*, **78** (18), 766–767.
Jones, A. (1988) The significant communication: a clinical study. *Community Psychiatric Nursing Journal*, **8** (4), 19–22.
Judkins, M. (1976) *Introspective dialogue technique*, Royal Free Hospital, London.
Kelly, G.E. (1955) *The psychology of personal constructs*, Volumes I and II, Norton, New York.
Kelly, G.E. (1963) *A theory of personality*, Norton Press, New York.
Keyser, D. (1986) Using learning contracts to support change in nursing organisations. *Nurse Education Today*, **6**, 103–108.
King, S. (1962) *Perceptions of illness and medical practice*, Russell Sage Foundation, New York.
Kirkpatrick, W.J.A. (1967) The in-and-out nurse. Some thoughts on the role of community psychiatric nursing and preparation required. *International Journal of Nursing Studies*, **4**, 225–231.
Landfield, A.W. (1971) *Personal construct systems in psychotherapy*, Rand McNally, New York.
Leopoldt, H. (1973) Psychiatric community nursing. *Health and Social Services Journal*, **83** (4324), 489–490.
Leopoldt, H. (1974) The role of the psychiatric community nurse in the therapeutic team. *Nursing Mirror*, **138** (5), 70–72.
Leopoldt, H. (1975) GP attachment and psychiatric domiciliary nursing. *Nursing Mirror*, **140** (7), 82–84.
Leopoldt, H. (1979a) Community psychiatric nursing – 1. *Nursing Times*, **75** (13), 53–56.
Leopoldt, H. (1979b) Community psychiatric nursing – 2. *Nursing Times*, **75** (14), 57–59.
Lifshitz, M. (1974) Quality professionals. Does training make a difference? A personal construct theory. *British Journal of Social and Clinical Psychology*, **13**, 183–189.
Luther, D.C. and Wolfe, M.J. (1980) Toward a partnership in learning. *Nursing Outlook*, December, 745–750.
Maisey, M. (1975) Hospital based psychiatric nursing in the community. *Nursing Times*, **71** (9), 354–355.
MacDonald, D.J. (1972) Psychiatric nursing in the community. *Nursing Times*, **68** (3), 80–83.
Marais, R.A. (1976) Community psychiatric nursing – an alternative to hospitalisation. *Nursing Times*, **72** (44), 1708–1717.

May, A.R. (1965a) Psychiatry within the general hospital. *Nursing Mirror*, **121** (3157), 427–432.

May, A.R. (1965b) Psychiatry within the general hospital. *Nursing Mirror*, **121** (3158), 461–465.

McCall, G. and Simmons, J.L. (1969) *Issues in participant Observation: a text and reader*, Addison Wesley, Massachusetts.

Nickerson, A. (1972) Psychiatric community nurses in Edinburgh. *Nursing Times*, **68** (10), 289–291.

Peplau, H.E. (1988) *Interpersonal relations in nursing*, 2nd edn, Macmillan, London.

Persaud, T. (1985) The general student in the community. *Community Psychiatric Nursing Journal*, **5** (1), 6–10.

Philip, A.E. and McCulloch, J.W. (1968) Personal construct theory and social work practice. *British Journal of Social and Clinical Psychology*, **7**, 115–121.

Pollock, L.C. (1986) An introduction to the use of repertory grid technique as a research method and clinical tool for psychiatric nurses. *Journal of Advanced Nursing*, **11**, 439–445.

Pollock, L.C. (1987) *Community psychiatric nursing explained: an analysis of the views of patients, carers and nurses*, PhD Thesis, Edinburgh University, Edinburgh.

Pollock, L.C. (1988a) The work of community psychiatric nursing. *Journal of Advanced Nursing*, **13**, 537–545.

Pollock, L.C. (1988b) The future work of community psychiatric nursing. *Community Psychiatric Nursing Journal*, **8** (5), 5–13.

Pollock, L.C. (1989) *Community psychiatric nursing – the myth and the reality*, Scutari Press, London.

Pullen, I. and Gilbert, M.A. (1979a) Crisis team turns chaos into relief. *Nursing Mirror*, **149** (14), 34–35.

Pullen, I. and Gilbert, M.A. (1979b) When crisis hits the home. *Nursing Mirror*, **149** (13), 30–32.

Richards, D.A., Butterworth, G. and Shrubb, S. (1988) Outcome measures in community psychiatric nursing: a pilot study. *Community Psychiatric Nursing Journal*, **8** (6), 7–16.

Ritson, B. (1977) Psychiatry and the community. *Contact*, **2**, 27–31.

Roberts, L. (1976) The community psychiatric nurse. *Nursing Times*, **72** (51), 2020–2021.

Sencicle, L. (1981) Which way the CPN? *Community Psychiatric Nurses' Association Journal*, **2** (1), 12–13.

Sharpe, D. (1975) Role of the community psychiatric nurse. *Nursing Mirror*, **141** (16), 60–62.

Sharpe, D. (1980) Figures tell their own story. *Nursing Mirror*, **150** (2), 34–36.

Sharpe, D. (1982) GP's views of community psychiatric nursing. *Nursing Times*, **78** (40), 1664–1666.

Shires, J. (1977) A travelling day hospital – an experiment in rural community care. *Social Work Today*, **8** (24), 16–18.

Simmons, S. and Brooker, C. (1986) *Community psychiatric nursing: a social perspective*, Heinemann, London.

Slater, P. (1976) *Explorations of Interpersonal Space*, Volume 1, John Wiley, Chichester.

Stewart, V. and Stewart, A. (1981) *Business application of repertory grid*, McGraw-Hill, London.

Stobie, E. and Hopkins, D. (1972a) Crisis intervention: 1 – a community psychiatric nurse in a rural area. *Nursing Times*, **68** (43), 165–168.

Stobie, E. and Hopkins, D. (1972b) Crisis intervention: 2 – *Nursing Times*, **68** (43), 169–172.

Suchman, E.A. (1967) *Evaluative Research*, Russell Sage Foundation, New York.

Warren, J. (1971) Long acting phenothiazine injections given by psychiatric nurses in the community. *Nursing Times*, **67** (36), 141–143.

Weeks, K. and Greene, J. (1966) Nursing after care in psychiatry. *Nursing Times*, **65** (51), 1629.

Willey, R. (1969) Nursing after care in psychiatry. *Nursing Times*, **65** (51), 1629.

Williamson, F. (1982) The nursing process in a community psychiatric nursing service. *Nursing Times*, **78** (1), 1–3.

Wright, C. (1955) Evaluating mass media campaigns. *International Social Science Bulletin*, **7**, 3.

Wright, K.J.T. (1970) Exploring the uniqueness of common complaints. *British Journal of Medical Psychology*, **43**, 221–232.

CHAPTER SEVEN

Evaluation of community psychiatric nursing in general practice

Jan Illing, Chris Drinkwater, Tony Rogerson, Don Forster, and Peter Rutherford

SUMMARY

A pilot study was carried out in Newcastle to evaluate the effect of placing a community psychiatric nurse (CPN) in a general medical practice. The aims were to find out what impact, if any, a CPN would have on both the patient population and behaviour of the other professionals within the practice, by comparing the following different models and degrees of contact with a CPN: attached (full-time in practice); aligned (sessional work in practice); and a comparison model (involving referral to a team of CPNs located at the DGH). A variety of methods were used to measure the effects; they included surveys of both the GPs' and patients' views, collecting information on who the CPN clients were and type of CPN intervention received, reasons for referral, and data on the amount of psychotropic drugs prescribed, using both cross-sectional and prospective designs. The results indicate that both the GPs and the patients valued having a CPN in the practice, that the greater the CPN contact with the practice the higher the number of CPN referrals. Over half of the patients referred to CPNs were not prescribed psychotropic drugs, suggesting CPNs were viewed as an alternative to drugs. The CPNs also appeared to have little influence on the wide range of prescribing.

INTRODUCTION

Since the late 1950s there has been a shift in emphasis in the field of the mental health services, from institutional care to community-oriented care.

This shift has been brought about by two sets of factors: negative factors associated with institutional care, and positive factors seen to be associated with community care.

The negative factors have been the increasing recognition of the damaging effects that, even with the best intentions, institutionalization has had on individuals (Martin, J.P., 1984). In the very worst cases this has led to neglect and even to physical harm being done to patients, resulting in a spate of formal enquiries into certain psychiatric hospitals in the 1960s and 1970s. Thus, apart from any intrinsic virtues that community care might have, it came to be seen as the means of solving the problems of large institutions. The largely untested positive effects of community care were that it would provide small-scale, personal care which was non-stigmatizing and valued individual autonomy. Two other important assumptions were often made: firstly, that care of the mentally ill would become a community responsibility; and secondly, that community care would be cheaper than institutional care. In an era of cost limits and finite resources there are increasing demands to test this second assumption, and increasingly the burden of evaluation is falling on community services, including community psychiatric nurses (CPNs).

Although mental health nurses have been working in the community since the early 1950s (May and Moore, 1963), a stimulus to expansion came about when a gap in the provision of care for the mentally ill in the community was created, by the establishment of generic departments of social work following the Seebohm Report (HMSO, 1968). Social workers were now to work with all types of clients and the specialism of mental health was redundant (Martin, F.M., 1984). In the period 1980–1985, the number of CPNs grew by 65%, from 1667 to 2758 (Brooker, 1987). This expansion was taking place up until the early 1980s in the context of scant research and analysis being carried out into CPN roles and work. Some of the dominant general themes for evaluation that have been identified are:

1. What is the range of skills that CPNs are required to exhibit in their day-to-day work? For example, should their work focus on primary prevention, secondary prevention or tertiary prevention? Each of these can be subdivided into a wide variety of detailed tasks but broadly speaking the question is whether CPNs practise generically using a number of methods across a range of tasks or specialize using a limited number of methods on a restricted range of diagnoses or problems.

2. To what extent are the role and function of CPNs influenced by the setting in which they work and the associated managerial arrange-ments? This debate has centred around comparisons between CPNs being based in primary care or being based in psychiatric institutions

(Brooker and Simmons, 1985; Skidmore, 1986).
3. How effective is community psychiatric nursing care? Evaluations using randomized trials in this field are few, though Paykel *et al.* (1982) showed no significant difference in neurotic patients allocated to routine psychiatric follow-up in out-patient clinics or community psychiatric nursing care. The outcome measures used were symptom relief, social adjustment and family burden. Importantly, however, the patients preferred the community psychiatric nursing care to the routine psychiatric follow-up. This study referred to restricted diagnostic categories. It remains to be seen if CPNs are effective across the range of diagnoses or problems they may encounter in their clientele.
4. How efficient is community psychiatric nursing care? Mangen *et al.* (1983) in a cost-effective analysis of the randomized controlled trial noted above, concluded that over the 18-month study period community psychiatric nursing care was a cheaper alternative to routine out-patient care in terms of direct costs. Nevertheless, using the psychiatric case register at Salford, Wooff, Freeman and Fryers (1983) have shown that the development and use of community psychiatric nursing services in the period 1968–1978 hardly affected the use by patients of other psychiatric services.

Clearly, all of the general evaluation themes noted above overlap. Yet it is against this background that the specific objectives and methods for the Newcastle pilot study were planned.

THE NEWCASTLE PILOT STUDY

The aim of this project was to try to evaluate the effect of placing a CPN in a general practice.

Design

The results presented in this chapter were collected as part of a before-and-after study. This was a quasi-experimental design (Cambell and Stanley, 1963), in that whilst it was possible to have a comparison group that received no intervention and compare it to an intervention group it was not possible (as is common in much health service research) to randomly allocate patients, CPNs and general practitioners (GPs) to different practices. The study involved comparing a number of measures over the 12-month period prior to CPN input with the same measures over a 12-month period of CPN input, in three groups of general practices. The practice groups all have equal patient list size of approximately 10000 patients and are based in the west of the city of Newcastle upon Tyne (with the exception of a third of the patients in one practice that had a branch surgery located in the north of the city). The following measures were used:

1. a survey of GPs, this included GPs in the CPN study and all other GPs in the same health services sector. The survey focused on views of mental health services;
2. collection of data on the type of patients seen by the CPNs;
3. a postal survey of the CPN clients;
4. a survey of new referrals to out-patient clinics;
5. a comparison of the amount of psychotropic drugs prescribed in the two 12-month periods;
6. a comparison of the number of referrals to out-patient clinics and admissions to hospital in the two 12-month periods.

Analysis of the data was carried out using the Minesota Terminal System computer, located at the University of Newcastle. The data were analysed using cross tabulations and correlation tests.

The study was carried out in a deprived area, exemplified by 40% unemployment, 21% single-parent families and 47% council rented housing (Newcastle upon Tyne Household Survey, 1986). The practices were allocated to one of three types of community psychiatric nursing service:

1. *Attachment.* Having a CPN attached to the practice. In this study attachment was defined as working full-time for the practice and only working with patients from that practice. In fact the CPN worked seven sessions in the practice (one session being either a morning or afternoon) the remaining time was spent on research.
2. *Alignment.* Having a CPN aligned to the practice. In this study having an aligned CPN meant that the practice was given a named CPN to contact when making referrals. The CPN provided a service of two hours in the practice on a fortnightly basis.
3. *Comparison.* The third type of service to be examined by this study was the one that was already in existence and in which there was no intervention by this study. The aim of including this group was to compare the 'new' services with that which was already in operation. In this case, the community psychiatric nursing service available to GPs in sector four of the Newcastle Mental Health Unit was by direct referral to a team of CPNs who were based at the district general hospital, located in the west of the city. Referrals were then allocated to individual CPNs. The GPs would have no control over who would deal with the referral, nor were they likely to deal regularly with the same CPN. This was the mechanism in effect for all three groups of practices in the 'before' period of the study.

There are many measures one might take in order to try to evaluate the effect of placing a CPN in a general practice. This study used several different measurements in an attempt to answer the following questions.

1. Does the frequency of referrals to psychiatrists at out-patients change? If referrals decrease, this may be because the CPN is used by the practice to help identify and screen off those clients who need to be referred to a psychiatrist; the remaining clients may then be treated by the CPN. If, however, the referrals increase, this may be brought about by the presence of a mental health specialist in the practice increasing the GPs' awareness of mental health problems. It is estimated that between 30% and 50% of emotional problems are not recognized by the GP (Marks, Goldberg and Hillier, 1979; Bordman, 1978). Strathdee and Williams (1986) have reported that one of the benefits of having a psychiatrist in the practice was that it increased awareness of mental health. It seems feasible, therefore, to ask whether a CPN might perform a similar task, and thus lead to more mentally ill patients being identified.

2. Does the frequency of hospital admissions to psychiatric hospitals change? CPNs might have an impact on the number of admissions to hospital if by their intervention, whether direct or indirect, better care were to be provided for the patient in the community or if due to intervention from CPNs being provided at an early stage in the patients disorder, fewer problems were to escalate to a stage where hospitalization became necessary. Alternatively, the CPN might uncover more sickness and indeed might recommend a period in hospital (Hunter, 1974).

3. Does the amount and cost of prescriptions for psychotropic medication change? If the CPN is seen to offer an alternative to drug treatments, i.e. talking treatments, it is likely that the amount of psychotropic medication will decline. Also the presence of the CPN may raise awareness of some of the disadvantages of psychotropic medication in the long term. If prescriptions are found to increase, however, there is not only the possibility that more patients are being identified, but also disillusionment with alternative treatments, including the effectiveness of CPNs!

4. Will GPs and clients value this service and prefer it to existing services? The study by Paykel *et al.* (1982) suggested that clients prefer the community psychiatric nursing service to the alternative of seeing a psychiatrist at the out-patient clinic. The users' view of the service must be one of the important measures in determining its value.

5. How many and what type of patients do CPNs see under different referral conditions? One of the arguments used for not placing mental health specialists in the community is a concern that GPs change their referral patterns and instead of referring the same type of patients who would have been referred to the hospital services, a new category of patients are referred. Such patients have been termed the 'worried well'.

The concern centres on whether this category of patients will be identified or not; but the other side to this argument is that if they are identified and referred, are such referrals appropriate or not? This raises the question of whether or not there is unmet need. This study aimed to identify the type of patients seen by the CPN.

THE GP SURVEY

An important element of this study was the exploration of the primary care environment in which the attached and aligned CPNs were based. Our hypothesis was that the attached and aligned CPNs would develop different working relationships with primary care teams and that this would affect their ability to influence the team and be reflected in the range and number of referrals seen and in their pattern of work. White (1986) carried out a study to examine the factors that influence GPs in their decision to refer to a CPN. White concluded that the largest and most important variable was the idiosyncrasies of each GP and the individual nature of the relationships formed between GPs and CPNs.

As we considered that the structure of the existing primary health care team, and the background and attitudes of the GPs were important variables, that might influence the success of attachment or alignment, we carried out an interview survey of all the GPs who have practices within the boundaries of sector four of the Newcastle Mental Health Unit. This survey aimed to explore the following variables which might influence our overall hypotheses.

1. What is the GP's attitude to mental health problems?
2. How satisfied is the GP with existing psychiatric services?
3. What is the effect of the different training and experience of GPs?
4. What are the GP's views of teams and team-work?

Fifty-one GPs, including the 16 GPs who were in one of the three types of CPN service to be examined, were sent an introductory letter by the General Manager of the Newcastle Mental Health Unit. The letter informed the GPs that a survey was to be carried out and that the views of GPs, as the main providers of mental health care in the community, were being sought. The letter was then followed up by a telephone call to arrange a convenient time to visit. Interviews lasted between 20 and 60 minutes and were carried out by one of the authors between December 1987 and April 1988. Of the 51 GPs identified in sector four, 90% ($n=46$) took part in the survey. This high response rate was achieved by making, on average, as many as half a dozen telephone calls, first to speak to and then to arrange an interview with the GP. Of the remaining five GPs, two refused to be interviewed and the other three were not available due to factors such as illness. At least one GP was interviewed from each of the 20 practices in the sector. The sample included 14 female GPs and 32 male GPs. The age range was from 26 to 80 years, and the GPs qualified as doctors between 1926 and 1985.

Attitudes to mental health problems

There have been various attempts to measure the percentage of a GP's work-load that is taken up by emotional, psychiatric and psychological problems. These are confounded by the imprecision of defining a 'case'. Cartwright (1983), for instance, reports in her survey a perceived mental health work-load range of between 10% and 65%. This range is obviously a reflection of GPs' attitudes and aptitudes, but when cases are more objectively defined by instrument, such as the General Health Questionnaire (GHQ), there is evidence that GPs vary in their ability to identify them as such (Bordman, 1987; Marks, Goldberg and Hillier, 1979).

Eighty per cent ($n=38$) of the GPs reported spending 20% or more of their time on emotional, psychiatric and psychological problems. Of these the majority 65% ($n=30$) said that such work took up between 20% and 50% of their time. Forty-eight per cent ($n=22$) felt that they were spending about the right amount of time on these problems, 20% ($n=9$) felt they were spending too much time and 33% ($n=15$) felt they were spending too little time.

It has been suggested that pressure of time and disinterest in this area of work leads to limited assessment and management of mental health problems and to inappropriate prescriptions being given. A subsidiary aim of our study has been to see whether the attachment of a CPN alters prescribing patterns.

Views on existing mental health services

In order to discover their views of existing mental health services, GPs were asked to name the mental health services they were aware of and, if they had used that service, how satisfied they were with it. Hospital in-patient and out-patient services including the psychogeriatric unit and the regional drug and alcohol unit were the services mentioned most, followed by community psychiatric nursing services which were mentioned by 70% ($n=32$) of the GPs, of whom 39% ($n=18$) were satisfied, 11% ($n=5$) dissatisfied and 20% ($n=9$) neutral about the service.

They were also asked about the strengths and weaknesses of the mental health services. The most interesting findings were that although the service was perceived to be good for those who were clearly psychiatrically ill, they were said to be poor for clients with less clearly defined emotional and behavioural problems. Some typical comments were:

> Patients with neurotic type disorders, for example stress related, are not dealt with so good. I cannot possibly deal with all the counselling on my own.

> There is a lack of experienced psychotherapists and counsellors, because of this we are having to do this, but we are not trained!

This was also reflected in comments about lack of staff, particularly CPNs and psychologists for dealing with this area of work:

> One weakness in the present services for the mentally ill is not having CPNs in the primary health care team.

> There is not enough access to the psychologists.

The other major weaknesses identified by the GPs were poor communication, difficulty with admissions and sectorization.

In the context of this study sectorization is an interesting issue and reflects the different ways in which GPs and mental health units provide services. A GP's list is a reflection of historical tradition and consumer choice, and overrides geographical boundaries. This creates problems for GPs who often have patients living in more than one sector and it is not surprising that muddled communication can arise when GPs have to liaise with units with different policies. Mental health units have a choice of providing community mental health services by attachment or alignment of staff with general practices or by establishing their own community mental health centres.

The advantage of providing services through practices are that these are, and are likely to remain, the places where the vast majority of mental health problems are dealt with. The disadvantage is that it is less easy to tie staff to defined geographical areas with neatly defined packages of services that relate to demographic and morbidity features of the population. Community mental health centres can provide a package of services through a cohesive team, but it is likely that they will find it more difficult to establish fruitful working relationships with primary health care teams. It is also possible that the stigma of attending hospital psychiatric services will be transferred to the community mental health centre.

Different training and experience of GPs

Forty-six per cent ($n=21$) of the GPs had the qualification Member of the Royal College of General Practitioners (MRCGP). These GPs were more likely to have a professional in their practice who could offer some form of talking treatment such as a clinical psychologist, a counsellor or a CPN, 62% (13/21) compared to 24% (6/25) (this figure relates to the practice complement prior to the CPN input as a result of this study). When asked about any possible advantages that they could see to having a team, the GPs holding a MRCGP were significantly more likely to comment on the different skills a team can offer (p=0.04). This is particularly interesting in the light of the work carried out by White (1986). White discusses the notion that GPs delegate when they make a referral to a CPN, that had GPs the time they would have dealt with the problem themselves. The results from our study suggest that MRCGP holders do consider the CPNs to have different skills. In the present *ad hoc* situation it is possible that services go to those who make the most demands rather than those who have the most need, and that holders of the MRCGP are more likely to recognize the need for these services for their patients. They are also more likely to be successful in ensuring that their patients have access to these services, that they may not have either the skill or the time to provide themselves.

Fifty-nine per cent (n=27) of the GPs had some post-graduate training in mental health, for the most part this had been in hospital posts (59%, n=16/27). The remainder had spent some time learning to use a particular therapy to deal with a specific type of problem. Five of this group of GPs were involved in mental health work outside their practices (four in clinical posts and one in research). Forty-one per cent (n=19) of the GPs in sector four had no post-graduate training in mental health.

The needs and demands of mental health care in the community are both qualitatively and quantitatively different from hospital based care; the relevance of a post-graduate hospital post is therefore questionable. GPs deal with 90%–95% of psychiatric problems and refer only a small percentage to a psychiatrist (Shepherd and Clare, 1981). This then brings into question the relevance of psychiatric training in hospital. If they are to deal adequately with these problems they need both appropriate community based training and the support of CPNs.

GP's views of teams and team-work

Thirteen different professionals were identified as being either based in a general practice or were dropping in to see patients in a practice. All the GPs reported that there was a district nurse and a health visitor in the team (100%, n=46) and the majority reported the presence of a midwife (87%, n=40) and a practice nurse (85%, n=39). Social workers and psychologists were aligned with seven of the 20 practices. CPNs were the professionals who were next most common (ranking fifth), however this was only when the CPNs who had recently been allocated to practices as a result of this study were included, prior to this CPNs were in only two practices instead of five.

All 46 GPs (100%) said that they thought having a team was important. The most common reason given by 57% (*n*=26) of the GPs was that a team increased the range of skills available to patients. The next most popular reasons were providing support for one another (24%, *n*=11), generally providing a better service for the patients (22%, *n*=10) and increasing communication (20%, *n*=9), see Table 7.1. When asked about possible disadvantages of having a team, whilst a large number (37%, *n*=17) felt that there were none, the most common problem reported was difficulty of communication (30%, *n*=14).

When asked which professionals they would most like to add to their team, the most common answer (30%, *n*=14) was a social worker. This is interesting in view of the different philosophical bases and general lack of understanding of each others role (Huntingdon, 1981). A physiotherapist came next (26%, *n*=12), followed by a CPN (22%, *n*=10). Surprisingly, 26% (*n*=12) of GPs reported that they did not wish to add to their team, and a closer look at the professional make up of these practices revealed that the GPs who were satisfied with their professional complement, tended to be those who not only had the usual back-up but also had a social worker, a CPN, a psychologist and a psychiatrist. This suggests that once GPs have the resources they feel they need they do not continue to request more.

When GPs work with attached or aligned staff, it does not necessarily mean that they function as an effective team. Bond and Cartlidge (1986) have demonstrated that there are different levels of collaboration that measure team function. As an indirect measure of team-work, the GPs were asked about methods of communication within the team, referrals to

Table 7.1 GPs' views of the advantages of having a team

Advantages	n	%
Offer different skills	26	57
Provides support	11	24
Better for patient generally	10	22
Increases communication	9	20
Increases continuity	3	7
Faster problem solving	3	7
Reduces hospitalization	2	4

More than one advantage of having a team could be given.

team members and feedback. Our hypothesis was that GPs with a team-work approach would be more likely to work successfully with a CPN, and an effective team would hold regular meetings, refer patients frequently to other team members and receive good feedback.

Forty-three per cent ($n=20$) of the GPs reported that team meetings were held in their practice (meetings held in nine practices) but individual discussion was the most common form of communication used. The GPs who reported having team meetings were also more likely to report using the tea-break as another opportunity to discuss patients, indicating both good formal and informal communication systems; these GPs were also more likely to be working with a CPN. Practice size was related to the holding of team meetings as, of the eleven practices not holding team meetings, eight were single-handed GPs and the remaining three were partnerships of two GPs. Single-handed GPs were also the least likely to have any type of back-up service for counselling, only one of the eight single-handed GPs in the study had this support.

Referral behaviour of GPs

Referral rates by GPs to consultants have been shown to vary widely and this is not explicable by variations in patient characteristics, or by characteristics of the doctors such as age, experience or the possession of higher qualifications (Wilkin and Smith, 1987). It is likely that the same holds true for referrals to CPNs (White, 1986) and as an indirect and rather crude measure of referral behaviour all the GPs who took part in the survey were asked for their responses to two vignettes, previously used in a survey of GPs by Shepherd and Clare (1981).

The first vignette relates to a female patient who consults because her husband is having an affair. She is tearful, feels miserable, cannot sleep and cannot decide on any course of action. Forty-six per cent ($n=21$) of the GPs said they would treat her with drugs and, although 43% ($n=20$) of the GPs said they would not refer her, 57% ($n=26$) would refer her to a variety of agencies including marriage guidance, a CPN or a psychiatrist.

The second vignette refers to a young woman who complains she is having panic attacks since her husband, a regular soldier, was posted overseas. In this case 61% ($n=28$) of the GPs offered drug therapy and 93% ($n=43$) would consider referral. The three most popular choices for referral were a psychiatrist (37%, $n=17$), a psychologist (37%, $n=17$) and a CPN (20%, $n=9$). The wide variability of responses reinforces White's view that the idiosyncrasies of each GP may well affect the number of referrals to a CPN.

CLIENTS REFERRED TO THE CPNs DURING THE
12-MONTH STUDY PERIOD

There has been much interest in identifying where a CPN should be based in order to be most beneficial to both patients and other professionals. This debate has focused mainly on location in the community versus the hospital (Brooker and Simmons, 1985; Skidmore and Friend, 1986; Wooff *et al.* 1986). There is, however, another issue, namely whether a CPN service based part of the time or all of the time in a general practice is of most value. In relation to the first issue, does locating CPNs in the community divert patients from the traditional mental health services or does the CPN start to work with a new client group, who may, or may not have unmet needs? The second issue relates to the amount of work generated in a general practice for a CPN to be cost-effective and also whether the professional autonomy of the CPN is threatened in the general practice by becoming a member of a primary health care team. White (1986) discusses the views of Dingwall (1974), who dismisses the ambition of nurses to achieve professional autonomy as a pipe-dream, on the basis that they have their access to patients controlled by doctors. Skidmore and Friend (1985) in a study comparing the source of CPN referrals, commented that hospital doctors were more likely to suggest what CPN involvement should be, as compared with referrals from the primary health care team, which was less directive. However, if CPNs work full-time in general practice, is their autonomy likely to be eroded by the GP instead of the hospital consultant?

Five CPNs, two male and three female, were involved in providing a community psychiatric nursing service during the 12-month study period. Three of the CPNs were qualified in community psychiatric nursing. The attached CPN practice had two CPNs, one for four months and the other for the remaining eight months, who worked in a group practice containing five GPs. The aligned CPN practices had three CPNs who worked in three practices, that were of size three, two and two GPs. The comparison practice was a group practice containing four GPs. In the study year 107 patients were referred from 13 GPs, six GPs (including a trainee GP) who received an attached CPN service and seven GPs who were receiving an aligned service. Seventy-nine referrals were made from the CPN attached practice (an average of 13 referrals per GP) and 28 referrals were made from the CPN aligned practices (an average of 4 referrals per GP). In the comparison practice no referrals were made at all during the year. This was the case despite the fact that each practice was sent a letter from the CPN team, informing them that they could refer to CPNs who were now 'on site' i.e. based in the area at the district general hospital rather than at the psychiatric hospital on the other side of the city. Of the 107 referrals, 81 were seen by the CPNs and 26 did not turn up to any appointments (24%).

The number of clients who did not keep any appointments were not markedly different for each type of community psychiatric nursing service, 22% (*n*=17) and 32% (*n*=9) for attached and aligned respectively (see Table 7.2). This compares favourably with the 40% non-attendance for first appointments to psychiatrists at out-patient clinics reported by Carpenter *et al.* (1981).

The majority of clients referred were female (67%, *n*=72). The age of the clients ranged from 17 to 74 years, with the mean age for males being 41 years and 35 years for females. Of those whose marital status was known (*n*=85), 52% (*n*=44) were married or cohabiting, 28% (*n*=24) were divorced or separated, 19% (*n*=16) were single and 1% (*n*=1) was widowed. Where employment status was known (*n*=72), 58% (*n*=42) were unemployed (see Table 7.3). The type of accommodation was known for 66 clients, of whom only 6 lived in owner occupied property, 56 lived in council rented property and four lived in temporary accommodation.

The GPs were the main source of referrals to the CPNs (93%, *n*=99), the other referrals came from health visitors in the practice (5%, *n*=5) and a psychiatrist based at the district general hospital (2%, *n*=2). During the year the majority of clients referred were new referrals (94%, *n*=101), with only 4% (*n*=4) being re-referred to a CPN.

Although the bulk of the referrals were new to the CPNs, not all the patients were experiencing their first contact with a psychiatric agency. Of the 73 clients whose mental health history was known, 32% (*n*=23) had had previous psychiatric contact and at least 19% (*n*=14) had been admitted to a hospital for mental ill health.

When referring clients to the CPNs, GPs were asked to complete a referral form stating, amongst other things, what they believed the problem

Table 7.2 Number of referrals to the CPNs by type of community psychiatric nursing service

Type of CPN service	No. referrals made		No. clients who saw a CPN		No. clients who DNA*	
	n	%	*n*	%	*n*	%
Attached	79	100	62	78	17	22
Aligned	28	100	19	68	9	32
Comparison	0		0		0	
Totals	107		81		26	

*DNA: did not attend.

to be (more than one problem could be given). Anxiety was seen as a problem in more than half the cases (n=62), with the second and third most common problems being family and marital problems (n=35) and depression (n=22). These findings are consistent with previous research where anxiety and depression account for the problem most often seen in general practice (Cooper, 1972).

It is interesting that schizophrenia and manic depression were never stated as the problem and only once was psychosis named. When Paykel and Griffith (1983) carried out their study to examine hospital based community psychiatric nursing with neurotic patients, they commented that CPNs worked mainly with psychotic rather than neurotic patients; it is interesting that in this study the CPNs worked mainly with clients who would be described as having neurotic rather than psychotic symptoms. The reason behind referrals from the 'neurotic' population we felt was reflected in a view expressed earlier by the GPs, namely that they felt that the existing services were good for the clearly psychiatrically ill. This issue was raised in a follow-up interview with some of the GPs who had been involved in the study, the GPs confirmed our contention, one GP said '. . . they (the psychotic clients) were well dealt with I think, they usually had their own CPNs'.

Similarly, though reduced in number, anxiety was the problem the CPNs identified most often (n=37). It is noteworthy that the client's view of the problem was closer to the CPN's view than that of the GP, however, the CPN was required to provide the client's view of the problem, and the client's view is therefore open to bias from the CPN. There was an overall

Table 7.3 Characteristics of CPN clients

	Males	*Females*
Total no.*	32	72
Mean age	41	35
Married	10	34
Single	6	10
Divorced	8	16
Widowed	0	1
Employed[†]	4	20
Unemployed[†]	15	27

*There are 3 missing cases.
[†]Retired persons and students are not shown (n=6).

consensus on which were the most common problems: anxiety, depression, and family and marital problems (see Table 7.4).

Treatment options

A CPN working in a general practice may increase the range of treatment options available to the GPs. As already discussed, a significant number of GPs would have considered prescribing medication for the two patients represented in the vignettes; when the same cases were presented to the CPNs all thought medication was inappropriate. Interestingly, the GPs were aware of this as an issue and in a follow-up interview the GPs with the attached CPN said they felt they had used the CPN as an alternative to medication. One GP said: 'I think it's this business of offering something, something alternative to medication'. Another talked about the pressure on GPs to prescribe: 'You can spend so long talking to somebody telling them that tranquillizers aren't effective in sorting out their problems, they are not the answer, and they still go out the door saying, but you are not going to give me anything are you doctor?' Clearly, GPs are under pressure to 'do' something and it seems that, ideally, GPs want to offer an alternative to medication, but when there are no alternatives at hand, they find it difficult to appear not to care by not giving the patient anything.

Table 7.4 The problem as viewed by the GP, CPN and client

	GPs' view	CPNs' view	Clients' view
Anxiety	62	37	37
Depression	22	12	14
Schizophrenia/psychoses/manic depression	1	1	1
Personality problem	8	8	0
Marital/family	35	30	18
Obsessional states/phobias/compulsive states	10	10	6
Alcohol/drug problem	11	2	2
Benzodiazepine withdrawal	6	2	1
Bereavement/loss	8	7	4
Eating disorders	1	2	2
Interpersonal relations	12	6	6
Social problem	11	8	5
Total no. of problems	187	125	96

This impression gained more credence by the fact that 54% of the patients referred to the CPNs were not prescribed psychotropic medication (54 of the 100 patients who were known to have been prescribed drugs or not). There is also supporting evidence from the referral forms on which the GPs were asked to indicate what sort of intervention they expected the CPN to provide. The most popular reasons given for referring to the CPN were counselling (n=53), assessment (n=38) and anxiety management (n=29) (no percentage given as more than one category could be specified). When examining the interventions carried out by the CPNs the same three interventions were named most often and they accounted for 70% of CPN interventions.

The average length of an appointment with a CPN was three-quarters of an hour, this compares favourably with the average length of GP consultations, which has been reported to be between six and eight minutes, but rarely twelve minutes (Wilkin *et al.*, 1987). Therefore, when a GP offers the patient a referral to a CPN they are not only offering an alternative to drugs, they are also offering more time per consultation.

SOME IMPRESSIONS OF HOW THE ALIGNED CPN SERVICE COMPARED WITH THE ATTACHED

This section is headed impressions rather than conclusions to remind the reader of the limitations of the study, which must be viewed as a pilot. Nonetheless, without generalizing our findings, some important issues are raised by the study. The main factor that distinguishes the aligned from the attached CPN service is in the amount of contact the CPN has with the general practice. Looking at the results there does seem to be a relationship between amount of contact with the practice and the number of referrals made. The comparison group, that had no direct contact with CPNs, referred no one during the study period, the practice that had the most direct contact with CPNs referred most, with the aligned practice falling between these two in both the amount of contact with CPNs and the number of referrals made. The GPs said that knowing the person they were referring patients to influenced their likelihood of referral. Another aspect to this was that having a CPN in the team increased the ease of access to the service.

The question of cost-effectiveness is obviously one that interests the managers of health care services. We raised this question earlier in the context of whether there would be enough work to justify having an attached CPN or whether the aligned CPN is the best model. The number of referrals made to a CPN is a crude measure of the amount of need for a CPN in a general practice. The placement of a CPN can have many hidden benefits that indirectly lead to savings. For example the health visitor in the attached CPN practice said that the presence of the CPN in the practice increased her awareness of mental health and as a consequence she referred clients at an earlier stage than was her usual practice. Other savings relate to diverting patients away from more expensive treatments i.e. referral to out-patients and the need for admission into hospital. At the time of writing the results of this part of the study are still being processed, and are therefore not available for comment on. As regards the patients referred to the attached CPN, GPs reported viewing the CPN as an alternative to medication, this is reflected in the high percentage of patients who were referred to the CPN but were not on medication. On closer analysis of the results the practices that received the attached CPN were found to account for the bulk of patients not on drugs (88%, $n=48$). It might be the case that the more contact a practice has with a CPN, the more the CPN is perceived to be a real alternative to drugs.

Prescribing behaviour of the GPs

In order to assess whether CPNs had any effect on the prescribing behaviour of the GPs, we sought the consent of the GPs in the study for access to their personal prescribing data held by the Prescription Pricing Authority (PPA). All of the GPs except for one (who was in the comparison practice) gave their consent, and this enabled us to analyse their psychotropic prescribing by numbers of tablets of individual drugs for the two years of the study.

Our analysis was complicated by the fact that during the second year of the study the PPA changed from issuing monthly print-outs to quarterly print-outs as part of the change to the PACT (prescribing analyses and cost) information system. Fortunately, the quarterly analyses coincided with the termination date of our study. Electronic transfer of data was not possible so that data from the print-outs was laboriously coded and entered on the University of Newcastle main frame computer, and a program was designed which gave the total number of tablets prescribed by each doctor for the following British National Formulary (BNF) categories: hypnotics and anxiolytics, drugs used in psychoses and related disorders, antidepressants, central nervous system stimulants, appetite suppressants and drugs used in nausea and vertigo. The last group was used because it was felt that CPNs would be unlikely to have any effect on the prescribing of these drugs and they could therefore be used as a control group.

For this preliminary analysis of our results we have chosen to look at the three most commonly prescribed hypnotics, tranquillizers and antidepressants, on the basis that these are the three groups on which CPNs are most likely to have an influence. The results in Tables 7.5, 7.6 and 7.7 show that the prescribing of tranquillizers has declined over the two years of the study in all practices (except for Diazepam 2 mg which increased in the aligned practices). The change in the prescribing of hypnotics is very variable, in the attached practice there has been a decline apart from Temazepam 10 mg which has increased. The aligned practices show an increase for Temazepam 20 mg, while the comparison practice shows an increase in the mean number of tablets prescribed per doctor for both Nitrazepam 5 mg and Temazepam 10 mg. Antidepressant prescribing has risen by a proportionately similar amount in all three groups of practices.

As the period of study is a relatively short one, it is impossible to argue that any of these changes are due to the presence of a CPN. It is perhaps more likely that the most consistent result which is the overall increase in antidepressant prescribing is due to the fairly widespread communication of recent research findings about failure to diagnose depression by GPs (Freeling *et al.*, 1985).

The major finding that arises from these results is the wide range of prescribing between individual GPs. There is a sixteen-fold difference between the highest and lowest prescribers of Temazepam 20 mg. In the pre-intervention year, a twelve-fold difference in prescribing of Lorazepam 1 mg and a five-fold difference in prescribing of both Amitriptyline 25 mg and Dothiepin 25 mg.

Interestingly, the largest range is always within the aligned group of three separate practices, the comparison practice and the practice with an attached CPN having a much smaller range which suggests that there may be a practice style or consensus that influences an individual doctor's prescribing habits, as the GPs in the attached and comparison practices all work in one of two large group practices. The data also poses two other questions that have important implications for the distribution of CPNs in primary care settings and that would require further study.

1.   Do patients chose particular doctors to confide in and what is it about the attitudes, behaviour and consulting styles of these doctors that leads to this outcome?
2.   Is it possible to identify the diagnostic and treatment criteria which GPs use and to explore how these criteria match objective standards of psychiatric morbidity?

If the high prescribers are identifying appropriate cases but have little time to explore treatment options other than drugs, then they may benefit from community psychiatric nursing support. Conversely, if the low prescribers are failing to identify psychiatric morbidity within their population then there may be a need for an alternative pathway to psychiatric care. It is, however, just as possible that the high prescribers are inappropriately labelling and treating transient distress and social morbidity, and in this case a more direct educational initiative may be the best strategy for both

Table 7.5 Changes in three most commonly prescribed hypnotics, tranquillizers and antidepressants in the the practice with attached CPN for the pre-intervention and intervention year

Drug	Total no. of tablets		Mean no. of tablets per doctor		Range of tablets per doctor	
	Pre-intervention year	Intervention year	Pre-intervention year	Intervention year	Pre-intervention year	Intervention year
Hypnotics						
Nitrazepam 5 mg	32 270	29 575	6 454	5 915	3 138– 9 388	4 093– 7 669
Temazepam 10 mg	34 308	36 697	6 862	7 339	4 388–12 429	5 247– 9 472
Temazepam 20 mg	47 567	42 538	9 513	8 508	7 146–11 470	5 355–11 379
Tranquillizers						
Diazepam 2 mg	39 984	38 342	7 997	7 668	4 908–10 338	4 070–11 390
Diazepam 5 mg	38 648	33 751	7 730	6 750	4 817–12 167	4 504– 9 920
Lorazepam 1 mg	14 615	9 577	2 923	1 915	1 617– 3 740	1 135– 2 758
Antidepressants						
Amitriptyline 25 mg	15 892	20 216	3 178	4 043	2 296– 3 638	2 048– 7 383
Dothiepin 25 mg	21 103	23 373	4 221	4 675	2 883– 5 901	2 947– 6 175
Dothiepin 75 mg	23 577	18 659	4 715	3 732	2 283– 7 034	1 981– 6 194

Table 7.6 Changes in three most commonly prescribed hypnotics, tranquillizers and antidepressants in the practice with aligned CPN for the pre-intervention and intervention year

Drug	Total no. of tablets		Mean no. of tablets per doctor		Range of tablets per doctor	
	Pre-intervention year	Intervention year	Pre-intervention year	Intervention year	Pre-intervention year	Intervention year
Hypnotics						
Nitrazepam 5 mg	49 915	45 852	7 131	6 550	2 956–17 068	3 702–13 679
Temazepam 10 mg	45 820	44 041	6 546	6 292	1 726–15 158	2 902–11 908
Temazepam 20 mg	45 104	50 988	6 443	7 284	850–13 966	1 375–17 703
Tranquillizers						
Diazepam 2 mg	50 251	59 308	7 179	8 473	3 751–14 226	2 372–13 599
Diazepam 5 mg	34 404	30 146	4 915	4 307	1 699– 7 080	1 785– 8 329
Lorazepam 1 mg	12 219	9 804	1 746	1 401	480– 5 850	318– 3 954
Antidepressants						
Amitriptyline 25 mg	22 073	26 167	3 153	3 738	1 060– 5 616	1 080– 5 853
Dothiepin 25 mg	26 805	38 559	3 829	5 508	1 230– 6 870	2 041– 9 343
Dothiepin 75 mg	11 303	14 150	1 615	2 021	1 184– 2 239	943– 3 164

Table 7.7 Changes in three most commonly prescribed hypnotics, tranquillizers and antidepressants in the comparison practice for the pre-intervention and intervention year

Drug	Total no. of tablets		Mean no. of tablets per doctor		Range of tablets per doctor	
	Pre-intervention year	Intervention year*	Pre-intervention year	Intervention year	Pre-intervention year	Intervention year
Hypnotics						
Nitrazepam 5 mg	20 707	18 106	6 902	8 047	5 271–10 032	2 244– 7 849
Temazepam 10 mg	19 914	17 987	6 638	7 994	4 552– 8 129	6 529–10 410
Temazepam 20 mg	12 233	9 118	4 078	4 052	2 407– 5 325	2 880– 5 550
Tranquillizers						
Diazepam 2 mg	23 249	14 775	7 750	6 567	5 440–10 733	5 981– 7 847
Diazepam 5 mg	10 158	6 761	3 386	3 005	2 655– 5 793	1 861– 4 268
Lorazepam 1 mg	7 091	3 966	2 364	1 763	1 766– 3 148	1 496– 2 414
Antidepressants						
Amitriptyline 25 mg	13 940	12 361	4 647	5 494	3 930– 6 236	4 433– 6 494
Dothiepin 25 mg	14 084	15 672	4 695	6 965	2 998– 5 572	1 686– 6 670
Dothiepin 75 mg	7 585	8 154	2 528	3 624	2 196– 2 854	3 540– 3 768

*In this four-person group, one doctor refused access to prescribing data, so the total number of tablets reflects the prescribing of only three doctors. The number of tablets for the intervention year is lower because one of the doctors died early in this year and the mean has therefore been derived by dividing by 2.25.

groups. Without more detailed information about the individual doctor–patient contact and about the psychiatric morbidity within the populations they serve, it is not possible to answer any of these important questions.

PATIENT VIEWS OF THE COMMUNITY PSYCHIATRIC NURSING SERVICE

A survey of the views of users of our health services is thought to be an important element of the evaluation process, particularly when those services are undergoing change or experimentation as in this case (Paykel and Griffith, 1983). In order to compare the community psychiatric nursing service with that provided by out-patient clinics we carried out a small pilot survey of new referrals from GPs to the out-patient department at Newcastle General Hospital. Patients were identified by the receptionist at the out-patient clinic, and handed out self-completion questionnaires together with an explanatory letter. The patients were asked questions about the length of time they had waited to be seen and whether they would have preferred to have been seen in the community. Unfortunately, few new referrals were made during the time period set for carrying out this part of the study, together with this was the added complication of relying on a receptionist to identify the patients, hand out and collect in the questionnaires. During the six months of data collection only 18 questionnaires were completed and returned. This is a small and not necessarily representative sample, and unfortunately the same problems apply to the survey of CPN clients.

Over the 12-month period, the CPNs in this study saw a total of 81 clients, 62 by an attached CPN and 19 by an aligned CPN. Of these 81 clients, 69 were sent a postal questionnaire, the remaining 12 were not contacted for various reasons such as one patient died and one GP requested that a client was not sent a questionnaire as the client's family did not know about the CPN contact.

All of the remaining 69 clients were sent a postal questionnaire with an explanatory letter signed by their GP and a return envelope. Confidentiality of responses was stressed and no names were required in order to facilitate expression of both positive and negative views of the service received. This produced an initial response of 27% ($n=19$) which was increased to 45% ($n=31$) by sending out the questionnaire a second time. Of the questionnaires not completed, 10% ($n=7$) were returned unopened with no forwarding address. This latter figure is not surprising given the mobility of the population in this area which is approximately one third higher than the city average (Newcastle upon Tyne City Council, 1986). The results therefore relate to these 31 respondents.

As only 16% ($n=3$) of the aligned group completed the questionnaire against 50% (*n*=28) of the attached group it is not possible to make distinctions between these two types of service. It may be the case that the patients who were in the aligned practice were less satisfied with the service received given that greater difficulties have been reported with respect to the collection of information that reflects dissatisfaction with health services (Larsen *et al.*, 1979).

The questions asked fell into three sections. Firstly, those relating to the logistics of seeing a CPN such as how long they waited for an appointment, where and how often they were seen. Secondly, questions relating to the help given by the CPN, and finally, questions regarding overall satisfaction with the service.

Of the 31 respondents, 97% (*n*=30) had been referred by their GPs, the remaining client did not know who had made the referral. Eighty-four per cent (*n*=26) of respondents were seen within 14 days of being referred and of these 45% (*n*=14) were seen within seven days. Ninety per cent (*n*=28) expressed satisfaction with the speed of receiving a first appointment. On further examination 26% (*n*=8) said that the longer wait was acceptable and in fact they had expected it to be longer. It may be reasonable to assume that some clients were making comparisons with other health services (although only two respondents made this explicit). For example patients from the out-patients survey reported waiting twice as long (89%, 16/18 reported waiting 16 days or longer). Sixteen per cent (*n*=5) said they would have preferred to have been seen sooner, with one client commenting that the wait contributed to their anxiety. The question arises as to why CPNs can see clients quickly. Primary care is a demand-led service where rapid response rate is important, there are also fewer barriers between client and service than hospital based services and therefore perhaps more pressure to deal with the client's perceived needs.

Recent debate focuses on the optimum location of the CPN (McFadyen, 1985; Skidmore, 1986). Included in this issue should be the effect of the place in which the client is seen. In this survey 81% (*n*=25) of respondents saw the CPN in the surgery, with 16% (*n*=5) being seen at home and 3% (*n*=1) in a health clinic. Although only 16% (*n*=5) said they had been given a choice of where they could be seen, the number of clients who expressed satisfaction with the venue was very high at 84% (*n*=26). The most common reasons given for this were to do with convenience and familiarity of the location (32%, *n*=10), Oyebode *et al.* (1988) also report on the importance clients placed on being seen in familiar surroundings. Some respondents compared being seen in the surgery with going to hospital out-patient clinics and thus it is likely that there may be a number of clients who, although expressing satisfaction with being seen in the surgery, would have preferred to have been seen at home. The value placed by clients on domiciliary visits has been reported elsewhere (Paykel and

Griffiths, 1983). One person, however, stated that they were seen in the best place for them and another suggested that being seen in the surgery was therapeutic in that it motivated them to get out of the house. Despite the high reported levels of satisfaction here, there remain negative aspects of being seen in a surgery. Thirteen per cent ($n=4$) of respondents said they thought the situation in the surgery felt uncomfortable for reasons of formality and because the room available to the CPN was so small. It is of interest to report that 61% (11/18) of patients who responded to the out-patient survey, reported that given the choice they would have preferred to have been in the community rather than at hospital. The responses given were very similar to those reported by the CPN clients, for example feeling more at ease in familiar surroundings.

Clients were asked if, before being seen, they had any idea about what a CPN does. Seventy-seven per cent ($n=24$) reported that they did not know and only 19% ($n=6$) reported that they did. This draws to our attention the fact that new clients will probably be unaware of the role of the CPN, as CPNs, unlike social workers for example, do not receive much publicity. This lack of knowledge about CPNs may be an important factor associated with non-attendance by new referrals.

At the follow-up meeting with some of the GPs, they were asked how they introduced the idea of CPN referral to the client. It was quite clear from the responses that both GPs and other members of the practice avoided mentioning the word 'psychiatric' when discussing the CPN. Instead the CPN was introduced as 'a member of our team' or 'somebody in the practice'. The GPs stated they did not think that they had used the term community psychiatric nurse and although it was not a deliberate decision, all agreed that there was some stigma in the label 'psychiatric'. Similarly, Oyebode *et al.* (1988) quoted from patients who in their survey reported that they were not informed they were seeing a psychiatric nurse. From this one can start to understand why so few patients knew what a CPN did.

Clients were asked whether or not the CPN had helped them to under-stand their problems. Seventy-four per cent ($n=23$) reported that the CPN had helped, while 23% ($n=7$) reported that they had not. Of those who answered yes, 35% ($n=11$) commented that the CPN had explained their problems to them and they found this helpful and a further 19% ($n=6$) stated they had found the counselling helpful. It was noted that the clients who reported the help as not useful, offered explanations that were either unclear or vague. Again, this perhaps reflects a general reluctance to complain about health services (Godine, Pearce and Wilson, 1987). It is important however, to know about weaknesses as well as strengths and, as Paykel and Griffith report (1983), CPNs as well as psychiatrists could do better with respect to the amount and quality of information given to clients regarding their problems. One person implied that their under-standing of the problem remained different to that of the CPN, and another described how help in this area did not go far enough.

A question asking if the CPN provided the help they wanted produced similar results with 77% ($n=24$) saying yes and 19% ($n=6$) saying no. When asked about the help they received 84% ($n=26$) expressed satisfac-tion. Twenty-seven per cent ($n=7$) said the reason for this was that they felt the CPN understood their problem, with a further 27% ($n=7$) suggesting that the CPN had helped them to change or see things differ-ently. Of the few who gave reasons for dissatisfaction one suggested that there had been no change in their condition since seeing the CPN.

The final section of the survey attempted to rate overall satisfaction with the service received. Clients were asked whether, if they needed help in the future, they would like to be seen by a CPN again. Eighty-four per cent ($n=26$) responded positively, whilst 13% ($n=4$) responded negatively. When asked whether they would recommend seeing a CPN to a friend with similar problems, the same individuals answered in the same way. Similarly, on general satisfaction with the services, 84% ($n=26$) expressed satisfac-tion and 13% ($n=4$) expressed dissatisfaction. From these results it seems that clients generalize their experience of the service received in such a way as to influence possible use of the service in future.

When the criterion 'satisfaction' was broken down to examine specific aspects of the service the client was satisfied or dissatisfied with, 29% ($n=9$) described having someone to talk to or listen to them as being the most important element of the service. A further 16% ($n=5$) described the understanding or caring nature of the CPN as valuable and 13% ($n=4$) said that they were satisfied with everything. Thirty-two per cent ($n=10$) reported other elements that had given them satisfaction, which included being referred to a group, a relaxation tape and explanation of problems.

As may be expected, clients were less forthcoming about the parts of the service with which they were most dissatisfied and 77% ($n=24$) stated none or left this section blank. Ten per cent ($n=3$) said that they were disappointed at ending their sessions with the CPN, and one respondent stated that it did not go on long enough to solve their problems. Another respondent cited the lack of facilities in the surgery as an element of dissatisfaction and another described lack of encouragement and feedback from the CPN.

CONCLUSIONS

This is a preliminary report of a pilot study in which the collection and collation of data is not yet complete. The main reason for delay has been the difficulty in linking GPs names with out-patient and in-patient data.

Hopefully improved information systems will help to solve this problem for future researchers, but at present we are not able to make any comments on whether attached or aligned CPNs make any difference to the frequency of referrals to psychiatric out-patient clinics or to the frequency of admissions to psychiatric units.

As far as psychotropic medication is concerned there is little evidence that CPNs had any influence during the one year of the study on the wide range of prescribing. This wide range raises the interesting question of whether prescribing directly reflects psychiatric morbidity or whether it is entirely idiosyncratic. If high or low prescribing could be shown to have a direct relationship with morbidity measured against objective standards then this could prove a relatively simple way of deciding which practices in an area were most in need of community psychiatric nursing or other psychiatric support services. Both the GPs and the patients in the study valued having a CPN in the practice. The difference in the number of referrals between the attached, the aligned and the comparison practices strongly suggest that a high number of referrals correlates with an increased amount of interaction between the CPN and the practice. We are unable to say how these referrals would have been dealt with if access to a CPN had not been available and neither do we know whether these cases represent previously unreferred and possibly mild psychiatric morbidity or whether they represent severe morbidity referred at an earlier stage of presentation than would otherwise have been the case for a referral to consultant psychiatric care.

The fact that 54% of the patients referred to a CPN had not been prescribed psychotropic medication and that most cases were referred for counselling, assessment and anxiety management suggest that a number of referrals were cases which would previously have been dealt with by the GP. There is therefore an element of supply of the service (a CPN) creating the demand, a point explicitly made by one of the GPs in the attached group who stated that if they did not have an attached CPN they would 'simply put the lid back on the pot'. Whether or not this group represents psychiatric morbidity in terms of 'caseness', they may still suffer considerable emotional distress and be an important part of the GPs' work-load, and it is encouraging to see that the majority of patients (77%) who replied to the questionnaire felt that they had benefited from the service provided.

Apart from questions about the categorization of the referrals, the increased number of referrals from the attached practice has important implications for the provision of community mental health services which can either be provided through community mental health centres or by increased support to existing primary health care teams based on general practices. As a recent report, *Mental Health in Primary Care* (Good Practices in Mental Health, 1989), points out the general practice model which is based on specialists working in practices, builds on an existing network that is highly accessible, socially acceptable and currently deals with 90% of all mental health problems. It also has the important advantage of providing a direct link between general medical care and mental health care.

The results of this study, although it did not directly compare these two models would seem to suggest the general practice model is more favourable, if we assume that the higher level of referrals to the attached CPN reflects a more effective collaborative relationship. This, however, was only achieved because the CPN became a member of the primary health care team rather than remaining, like the aligned CPNs, part of a team at the Mental Health Unit.

Professional isolation was not a problem for the attached CPN because of the support provided by the research team. But if the model was to be generally applied then there would need to be effective administrative and professional mechanisms to prevent isolation. Consideration would also need to be given to the amount of time a CPN needed to devote to a practice in order to develop an effective collaborative relationship, as seven sessions per week to a population of 10000 may not be cost-effective. A more viable model may be an initial intensive involvement followed by a more limited but continuing commitment. A feedback meeting with the attached practice suggested that continuity with the same named individual was very important and that the change in the attached CPN after four months had been disruptive.

Future research

This study is a pilot and as such was aimed at identifying further areas of study. Community mental health care is an increasingly important issue and if resources are going to be effectively invested there is a need to directly compare the community mental health centre and the general practice models. This should be done over at least three years and should look more directly at what influences a GP in their decision to provide care themselves or to refer to a CPN or a consultant psychiatrist, as at present this is not at all clear. It is hoped that this would also shed some light on the meaning of the wide range of psychotropic prescribing by GPs.

There would also need to be more formal categorization of the patients seen by different agencies and more objective assessment of the effectiveness of any interventions. Finally, there would need to be some measure of whether an effective collaborative relationship resulting in attitudinal and behavioural change in both primary health care and mental health care professionals had developed.

ACKNOWLEDGEMENTS

The work reported here was funded by the Newcastle District Research Committee and the Mental Health Unit. We owe an immense debt to the cooperating GPs, CPNs and the patients. We would also like to acknowledge John Kennedy, Lecturer in the Department of Social Policy at Newcastle University for his help with computer programming.

REFERENCES

Bond, J. and Cartlidge, A.M. (1986) *Collaboration among professionals in the delivery of primary health care*, Report 30, University of Newcastle Health Care Research Unit, Newcastle upon Tyne.

Bordman, A. (1987) The general health questionnaire and the detection of emotional disorder by general practitioners. *British Journal of Psychiatry*, **151**, 373–381.

Brooker, C.G. (1987) An investigation into the factors influencing variation in the growth of community psychiatric nursing services. *Journal of Advanced Nursing*, **12**, 367–375.

Brooker, C.G. and Simmons, S.M. (1985) A study to compare two models of community psychiatric nursing care delivery. *Journal of Advanced Nursing*, **10**, 217–223.

Cambell, D.T. and Stanley, J.C. (1963) *Experimental and quasi-experimental designs for research*, Houghton Mifflin, Boston.

Carpenter, P.J., Morrow, G.R., Del Gaudio, A.C. and Ritzler, B.A. (1981) Who keeps the first out-patient appointment? *American Journal of Psychiatry*, **138**, 102–105.

Cartwright, A. (1983) *Health surveys in practice and in potential*, King Edwards Hospital Fund, London.

Cooper, B. (1972) Clinical and social aspects of chronic neurosis. *Proceeding of the Royal Society of Medicine*, **65**, 509–512.

Dingwall, R. (1974) Some sociological aspects of nursing research. *Sociological Review*, **22**, 1.

Freeling, P., Rao, B.M., Paykel, E.S., Sireling, L.I., Burton, R.H. (1985) Unrecognised depression in general practice. *British Medical Journal*, **290**, 1880–1883.

Good Practices in Mental Health, (1989) *Mental Health in Primary Care – A New Perspective*, London.

Godine, P., Pearce, I. and Wilson, I. (1987) Keeping the Customer Satisfied, *Nursing Times*, **83** (38), 35–37.

Hunter, P., (1974) Community psychiatric nursing in Britain: an historical review. *International Journal of Nursing Studies*, **11**, 223–233.

Huntingdon, J., (1981) *Social Work and General Medical Practice: Collaboration or Conflict*, Allen and Unwin, London.

HMSO (1968) *Report of the Committee on Local Authority and Allied Personal Social Services*, (Chairman F. Seebohm). Cmnd 3703, HMSO, London.

Larsen, D.L., Attkisson, C.C., Hargreaves, W.A. and Nguyen, T.D. (1979) Assessment of client/patient satisfaction: development of a general scale, *Evaluation and Program Planning*, **2**, 197–207.

Mangen, S.P., Paykel, E.S., Griffith, J.H. Birchell, A. and Mancini, P. (1983) Cost-effectiveness of community psychiatric nurse or out-patient psychiatrist care of neurotic patients. *Psychological Medicine*, **33**, 407–416.

Marks, J., Goldberg, D. and Hillier, V. (1979) Determinants of the ability of general practitioners to detect psychiatric illness. *Psychological Medicine*, **9**, 337–353.

Martin, F.M. (1984) *Between the Acts: Community Mental Health Services 1959–1983*. Nuffield Provincial Hospitals Trust, London.

Martin, J.P. (1984) *Hospitals in Trouble*, Blackwell Scientific, Oxford.

May, A.R. and Moore, S. (1963) The mental nurse in the community. *The Lancet*, **i**, 213–214.

McFadyen, J. (1985) Primary health care attachment *vs.* hospital attachment and generic prevention. *CPN Journal*, **5** (3), 31–37.

Newcastle upon Tyne City Council (1986) *City Profiles*, Results from the 1986 Household Survey, Policy Services Department, Newcastle upon Tyne City Council.

Oyebode, F., Gadd, E., Berry, D., Lynes, M. and Lashley, P. (1988) Community psychiatric nurses in primary care: consumer survey. *Psychological Bulletin*, **12** (11), 483–485.

Paykel, E.S. and Griffith, J.H. (1983) *Community Psychiatric Nursing for Neurotic Patients*, The Royal College of Nursing, London.

Paykel, E.S., Mangen, S.P., Griffith, J.H. and Burns, T.P. (1982) Community psychiatric nursing for neurotic patients: a controlled trial. *British Journal of Psychiatry*, **140**, 573–581.

Shepherd, M. and Clare, A. (1981) *Psychiatric Illness in General Practice*, Oxford University Press, Oxford.

Skidmore, D. (1986) The effectiveness of community psychiatric nursing teams and base-locations, in Brooking, J. (ed.) *Psychiatric Nursing Research*, John Wiley, New York.

Skidmore, D. and Friend, W. (1985) Should CPNs be in the primary health care team? *Nursing Times*, **9**, 310–312.

Strathdee, G. and Williams (1986) Patterns of collaboration, in Shepherd, G., Wilkinson, G. and Williams, P. (eds) *Mental Illness in Primary Care Settings*, Tavistock, London.

White, E. (1986) Factors influencing general practitioners to refer patients to community psychiatric nurses, in Brooking, J. (ed.) *Psychiatric Nursing Research*, John Wiley, New York.

Wilkin, D. and Smith, A.G. (1987) Variation in general practitioners' referral rates to consultants. *Journal of the Royal College of General Practitioners*, **37**, 350–353.

Wilkin, D., Hallam, L., Leavey, R. and Metcalfe, D. (1987) *Anatomy of Urban General Practice*, Tavistock, London.

Wooff, K., Freeman, H.L. and Fryers, T. (1983) Psychiatric service use in Salford. *British Journal of Psychiatry*, **142**, 588–597.

Wooff, K., Goldberg, D.P. and Fryers, T. (1986) Patients in receipt of community psychiatric nursing care in Salford 1976–82. *Psychological Medicine*, 407–414.

Wooff, K., Goldberg, D.P. and Fryers, T. (1988) The practice of community psychiatric nursing and mental health social work in Salford. *British Journal of Psychiatry*, **152**, 783–792.

CHAPTER EIGHT

Out-of-hours work by CPNs

Helen Lee

SUMMARY

The focus of this study is on the out-of-hours work carried out by a group of community psychiatric nurses (CPNs) working in the English Midlands. In order to place this in context, emergency psychiatric services in the UK are described, as are crisis intervention theory and practice. Finally, a description of the community psychiatric nursing service concerned is given, along with an account of the local factors which led to the study being undertaken.

BACKGROUND

Emergency psychiatric services in the UK

Health problems can arise at any time of the day or night, yet most health services are geared to provide the majority of their care during normal working hours. Clearly, there will be times when treatment for a health problem cannot wait and, in recognition of this, various arrangements have to be made for emergency care. Cooper (1979) describes the emergency cover provided by the UK health service with particular reference to emergency psychiatric care.

In the UK, virtually all individuals are registered with a general practitioner (GP), who should be the first point of contact for any type of medical problem. GPs are obliged to provide an emergency service during the daytime and also to provide emergency cover for their patients when they are off-duty at night and at weekends. Most GPs have an internal arrangement within their own partnership or group practice so that they can take it in turn to provide such cover (Anon., 1984). Alternatively, a deputizing service may be used, where the GP pays a privately financed organization to provide emergency medical cover (Bollam, McCarthy and Modell, 1988).

174

GPs can call out hospital consultants to see a patient at home urgently, if they need specialist advice. In most districts, consultant psychiatrists take part in a 24-hour rota so that a domiciliary visit can be carried out within a day, if not sooner (Cooper, 1979). Cooper describes how most consultant psychiatrists develop a close relationship with their local GPs and will offer urgent advice to them over the telephone. Many also agree to see patients at a few days or occasionally a few hours notice in an out-patient clinic, and will arrange an immediate admission if necessary.

In addition to the emergency provisions outlined above, each district general hospital has a casualty/accident and emergency department. Usually, a patient attending the casualty department is expected to have a referral letter from a GP but self-referrals are accepted where the problem is very urgent. Arrangements exist for a person presenting with an acute psychiatric problem to be seen by an on-call psychiatrist.

The success of this system of emergency care depends both upon the patient being registered with a GP and easy access, particularly outside normal surgery hours. It is therefore encouraging that over 95% of the UK population are registered with a GP (Fry, Brooks and McColl, 1984). The findings of two large surveys (Ritchie, Jacoby and Bone, 1981; Consumers' Association, 1987) are that the majority of people have satisfactory access to their GP outside normal working hours. However, these statistics may disguise a much bleaker picture for the mentally ill. Anecdotal evidence from community workers dealing with both the mentally ill and the homeless, suggests that a higher proportion of these groups are not registered with a GP and that many have particular difficulties in calling for help out of hours. For whatever reason, in spite of a seemingly comprehensive system of emergency psychiatric care, there appears to be a growing belief amongst mental health workers that an emergency psychiatric service of a different nature is required.

Crisis intervention

In recent years, the general public have begun to demand urgent help at times of emotional stress and illness and to feel that medical, psychiatric and social services are not meeting this need adequately. One possible response to this demand would be to try to improve existing services. However, an increasing number of mental health professionals and planners believe a different solution is required and are calling for the provision of crisis intervention teams (Szmukler, 1987).

Crisis intervention work developed in the USA during the 1960s when there was widespread growth of community mental health centres. The centres developed in response to an awareness of a huge gap in services for the mentally ill. Previously the only choice was between treatment in one of

the large state mental hospitals and privately financed individual psychotherapy. Cooper (1979) describes how mental health workers attached to
the community centres were faced with patients who wanted immediate
and practical help. The mental health workers' training in analytically
oriented psychotherapy left them ill equipped to deal with such problems
and many found that crisis theory and practice had more to offer. Crisis
intervention did not really take off in Europe until the early 1970s and this
may be because, in contrast to the USA, many European countries had
comprehensive medical and psychiatric services which were readily available to the public.

Caplan (1964) is widely acknowledged as the person who drew together
ideas concerning community health care and the management of acute
stress, to develop what has become known as crisis theory. Briefly, he
defined a crisis as a novel situation which an individual is unable to handle
with his existing coping and defence mechanisms. Caplan proposed that
crises present the individual with both the opportunity for personality
growth and the danger of increased vulnerability to mental disorder. In
Caplan's view there is a possibility of stress and trauma ultimately proving
helpful to the individual, because those who succeed in mastering a
distressing experience can be strengthened and become better able to deal
effectively with future difficulties. Thus, a crisis is seen as a turning point,
either toward or away from mental disorder. Caplan suggested that during
a crisis an individual experiences a heightened desire for help and is also
more susceptible to influence by others, thus providing:

> Care-giving persons with a remarkable opportunity to deploy their
> efforts to maximum advantage in influencing the mental health of others.

Crisis theory has become the basis for a collection of diverse activities
called 'crisis intervention' or 'crisis practice'. Szmukler (1987) summarizes
these as: stressing the importance of immediate aid; defining the presenting
problem as a crisis and paying special attention to the immediate pre-
cipitating factor(s); focusing the intervention on the here and now; using a
therapeutic style which is active and often directive in order to support the
client and help them develop problem-solving techniques; and providing
intensive but time-limited intervention using pharmacological means as an
adjunct where appropriate.

Cooper (1979) conducted a study for the World Health Organization, of
15 European crisis admission units and emergency psychiatric services, and
identified some of the problems which have arisen in the application of
crisis theory. The stereotypical patient implied in Caplan's theory is a
previously well adjusted individual, who needs constructive help during a
severe crisis. The staff of most of the units which Cooper visited expressed
disappointment that few patients they saw fitted this stereotype. Despite

this, most workers continued to follow the principles of crisis practice outlined above. Cooper also reported that the staff members were a highly select group who appeared particularly able to tolerate the unusual stresses of crisis work. On the basis of this study it would appear that the theoretical basis for crisis work may be seriously challenged in practice.

Confusingly, the term 'crisis intervention' is used in two ways. It is used precisely to describe the work carried out by a specialist, professional, multidisciplinary team, who base their intervention on the principles of crisis theory and practice. The term is also used more loosely, to describe the work carried out by community-oriented psychiatric services. Thus, CPNs can be described as being involved in crisis intervention work either because they are members of a crisis intervention team (at most, 4% of all CPNs, according to the 1985 Community Psychiatric Nurses' Association's national survey), or because all mental health workers are, in the loose sense, involved in crisis intervention work. Whilst CPNs belonging to the former group could be expected to have a sound understanding of crisis theory and crisis practice, it is likely that many in the latter group do not.

Caplan (1964) repeatedly stressed that crisis intervention should only be one part of a comprehensive network of services for those with a mental illness; and Szmukler (1987) argues that the narrow model of crisis theory cannot be applied across the board in emergency psychiatry. Nevertheless, many mental health workers continue to believe that the increasing demand made by the general public for urgent help, at times of acute stress and illness, would best be met by establishing more crisis intervention teams.

An alternative approach is currently being investigated at the Maudsley Hospital in London (Marks, Connolly and Muijen, 1988), where an attempt is being made to replicate controlled studies from the USA and Australia (Stein and Test, 1980; Fenton *et al.*, 1982; Hoult, Rosen and Reynolds, 1984). These studies have shown that people with serious mental illness (SMI), such as schizophrenia, or severe affective disorder, can be treated effectively with a package of community based care which combines problem-oriented crisis intervention with ongoing aid throughout illness. In the Maudsley study, a group of 200 people with SMI, judged by a psychiatrist to require immediate admission, are being randomly assigned to either standard in-patient care or to the 'daily living programme' (DLP). The DLP provides a comprehensive service including 24-hour access for crisis resolution (at home, work or elsewhere if necessary), out-patient clinics, some long- and short-term in-patient facilities, day care, and specialized living and work aids. Continuing support is given to the patients, to their families and to all those who have regular contact with them. Programmes are individually tailored to meet each patient's particular needs, and determined follow-up is undertaken to prevent relapse.

The project staff comprises of eight nurses, a social worker and a training psychiatrist. The authors have devised a multidisciplinary training course in DLP for mental health care providers and hope to produce guidelines about how to train staff in such care. If the results of previous studies are replicated, then, compared with standard in-patient care, treatment based mainly outside hospital will yield similar or superior outcomes on various measures. This would have far-reaching implications for the training and practice of all those involved in community psychiatric care.

Out-of-hours work by CPNs

Most community psychiatric nursing services in the UK provide the bulk of their care between the hours of 9.00a.m.–5.00p.m. More recently, there has been a move towards working outside of these hours. Nurses employed by the National Health Service (NHS) are paid at a higher rate after a certain time in the evening and at weekends and therefore out-of-hours work is more expensive.

Parnell (1978) carried out an extensive survey of community psychiatric nursing services in 1975 and found that few services were available at weekends and few had nurses working on call. By 1985, when the CPNA conducted a national survey, the picture had changed, with nearly half of the community psychiatric nursing services providing some kind of out-of-hours service (CPNA, 1985). The type of service offered was found to vary. For some, out-of-hours cover was provided on an *ad hoc* basis and was determined by individual client need. A number had one CPN working a rota which provided daytime cover at the weekend. Other services provided an on-call service, which ranged from being evenings only, to a full 24-hour, seven-day-a-week service. Unpublished data from this survey showed that approximately one third provided some kind of weekday evening cover and about half provided a weekend daytime service (Purnell, 1988, personal communication). Some of the out-of-hours work was of a planned nature, for example providing evening or weekend appointments for clients who presumably were working during office hours. However, it would appear that most out-of-hours services were organized to deal with emergency or crisis calls only.

Little other published information about out-of-hours work by CPNs is available, apart from a survey of weekend working by nurses in the North and West Region (McKendrick, 1984). This work is highly relevant to the present study and will be described in some detail.

McKendrick, a nurse manager of an expanding team of CPNs, questioned whether they ought to extend the hours they worked. He was concerned to provide both an optimum service and one that used resources economically, and was anxious that any extension in service should complement rather than replace existing emergency provision. In order to help him reach his decision he undertook a survey of 20 community psychiatric nursing services. Of these, he found that seven (35%) provided a weekend service. Six had a CPN working at the weekend on a rota basis, taking days off during the week, whilst one had a nurse on call working overtime. Five of the seven services undertook planned visits as well as providing emergency cover. Those providing emergency cover were asked for details of all CPN visits undertaken during a particular month. It was found that only 4.6% of 3632 visits were carried out at the weekend, and most of these were described as being of a routine nature. McKendrick concluded that undertaking routine weekend visits is an expensive means of providing community psychiatric care and one which may detract from the weekday service. He also thought that the case for CPNs working at the weekend had not been clearly demonstrated and suggested that:

> On call or unit based emergency teams may prove a better alternative to routine weekend cover, releasing resources for a more intensive weekday service, and providing a multi-disciplinary resource better able to give a true emergency service.

McKendrick clearly saw little point in paying CPNs extra money to work at the weekend in order to undertake routine work that, presumably, could wait for a weekday. He also suggested that a crisis intervention team may be a more appropriate way of dealing with emergencies at the weekend. Given the small number of emergency calls implied by his data, it might be difficult to justify the cost of such a service.

Community psychiatric nursing in the study area

At the time of the study, many of the CPNs were working within teams which provided a 'specialist' service such as rehabilitation, or care of the elderly mentally ill. Approximately half worked 'generically', within one of six sector teams, each of which provided a general acute psychiatric service to a geographical area. The study is concerned with out-of-hours work undertaken by these sector team community psychiatric nurses. The area had a resident population of over 600000 and the majority of these lived in a city or its immediate vicinity.

In line with Government policy, there was a strong commitment within the local psychiatric service to provide care in the community in, or near to, the individual's home. The development of sector teams over the previous few years, had been part of an attempt to make the service more community oriented.

Sector team personnel included psychiatrists, a clinical nurse manager, day hospital and ward nursing staff, CPNs, social workers, secretarial and administrative staff and, in some teams, a psychologist and a community occupational therapist. Most of the teams had bases outside the hospitals and worked from premises within the geographical area they served, although they continued to have access to in-patient beds at either a large psychiatric hospital or at one of the city's district general hospitals.

Referrals to the sector teams came initially to the consultant psychiatrists and were then discussed at a multidisciplinary referral meeting. Clients were then allocated to an appropriate worker. Thus, whilst CPNs might undertake initial assessments, they did not accept direct primary health care referrals. Occasionally, urgent referrals might be taken on directly by a team member but they were discussed at the next referral meeting.

Out-of-hours provision for the mentally ill in the study area

Mentally ill individuals needing psychiatric help outside of normal working hours, were advised first to contact their general practitioner. A duty psychiatrist was always available to provide specialist help when necessary. Both hospitals had a rota system whereby a junior psychiatrist, a senior registrar and/or a consultant psychiatrist were on call 24-hours a day, seven days a week. One of the senior doctors would undertake a visit to an individual's home at short notice, if it was considered to be necessary. In addition, a separately staffed team of social workers was available outside office hours to deal with mental health emergencies. In practice their involvement was limited to cases where compulsory admission to hospital was being considered.

In the past, generic CPNs had worked at the weekend but this service had been withdrawn by nursing management because it was thought to be under used and too expensive. Unfortunately, the researcher was unable to find any documentation of this earlier service. The community nurses in some of the specialist teams, such as Rehabilitation and Care of the Elderly, worked at the weekend. The sector CPNs were doing some out-of-hours work on an *ad hoc* basis, when the study began.

The impetus for change

In the year prior to the study a document was published outlining plans to close one of the local psychiatric hospitals the following year. During the consultation process, members of the public called for an extended community psychiatric nursing service. A recent inquiry held at the local psychiatric hospital had also called for the re-introduction of an out-of-hours and weekend emergency on-call community psychiatric nursing service. Pressure had also come directly from some of the clients. Munton

(1989) undertook a project in the same health district and invited evaluation feedback from a small group of clients who had been discharged from a period of CPN intervention. She also met with a number of local consumer groups and asked for any comments about members' experiences with CPNs. Munton reports that members of the Manic Depressive Fellowship, the National Schizophrenia Fellowship and the Patients' Council all suggested that CPNs should be available outside of normal office hours.

Sector team personnel disagreed about the best way to respond to the pressure for change. Some argued that an extension of the community psychiatric nursing services might be an inappropriate response to the real need for additional services to deal with emergencies or to the need to extend the non-emergency support provided by the sector teams. Some were in favour of developing a district-wide crisis intervention service. It was eventually decided that an out-of-hours service should be provided by the sector team CPNs for a trial period. This service became the basis for the present study.

THE STUDY

Funding was made available by the Health Authority's Mental Illness Unit for a part-time research nurse to be employed for a six-month period. The researcher's brief was to work with the sector team CPNs in order to facilitate the setting up of a trial out-of-hours service. The use of the service was to be monitored closely.

The original research question was whether a community psychiatric nursing out-of-hours service was needed. Further questions arose: Why was the service needed? Could the need be met in any other way? Could the unit afford such a service? Should it be made a priority? It proved difficult to design a study which would provide adequate answers. One approach would have been to talk to potential users of the service – the consumers, their carers and front-line professionals such as GPs, social workers and hostel staff. An attempt could also have been made to measure the efficacy of the service. A major decision had already been taken before the researcher was appointed: the management had decided that a trial service was to be implemented. Due to limited resources it was felt to be impossible to investigate the consumer view any further and it was decided to focus on describing the use of the service during the trial period and also on describing the attitudes of the nurses and the doctors involved. It was not possible to undertake a pilot study, nor to allow for a period of 'settling down' before collecting data from the trial service. This was because of pressure for rapid planning and implementation. Despite these constraints, it was thought important to undertake the study. Milne (1987) discusses the difficulties of undertaking applied research in the field of mental health practice. He argues that service development is enhanced by research, even when it is imprecise and lacking in rigour. He views each attempt at studying a problem, as a step towards the next more careful study, in a process of successive approximation to basic research standards. All those involved in the study were aware of its serious limitations, but ultimately shared Milne's pragmatic approach: 'We must do the best we can with what is available to us'.

Aims and objectives

The aims of the study were:

1. To describe the amount of out-of-hours work which was already being carried out by the CPNs.
2. To monitor the use of the trial service.
3. To describe the attitudes of the nurses and doctors both to the trial service and to a possible future out-of-hours service.

The specific objectives were:

1. To describe the amount and nature of work undertaken outside normal office hours, by the CPNs, in a three-month period before the trial began.
2. To facilitate the planning, organization and implementation of a trial CPN out-of-hours service and to publicize the service to potential users.
3. To collect information about each referral to the service, in order to indicate the amount and type of work undertaken and also whether the nurses thought the work appropriate.
4. To collect information about any occasion when a psychiatrist felt there was a need for CPN involvement, which was not met by the trial service, i.e. a shortfall in service.
5. To identify the attitudes of the CPNs and the doctors to the trial service and to a possible future service.
6. To estimate the cost of the trial service.

Method

Information was collected retrospectively concerning the amount and nature of work carried out by CPNs after 5.00 p.m. Monday–Friday and at weekends, for a period of twelve weeks prior to the trial. Opinions of whether service should be extended were also sought. Twenty-one CPNs were asked to complete pre-coded postal questionnaires (see Appendix).

During the subsequent 12-week trial period, data was collected concerning the number and details of all referrals made to the service, the CPNs' action and their opinion about whether the referral was appropriate. The CPNs recorded data on a pre-coded sheet. The number and details of all occasions of a shortfall in service were recorded by participating doctors. During the last few weeks of the trial period, the researcher conducted semi-structured interviews with all the CPNs attached to the sector teams ($n=26$) and a random sample ($n=32$) of the total number of psychiatrists who worked at the weekend during the trial period ($n=45$). Opinions were sought about the organization and implementation of the trial service and a possible future service. Assurances of confidentiality were given to all participants and it was not necessary to seek ethical clearance for the study since client–contact information was anonymous. Research supervision was provided by staff at the local university.

The trial service. A working party was formed in order to plan the trial service. Membership comprised of CPN representatives, their nursing managers and the researcher. The CPNs agreed to provide an extended service between the hours of 9.00 a.m.–5.00 p.m. on Saturdays, Sundays and bank holidays during the 12-week trial period. They saw less need for a service after 5 pm during the week and decided against this. Two CPNs were on call at the weekend, one providing nursing cover for the three sectors to the north of the city and the other providing cover to the three sectors to the south. Referrals were to be made by one of the senior psychiatrists on call. The hospital switchboard staff contacted the CPNs at home or by radiopager. The CPNs chose to work overtime in order that the operation of the trial did not interfere with their usual weekday work. GPs, clients and their relatives did not have direct access to the service.

The CPNs considered that the aim of the service was to extend their existing work to provide emergency cover at the weekend to those clients who were currently known to the sector team staff. They decided not to undertake planned or routine visits and to exclude clients newly referred to the service, past clients and clients under the care of one of the specialist teams. The CPNs saw themselves as offering:

1. telephone advice/support/counselling;
2. an assessment and/or nursing intervention;
3. a joint assessment/intervention with a CPN colleague, duty psychiatrist, duty social worker, etc.

The unit managers and medical staff were consulted and agreed to the implementation of the proposed service for a trial period, although concern was voiced about the 'restrictive' nature of the cover being offered by the CPNs.

Results

Of the 21 questionnaires concerning out-of-hours work prior to the trial, 20 were returned, giving a 95% response rate. During the three months, the majority of CPNs (79%) had seen clients after 5.00 p.m. during the week and many (60%) had regular work commitments outside normal working hours. Only one CPN had seen a client at the weekend. Whilst most CPNs had been involved in evening work, this was an infrequent occurrence. The majority (70%) worked late on less than one occasion per week. Most of the evening work involved direct client contact, but a number of CPNs (35%) attended clinical case discussions and professional meetings after 5.00 p.m. Over half (60%) of the CPNs thought that they should not extend the hours they were available to clients (see Table 8.1). Several commented that by arranging their own timetable and being flexible about the hours they worked, they were already providing an adequate service to their clients. One CPN believed that where there was a real need for out-of-hours care; it already existed, since specialist CPNs in both rehabilitation and care of the elderly, worked at weekends. Several CPNs thought that they would be of limited use out-of-hours because they did not have any statutory powers under the Mental Health Act (1983). A number also commented that a previous weekend service had been withdrawn because it was thought to be too expensive.

During the subsequent 12-week trial period, which included two bank holidays and one statutory holiday, there were a total of 26 referrals to the service. Of these, 21 were from the northern sectors and five from the southern sectors. Most referrals (69%) were received on a Saturday and the largest number were on the Saturday of the four-day weekend. Half of the clients were already being seen by either a sector team psychiatrist or a

Table 8.1 CPNs' pre-trial opinion about whether sector CPNs should extend their hours

Response	CPNs	
	no.	%
Yes	3	15
No	12	60
Not sure	1	5
No reply	4	20
Total	20	100

CPN on a regular basis. Individuals were referred for a variety of reasons (see Table 8.2). The largest group were those considered to be a suicide risk. Over half (14) of all those referred were known to be suffering from a long-term mental illness.

The CPNs carried out unaccompanied home visits in response to more than half (15) of the referrals. Six of the referrals were dealt with over the telephone, and two joint visits were undertaken, both with a duty psychiatrist. Limited data was collected about subsequent care, but it is known that the CPNs referred eleven of the clients to other agencies, immediately after they had intervened. Six clients were referred back to the duty psychiatrist, two to their general practitioner, one to the accident and emergency department and one to a specialist CPN. Four were known to have been subsequently admitted to hospital. Following each period on call, the duty CPNs passed on details of any clients who had been referred to sector team personnel who were thus able to plan follow-up care if necessary. The nurses were asked to estimate the total time spent dealing with referrals including telephone contact, direct client contact and time spent on administration. They reported taking between fifteen minutes and over six hours dealing with each referral, the average being one hour forty minutes. Half of the referrals were judged by the CPNs to be appropriate, ten (39%) were considered inappropriate and there was uncertainty about the remainder (11%). Neither the CPN nor the client were identified on the data forms, so it is impossible to examine whether there was a relationship between the CPNs who felt positively about the service and judgements concerning the appropriateness of referrals. During the 12-week period one incident of shortfall in service was recorded. The client concerned

Table 8.2 Clients' main problem/duty psychiatrists' reasons for request for help

Problem	No. of clients
Threatened suicide	6
Disturbed/bizarre behaviour	5
Depressed (no mention of suicidal behaviour)	4
Family/hostel worker unable to cope	4
Medication problems	2
Other	4
Not known	1
Total	26

needed specialist help and came from outside the catchment area.

Quarterly running costs were estimated at £2500, including items such as overtime payments, and telephone and radiopager rental, therefore each referral cost approximately £100. However, this did not take into account any possible savings made, for example by avoiding hospital admission.

Twenty-six CPNs were interviewed, the increase in number being due to nurses returning from a course, from maternity leave and new appointments; 22 CPNs had been on call during the trial period. Thirty-two of the 45 doctors who had contributed to the weekend rota were interviewed; 34 had been approached.

Fourteen of the CPNs had received a referral and 13 of the doctors had been involved in making a referral to them. This sub-sample was asked a number of questions concerning the operation of the trial service. None of the CPNs reported being concerned for their own safety whilst on call and none made contact with the other CPN who was on call for advice or support. Several ($n=6$) had sought advice or support from either the duty clinical nurse manager or the duty psychiatrist. Three found difficulty in covering unfamiliar sectors of the city and three thought the lack of access to patients' notes caused some problems. Over two-thirds of the CPNs were satisfied with their contact with the duty psychiatrists and all the doctors who had direct contact with the CPNs were satisfied with this contact. Only one doctor reported a CPN being reluctant to take on work that the doctor believed to be appropriate, whereas nearly half of the CPNs who received a referral said that they experienced pressure to accept work that they felt to be inappropriate.

All of those interviewed were asked about the overall organization of the trial service. Almost all of the CPNs (89%) and over half of the doctors (57%) said they were generally satisfied with the criteria for accepting referrals that had been drawn up by the working party. Many of the CPNs commented upon the need for flexible interpretation, although several believed that it was important to 'lay down the rules'. One CPN commented:

> It is my personal opinion that the criteria should be very strict but then the individual CPN can use their discretion and be given room to manoeuvre. They were a way of being able to fend things off and have a discussion about each client.

The doctors found the referral criteria limiting and a sizeable minority (20%) reported dissatisfaction. Many were concerned that new patients, who had been assessed by the duty psychiatrist, could not be referred if the policy was strictly adhered to. One doctor said that the criteria were: 'Too restricting, but in practice there was some flexibility'.

Two-thirds of the CPNs agreed with the decision to restrict the service to clients who were currently known to one of the sector teams whereas the majority (72%) of the doctors disagreed. One doctor said:

A lot of [new] referrals at the weekend are of people who are distressed and needing a chat and reassurance, and CPNs could be very helpful to these people.

The CPNs and doctors also disagreed about whether CPNs should have been prepared to undertake planned visits. Interpretation of 'planned visit' varied, but to most people this included both routine visits and fairly urgent visits which were considered necessary before the start of the on-call period. An example of the latter would be if a sector team member became concerned about a client during the week and thought they would benefit from a visit at the weekend. Most of the doctors (71%) thought that the CPNs should have been prepared to visit clients who were either causing worry to sector team members, or who were first seen by a psychiatrist on a Friday and who needed support until they could be seen again on Monday. On the other hand, few of the doctors were in favour of the CPNs undertaking routine weekend work. Some of the comments made by doctors were:

It is disappointing they were not prepared to do it [planned visits] but I can understand their reticence ... it would be nice to have that service for both emergency and routine planned visits, in an ideal world.

It would be useful if people seen on a Friday could be seen over the weekend, but that might be determined to be a luxury service.

The CPNs were less clear about planned visits. Just over half (52%) said they would not have been prepared to undertake planned visits, a quarter would have done and the remainder were unsure. Five of the six nurses who said they would have done planned visits, worked in the northern sectors. Some comments were:

Had I been prepared to [do planned visits] I would have found myself busy on both days and where would I have had time for emergency work?

I think if patients need that amount of care then it should be done by their usual CPN or the GP should do it.

From a personal point of view it was fine not to do them, but from the patients point of view perhaps we needed them.

The majority of the doctors (84%) and CPNs (92%) were in favour of calls being initially screened by the duty psychiatrist. Most CPNs saw this as fitting in with their usual practice and providing them with medical 'cover', whilst the psychiatrists saw themselves as screening out inappropriate calls, particularly from GPs. Over half (56%) of those interviewed thought the trial period was the right length of time, but many (40%) thought it was too short. The doctors were more likely to believe that it was too short and many commented that they were only on duty at the weekend once or twice during the trial period and had little chance to become familiar with the operational policy. There were similarly divided opinions about the decision to restrict the service to between the hours of 9.00 a.m.–5.00 p.m. Many of the CPNs commented that whilst ideally they would have liked 24-hour cover, in practice they needed to limit the hours they worked. Some of the doctors thought that most calls outside these hours would be inappropriate for community psychiatric nursing intervention, in that they tended to be of a more 'serious' nature, requiring a psychiatrist's opinion. In contrast, a number of doctors thought that the CPN might be needed most in the evening or at night. Few of the nurses (14%) thought that their usual weekday work had been disrupted by working overtime at the weekend. Several commented that this might have been different had they been called out more.

Many of the CPNs expressed hostility towards the management. They felt that there had been insufficient initial consultation and many believed they had no real choice over whether to participate in the trial. One CPN said:

> CPNs were bulldozed into it, we made our position known from the outset and we knew more or less that there wasn't a need.

Many of the CPNs said they were pleased that a research worker was appointed and thought that the working party represented them well. Doctors were generally less clear about the workings of the service and a number would have liked to have been better informed. In particular they would have liked more opportunity for discussion with the CPNs and the research worker before the trial began, and would have liked a clearer and more concise statement concerning who they could refer.

All the staff were asked whether, in their opinion, a community psychiatric nursing out-of-hours service should be set up on a more permanent basis. Details of the replies are given in Table 8.3. Two-thirds of the doctors were in favour, although many qualified this by saying it would have to be considered in the context of other demands on resources and they would not personally give it top priority. Only one-quarter of the CPNs were in favour of a permanent service and nearly half were against the idea. The latter group were not convinced that there was a need to extend their hours, whilst those in favour saw a need and thought a future service should be more flexible and comprehensive. Staff were asked whether they would want future out-of-hours work to be organized in a

Table 8.3 Opinions about whether a more permanent CPN out-of-hours service should be set up

| | Doctors (%) | | | CPNs (%) | | |
	North	South	All	North	South	All
Yes	72	61	66	43	8	27
No	14	28	22	21	75	46
Not sure	14	11	12	36	17	27
	(n=14)	(n=18)	(n=32)	(n=14)	(n=12)	(n=26)

different way. Most of the CPNs (69%) wanted to involve all members of the multidisciplinary team in manning the service. Almost all the doctors (91%) thought the referral criteria should change and just under half (46%) of the CPNs agreed with them. The two most commonly desired changes were to allow urgent planned visits and to accept new clients. A considerable number of both CPNs and doctors thought that 24-hour cover was desirable and a number were in favour of having a multidisciplinary crisis intervention team.

There were no large differences of opinion between the doctors working in the north and south of the city. However, amongst the CPNs there were some marked differences, those working in the northern sectors being generally more keen to see hours extended and the range of services broadened.

Discussion

During the initial stages of the project most of the CPNs were resistant to the idea of providing an extended community psychiatric nursing service. Many believed that the demand was limited and that the current emergency services met any need adequately. They stated that, when necessary, they saw their clients in the evenings and at the weekend. They were therefore reluctant to give up any more of their free time. Many were hostile towards the management for imposing the trial upon them without adequate consultation. It is remarkable that, in spite of these feelings, the CPNs were willing to plan and implement a trial service in such a short space of time. However, there can be no doubt that these negative feelings influenced the kind of service eventually offered. Another influential factor was the difference in the working practice of the six sector teams. It was necessary to reach some consensus in order to operate the trial and this was mainly achieved by discovering the 'lowest common denominator' between the teams. The resulting practice was thought to be too limiting and too restrictive by some of the nurses and many of the doctors, one of whom commented: "Who is it that we are supposed to be able to refer? So many people seem to be excluded."

The first part of the study focused on the out-of-hours work which was already being carried out by the CPNs on an *ad hoc* basis. Most CPNs spent time one evening a week seeing clients, but rarely saw clients at the weekend. Bearing in mind that the reporting period may not have been truly representative, this finding can be interpreted in several ways. It may reflect an effective service that managed to contain most problems within normal working hours and that met the exceptional need for out-of-hours work. On the other hand, it may indicate that the CPNs were unwilling to undertake more than a limited amount of work outside of normal office hours. It would appear that the needs of working clients were being accommodated because evening appointments were usually available, but out-of-hours visits in response to urgent calls were rare.

In the trial service, referrals averaged two per weekend. It could be argued that had the duration been longer, this rate would have increased as people became more familiar with the service. However, the number of referrals did not increase in the second half of the trial period, which one might have expected were this the case. In order to gain a more accurate picture of need it would have been necessary to publicize the service more widely than was possible in the time provided. It is not possible to know from this study how many people may have felt reassured in the knowledge that CPNs were available at the weekend. Clients often report feeling safer knowing that help is at hand, even if they never call upon it. The same may apply to other professionals; during the interviews a number of the doctors specifically mentioned feeling reassured knowing that a CPN was on call. In one instance, a doctor who was new to the district found it helpful to have an experienced CPN available to give practical advice, in another, the duty CPN was familiar with a particular client and was able to give the duty psychiatrist valuable background information.

It is interesting to speculate about why so many more referrals were made to the CPNs working in the northern sectors. Many of the staff interviewed had their own hypotheses but no generally agreed explanation emerged. Several people commented that working practices differed between the north and south. Before the trial service began there had been no particular difference between the attitudes of the CPNs in the north and south towards extending their service, whereas a marked difference was found when the CPNs were interviewed at the end of the trial. It is very likely that CPNs were influenced by the number of referrals received, those in the north, who received many more referrals, were more likely to believe that a permanent service was needed than those in the south who received far less.

It is difficult to know how to interpret the finding that only half of the referrals were seen as appropriate by the CPNs. It would have been more useful to ask the CPNs to make this judgement both on receipt of the referral and then following their intervention, and also to collect more detailed information about subsequent care. It would also have been helpful to have comparative data about referrals received by the sector teams during the week and by the medical staff at the weekend. Nevertheless, it is striking that so many CPNs reported being pressurized by the doctors to take what they considered to be inappropriate work. This finding supports the view that the CPNs and doctors had differing opinions about what the trial service was able to offer clients. It would also suggest that CPNs and doctors would be wise to reach agreement about what constitutes an appropriate referral prior to implementing a permanent service. CPNs may have judged some of the referrals to be inappropriate because they felt they were being asked to undertake work for which they felt inadequately trained. Before the trial began, a number of CPNs had been apprehensive about participating because they believed that they would have to deal with clients whom they had not met before and who were in crisis. They felt that this would require a style of intervention which was unfamiliar to them, since they did not usually undertake initial assessments. CPNs participating in out-of-hours work in the future may need further training in order to undertake this role.

Before the trial began, many of the doctors commented that the proposed service was too restrictive and for this reason they were asked to document any shortfall in service. The fact that only one incident was reported is encouraging. There may have been under-reporting, (one doctor spoke during his interview about two incidents that he had failed to report), but it seems reasonable to conclude that the trial service largely met any need that arose at the weekend which was brought to the duty doctor's attention. It would have been useful to ask the doctors to document each referral received at weekends in order to examine their nature and the proportion that were considered appropriate for a nursing intervention.

Overall, both groups were satisfied with the trial service although they would wish to make certain changes if one were to be established permanently. The CPNs wanted a multidisciplinary work-force and the system of payment to change, whilst the doctors wanted to broaden the referral criteria. A major theme arising from the interviewing was that there was a lack of agreement about the aim of the trial service. There was confusion as to whether it was to improve the existing emergency services or if it was an attempt to offer something new. There was also confusion about the role of the CPN working at the weekend, opinions differed as to whether the CPNs were essentially working alongside and offering support to the doctors who were on call, or offering something new and distinct. Several factors probably contributed to this confusion. The CPNs felt that the decision to implement a trial service was taken precipitously and without their agreement. Possibly because of this, the working party concentrated on how the service should work rather than why the service should exist. There was also pressure to start the trial as quickly as possible, which limited the time for discussion amongst the nurses and also for consultation with the multidisciplinary team.

CONCLUSION

What are the implications of this study, both for CPNs in the study area, and beyond? Few definitive conclusions can be drawn from a small study carried out under such particular local conditions. Nevertheless, in the process of conducting the study a number of important issues were highlighted and it is useful to consider these in view of the growing national debate concerning out-of-hours psychiatric provision.

There can be no doubt that, as the move towards community care continues, increasing numbers of community psychiatric nursing services are going to be faced with the issue of extending their hours. How should CPNs respond? From the experience of this study, it would appear that CPN teams would be wise to begin to debate the issue amongst themselves and to enter into discussion with other mental health workers and consumers about what can be done to improve existing services. Failure to do this could mean that CPN teams will be forced by their managers to increase the hours they work without full consideration of either the rationale behind, or the implications of, such a decision. If CPNs believe that an extended service is unnecessary they need to be able to argue their case convincingly. In the study area, CPNs working with the elderly mentally ill and the rehabilitation services had seen a need for a weekend service and had organized their work to meet this. Presumably they believed that they were able to offer care at the weekend that was otherwise unavailable. It may well be that only specific client groups need such extended care and if this is the case these groups should be identified.

A number of the CPNs interviewed in this study said they suspected that a weekend service was needed but for personal reasons felt unable or unwilling to work at the weekend. Many nurses are attracted to work in the community because it enables them to have evenings and weekends free and this is entirely reasonable. There is a danger, however, that CPNs could turn a blind eye to a growing need because it may have unpleasant personal implications. Some district nursing services have overcome similar problems by recruiting those nurses who want to work different hours to a separate twilight and weekend service (Hornby, 1976; Sims, 1981). If CPNs are to increase the hours they work they will either have to spread themselves more thinly during normal working hours, with all the implications this has for multidisciplinary work, or their work-force will have to be increased. The CPNs in this study agreed to work overtime at the weekend for the three-month period in order that their usual weekday work was not disrupted. Such a system would probably be unsatisfactory in the long-term and alternatives would need to be considered.

Further attention needs to be given to the nature of help which appears to be required out of hours. This is an area ripe for further research. A growing number of mental health workers have argued that more crisis intervention teams should be created. There are two main problems with this. Firstly, it would appear that in practice crisis theory has been shown to have serious flaws. Secondly, it may well be that emergency care for people with acute psychiatric problems that arise out of hours is already adequate in this country, therefore, the gap in services that is being increasingly identified is for more low-key, supportive work that aims to prevent crises from occurring. Little out-of-hours help is available for people with less acute mental health problems. During public holidays routine psychiatric services can be closed for up to four days and this can be a long time for clients to manage without support. It is interesting to note that most referrals to the trial service came over one such long weekend. It is well recognized that people with enduring mental health problems tend to have difficulty integrating with neighbours and using local social facilities such as pubs and clubs (Goldie, 1988). In view of this, perhaps more consideration should be given to increasing the availability of social facilities out of hours. This could be achieved either by providing more social clubs and 'drop-ins' that are geared to meet the specific needs of this group of people or, perhaps more imaginatively, as Goldie suggests, by providing staff who would be available to accompany clients to local pubs and clubs in order to assist their integration into their neighbourhood.

In a recent study (Marsh, Horne and Channing, 1987) it was reported that 59% of calls made to an urban general practice during one year were managed by telephone advice. It may well be that many mental health problems arising out of hours could also be dealt with in this way.

To conclude, this study has raised many more questions than it has answered. Information is now available about one particular out-of-hours service, how it was used, what it cost, and the attitudes of the staff who helped to run it. Several recommendations follow. Further research into out-of-hours work should be undertaken with an emphasis on identifying what the consumer wants from an extended service. The fundamental issue concerning the aim of any future service needs to be addressed. Mental health workers need to engage in detailed discussion about how their service could best be extended in the light of their operational policy, and whether out-of-hours work should have financial priority. It is vital that any future service is designed in such a way that the professionals involved believe it is attempting to meet an identified need and deserves their active cooperation.

ACKNOWLEDGEMENTS

I am grateful to Dr P. Hawthorne, Professor J. Cooper, Dr B. Payman, Ms F. Cheater and Dr A. Lee for their help and support.

APPENDIX – POSTAL QUESTIONNAIRE

Out-of-hours work by sector community psychiatric nurses

Please circle answer, or fill in space provided, as appropriate.

1. In which sector do you work?

    (a) Sector A
    (b) Sector B
    (c) Sector C
    (d) Sector D
    (e) Sector E
    (f) Sector F

The following questions concern the 12-week period Monday 4 January–Sunday 27 March 1988.

2. During this period, did you see any clients/family members after 5pm Monday–Friday on any occasion?

    (a) Yes
    (b) No

If *Yes*, please answer Question 3 otherwise skip to Question 4.

3. (a) Please could you state on how many weekdays within the above period you saw clients/family members after 5pm?
        _____ days

    (b) Could you estimate how many hours of work in total this involved?
        _____ hours (to the nearest hour)

(c) Could you estimate how many clients/family members you saw after 5pm Monday–Friday during that period?

_____

4. During the specified 12-week period, did you see clients/family members at the weekend?

   (a) Yes
   (b) No

If *Yes* please answer Question 5 otherwise skip to Question 6.

5. (a) Please could you state on how many weekend days you saw clients/family members?

   _____ days

   (b) Could you estimate how many hours of work in total this involved?

   _____ hours (to the nearest hour)

   (c) Could you estimate how many clients/family members you saw at weekends?

   _____

6. Do you have any regular work commitments outside of the hours of 9am–5pm Monday–Friday?

   (a) Yes
   (b) No

If *Yes*, please give brief details below including type of work (e.g. group, social club), frequency (e.g. weekly, monthly) and duration.

7. In your opinion, should the sector community psychiatric nurses extend the hours that they are available to clients?

   (a) Yes
   (b) No
   (c) Don't know

Finally, thank you very much for completing this questionnaire. The space below is for you to add any comments should you wish to do so.

THANK YOU AGAIN.

REFERENCES

Anon. (1984) Survey of GPs attitudes to out-of-hours cover. *British Medical Journal,* **288**, 1627.

Bollam, M., McCarthy, M. and Modell, M. (1988) Patient's assessment of out-of-hours care in general practice. *British Medical Journal,* **296**, 829–32.

Caplan, G. (1964) *Principles of Preventative Psychiatry,* Tavistock, London.

Community Psychiatric Nurses' Association (1985) *The 1985 CPNA National Survey Update,* CPNA, Bristol.

Consumers' Association (1987) Making your doctor better. *Which?* May, 230–3.

Cooper, J.E. (1979) *Crisis admission units and emergency psychiatric services – report on a study,* Public Health in Europe, no. 11, Regional Office for Europe, World Health Organization, Copenhagen.

Fenton, F.R., Tessier, L., Struening, E.L., Smith, F.A. and Benoit, C. (1982) *Home and Hospital Psychiatric Treatment,* Croom Helm, London.

Fry, J., Brooks, D. and McColl, I. (1984) *NHS Data Book,* MTP Press, Lancaster.

Goldie, N. (1988) *'I hated it there, but I miss the people' a study of what has happened to a group of ex-long stay patients from Claybury Hospital,* Health and Social Services Research Unit Research Paper no. 1, South Bank Polytechnic, London.

Hornby, A. (1976) 24-hour community nursing – a pilot scheme in the Lancaster area. *Nursing Times,* March 18, 428–9.

Hoult, J., Rosen, A. and Reynolds, I. (1984) Community orientated treatment compared to psychiatric hospital orientated treatment. *Social Science and Medicine,* **18**, 1005–10.

Marks, I., Connolly, J. and Muijen, M. (1988) The Maudsley daily living programme – a controlled cost-effectiveness study of community-based versus standard in-patient care of serious mental illness. *Bulletin of the Royal College of Psychiatrists,* **12**, January.

Marsh, G.N., Horne, R.A. and Channing, D.M. (1987) A study of telephone advice in managing out-of-hours calls. *Journal of the Royal College of General Practitioners,* July, 301–4.

McKendrick, D. (1984) Weekend working: a survey of CPNs in the North and West Region. *Community Psychiatric Nursing Journal,* **4**, **6**, 7–12.

Milne, D. (ed.) (1987) *Evaluating Mental Health Practice: methods and applications,* Croom Helm, London.

Munton, R.A. (1989) What aspect(s) of community psychiatric nursing does the client find satisfactory? in Brooker, C. (ed.), *Community Psychiatric Nursing: a research perspective,* Chapman and Hall, London.

Parnell, J.W. (1978) *Community psychiatric nurses – a descriptive study,* The Queen's Nursing Institute, London.

Ritchie, J., Jacoby, A. and Bone, M. (1981) *Access to primary health care,* HMSO, London.

Sims, R. (1981) A community night nursing service in Essex. *Nursing Times,* **77** (34), 133–135.

Stein, L.I. and Test, M.A. (1980) Alternative to mental hospital treatment. *Archives of General Psychiatry,* **37**, 392–405.

Szmukler, G.I. (1987) The place of crisis intervention in psychiatry. *Australian and New Zealand Journal of Psychiatry,* **21**, 24–34.

CHAPTER NINE

Psychiatrists' influence on the development of community psychiatric nursing services

Edward White

SUMMARY

Radical changes have recently been made to the way in which mental health services are delivered. Many psychiatrists, however, are reported as being doubtful about or even openly hostile to such developments. It has also been observed that community psychiatric nurses (CPNs) are already regarded as probably being the most important single professional in the process of moving the care of mental illness into the community. Consultant psychiatrists are reported to be unduly anxious about the development of community psychiatric nursing services and have felt the need both to control and restrict their development.

The present study has shown that the proportion of referrals received by CPNs from psychiatrists was found to have halved over the last decade. This was indicative of a closer identification of CPNs with general practitioners (GPs) which psychiatrists have found largely unwelcome. The majority of psychiatrists were generally not found to be in sympathy with the ambitions of local community psychiatric nursing services and positive relationships with psychiatrists were found to be in the minority. The strategies employed to accommodate the interests of psychiatrists are illustrated, as are the latent tensions that underlie the accomplishments of the existing community psychiatric nursing services.

INTRODUCTION

The current developments in community based mental health services, together with the reduction and eventual closure of large psychiatric

197

hospitals may provide the most radical change in mental health care over the past four decades. However, it has been observed (Sturt and Waters, 1985) that many psychiatrists are doubtful about, or even openly hostile to such developments and many hospitals continue to function as if nothing will change. Morrison (1985) has asserted that psychiatrists ought to feel freer outside the walls of institutions, but found it was all too common for them to retreat from what they perceived to be a hostile society and yearn for the days when psychiatrists were both feared and respected. Consultant psychiatrists are presently being asked to contribute to the planning of psychiatric services for community psychiatry and a recent *Lancet* leader (Anon., 1985) argued that they must do this rather than risk their own credibility in rearguard action that would fail. The traditional role of the psychiatrist is thus being threatened and the response to such a threat would determine their contribution to psychiatric care in the future.

Simultaneously, it has been increasingly acknowledged that CPNs, despite a relatively short history, have already been regarded as probably being the most important single professional in the process of moving the care of mental illness into the community (Horrocks, 1985). The Health Advisory Service (Baker *et al.*, 1985) recently reported, however, that some hospital consultant psychiatrists were unduly anxious about the development of community psychiatric nursing services and felt the need both to control and restrict their development. Many feared that if a CPN was not directly responsible to a consultant psychiatrist, errors would be made, inappropriate patients would be treated and resources wasted. No evidence was observed to support the claim, though the Health Advisory Service found that such anxieties frequently surfaced amongst consultant psychiatrists.

Corrigan and Soni (1977) have argued that in a situation where a comprehensive programme of community care was not favoured, the psychiatric team was extremely hierarchical and the function of the CPN may not even develop past the mere giving of psychotropic injections to patients who did not attend clinics. The authors felt that under such circumstances the usefulness of CPNs might prove 'extremely limited'. Leopoldt (1975) reflected an earlier World Health Organization (1967) prediction (that has been more recently elaborated on by Carr, Butterworth and Hodges (1980), Williamson, Little and Lindsay (1981) and Brooker and Simmons (1985)) in which he argued that in broad terms two basic lines of community psychiatric nursing organization could develop. In the first, the organization would remain firmly linked to its place of origin, the psychiatric hospital, unit or day hospital. The CPNs would continue to work within hospital treatment teams and receive referrals exclusively from psychiatrists. In the second, CPNs would become attached to health centres on a full-time basis, much in the manner of health visitors and district nurses. Whilst other CPN organizational permutations have been described (White and Mangan, 1981), Parnell (1978) found early movement toward the second of Leopoldt's possibilities. Indeed, the trend since her 1975–1976 fieldwork has moved markedly toward a closer identification with primary care givers (Shaw, 1975; Harker, Leopoldt and Robinson, 1976; Corser and Ryer, 1977; Sencicle, 1981).

This movement, however, has not been without expressions of caution or, indeed, opposition (Petroyiannaki and Raymond, 1978). A discussion document produced by a Working Party of the Social and Community Psychiatry Section of the Royal College of Psychiatrists (1980) recommended that:

> ... the CPN should be a member of the psychiatric team but should keep closely in touch with the primary health care workers and social workers in the community. Referrals by GPs and their colleagues to the CPN should be viewed as referrals to the psychiatric team and should be discussed in team meetings. When CPNs are a limited resource and demand is great, referrals may be best screened by the consultant psychiatrist, but where pressures are not so great direct referrals from GPs should be welcome.

An update of the Royal College of Psychiatrists' policy position has yet to be published (A.C. Brown, personal communication), despite the invitation offered by the Social Services Committee on Community care (1985) for a statement from the Royal College of Psychiatrists 'specifically encouraging the idea of direct referral from GPs to CPNs'. Although in evidence to the Committee, the Royal College of Psychiatrists (1985), was 'enthusiastic about the new philosophy of care', the Committee also found evidence that the attitudes or practices of some psychiatrists were less than supportive of the policy statement. Competing evidence was, for example, provided by the Association of County Councils (du Sautoy, 1985):

> One matter of great importance in the provision of community services for both the mentally handicapped and the mentally ill is the development of multi-disciplinary teams. Such teams require a willingness on the part of all parties to respect each other's particular knowledge, skill and competence. From this base, confidence in each of the other facilitates the necessary degree of partnership essential to such team operation. Tragically there are many examples of failure, and the greatest obstacle arises from intransigent psychiatrists. The Committee needs to be aware of this situation.

The Committee thus echoed recent *Lancet* articles, referred to earlier, to report 'that in certain respects some psychiatrists were resisting the implementation of community care policies and that their style of work hindered the introduction of new approaches to care'.

Given (a) the development of the scenario above, in which the shift of mental health service provision has been away from psychiatric hospital environs towards the development of a system of care provided in a range of community settings; (b) the key part of CPNs in the new style service and (c) the apparent concern of psychiatrists with both; it was thus theoretically interesting to attempt an exploratory examination of psychiatrist-influence on community psychiatric service planning and development, and the implication of such influence for community psychiatric nursing services. An enquiry to the Social Sciences Research Council Survey Archive at Essex University, England, confirmed that the present survey had not been undertaken before.

The study, thus, had two broad ambitions at the outset:

1. To seek information from CPN managers regarding changes in service provision and the influence of psychiatrists on service plans which affected community psychiatric nursing service developments.
2. To seek information regarding the strategies adopted for the accommodation of such influence.

In the search for an explanation for the growth in the total CPN work-force between 1980 and 1985, Simmons and Brooker (1986) speculated, on the basis of some small-scale qualitative work (Brooker, 1985), that, amongst other possible explanatory factors, service expansion was dependent upon local relationships with consultant psychiatrists. A subsidiary ambition of the present study was, therefore, to examine the relationship between numeric growth in the CPN work-force and local CPN/doctor relations, for not only was that indicated from Brooker's account, but there were also theoretical grounds to locate the study within the context of the sociology of the professions.

THEORETICAL FRAMEWORK

The first English Act regulating the practice of medicine was issued by Henry VIII in 1508. Nine years later his personal physician, Thomas Linnacre, was granted a charter to constitute the Royal College of Physicians which enjoyed the sole privilege of licensing physicians within a seven mile radius of London. In one form or another State regulation of the practice of medicine has continued since that date. The 1858 Medical Act, a response to the *laissez-faire* politics of the period, removed that restriction on the practice of medicine but left the Royal College with its monopoly right to license physicians. This, together with a clause permitting only licensed physicians to be employed by the State, effectively strengthened the profession and left it well placed to capitalize on the growing involvement of the State in the delivery of health care (Hart, 1983).

The ideology of medical practices has embodied all of the classical traits associated with professionalism. The doctor's right to clinical autonomy was the fighting slogan of the profession in its struggle to resist incorporation in the State secretariat when the National Health Service was established in 1948. The compromise which the profession reached with Aneurin Bevan, then Labour Minister of Health, involved salaried employment for hospital staff and fee-paid independence for GPs, 'stuffing their mouths with gold' as Bevan put it. Such an economic arrangement has shown no tendency to diminish the profession's right to self control, nor to shift power and resources away from the privileged hospital sector to the less well endowed system of primary care.

Sociological interest in the analysis of the medical profession and in health policy has been most in evidence in the USA and research in the sociology of the professions, Dingwall (1983) noted, was largely founded on the contributions of two people – Talcott Parsons and Everett Hughes. Parsons (1951) drew upon his own earlier empirical field study of medical practice to illustrate the abstract model of social structure in *The Social System* and this was the context in which the sick role concept was developed. Modern medicine provided Parsons with an example of occupational specialization involving the application of scientific knowledge. Parsons recognized the power of medicine as an agency of social control but attributed the source of the profession's influence to technical rather than ideological factors. For Hughes (1958) the division of labour was at the heart of his interest in the professions and two concepts were particularly important: licence and mandate. He regarded the case of professions as the prime illustration of the possible legal, intellectual and moral scope of a mandate. Not only did professions presume to tell the rest of society what was good and right for it, they could also set the very terms for thinking about problems which fell in their domain.

> Professionals profess. They profess to know better than others the nature of certain matters and to know better than their clients what ails them or their affairs.
>
> (Hughes, 1963)

Professionalization, then, can be viewed as a dynamic process by which occupational control is achieved and maintained. To achieve and maintain such control can be problematic, hence professions must continually profess to their clientele, to laypersons in general, to rival and fellow occupational groups and to the State. Professionalism can also be viewed as ideology for the advancement of particular, collective aims and interests of other groups. Hence, as Beeby (1986) has argued, 'professionalism' has entered the political vocabulary of the wide range of occupational groups competing for status and income, and is used as an evaluative term even by occupational groups which have not achieved, and are unlikely to achieve, control over their occupational tasks. It was where such groups were in conflict over occupational control that elements of the ideology of professionalism were most clearly expressed.

Freidson (1970) discussed the notion of 'professional dominance' with reference to the medical profession's dominant role *vis-à-vis* 'paramedical' occupations, such as nursing:

> By the twentieth century the medical profession was at last able to establish a secure mandate to provide the central health service ... nursing, maintained an ancient function, while being brought firmly under medical control....

The shift of Government policy in favour of the provision of psychiatric care in community settings, reflected by the 1959 Mental Health Act, was confirmed by the 1962 Hospital Plan which proposed to run down the mental hospitals and to develop instead acute psychiatric units in district general hospitals. The latter was to cater for all medical specialities and specialized hospitals were to be phased out. For psychiatry, the objective was to provide a short-stay in-patient service for acutely ill patients only; a system which would work only in conjunction with well coordinated out-patient, day care and community mental health services. By 1975, the publication of the White Paper, Better Services for the Mentally Ill (Department of Health and Social Security, 1975), expressed disappointment at the relative failure of alternatives to hospital care to develop on a wide scale and acknowledged that achievement of the White Paper's goals would take many years. The possibility that mental health care might be expanded into the community beyond psychiatrists' ability to control it (Beeby, 1986), has been largely averted as subsequent spending restrictions have prevented the wholesale development of community care.

Nevertheless, acute units were introduced in the district general hospitals which, as Baruch and Treacher (1978) observed, were being developed irrespective of the development of community services and despite Carr's (1979) evidence to show that such a setting was unsuitable for psychiatric nurses to practice in. Situating mental health care within a general hospital context moreover emphasized the primacy of the medical approach to 'mental illness' by placing the treatment of physical and psychological symptoms on an equal footing.

> Psychiatry is to join the rest of medicine ... since the treatment of psychoneurosis, neurosis and schizophrenia have been entirely changed by the drug revolution. People go into hospital with mental disorders

and they are cured, and that is why we want to bring this branch of medicine into the scope of the 230 district general hospitals that are planned for England and Wales.

(Joseph, 1971)

This was one aspect of a general trend of re-emphasis by the medical profession of the essentially organic nature of 'mental illness'. Beeby (1986) argued:

... A psychotherapy can be specific to an individual practitioner in a way that, say, chemotherapy cannot, since doses and combinations of drugs are governed, to an extent, by technical rules. Thus in a pro-fessional–client relationship involving a particular combination of physical and psychotherapeutic methods, it is the psychotherapeutic element which distinguishes the individual relationship, and it is this psychotherapeutic ability which psychiatrists can profess with least confidence and conviction. It is therefore a 'danger area' in terms of maintaining occupational control.

Carr, Butterworth and Hodges (1980) had earlier rehearsed a very similar argument for CPNs:

... the generalist role of the CPN does not call for the same sort of formal delegation that is necessary for general nurses, because the doctor cannot lay claim, in the area of mental illness/handicap, to the sole exercise of these functions by custom and practice. Such a claim would indubitably be hotly disputed by analysists, psychologists and social workers to name but a few.

Thus, while attempting to earth a discussion of the following empirical findings within the theoretical context of the sociology of the professions, permutations of inter- and intradisciplinary relations have been acknowl-edged. For as Sladden (1979) observed:

Serious conflict between doctors and nurses is unlikely so long as existing status distinctions remain unchallenged, and values and perspectives derived from their common clinical background are shared. Difficulties may arise, however, if doctors disagree among themselves about what is expected of a community psychiatric nurse.

METHODOLOGY

A national postal survey of community psychiatric nursing services of all 192 district health authorities in England was undertaken. Evidence has shown that postal surveys that have clear aims and that are well designed produce high response rates especially in the health service field when the topic is understood by the respondent as being of high professional interest (Oppenheim, 1966; Dunnell and Dobbs, 1982; Cartwright, 1978), and Brook (1982) has discussed the prevention of interviewer-bias variability. The level of detail that can be achieved may also be enhanced because the respondent has time to research the answer to the questions posed – a desirable attribute for the present study in which the canvass of service-provider experience was welcomed. Postal surveys are considerably less expensive than a large number of personal interviews and can obtain large amounts of data in a relatively short time (McNeill, 1985). Limited finance and time have been acknowledged as restrictions of the present study.

Postal questionnaires, however, may cause difficulties if the survey instrument is ambiguous or vague. Moser and Kalton (1971) cautioned that such instruments were subject to low response rates if they were too complicated to complete, or did not contain simple, straightforward, printed instructions and definitions. Efforts were made, in this study, to minimize the frequency of question-routing instructions. Careful pre-testing and pilot work with non-intended respondents was undertaken and minor modifications made to the structure of the instruments.

A weakness of self-completion mail surveys is that they are sometimes unsuitable for asking open-ended questions of the sort used in attitude research. Because of the remoteness of the method, no opportunity existed for the researcher to probe closely the respondent's opinion or to follow a fruitful, though unplanned, enquiry. Marsh (1982) observed that, over the years, there had developed a practice termed 'facesheet sociology' which, she argued, used a rather mechanical algorithm for coming up with socio-logical explanations. Thus, to complement the numerical analysis, six purposive interviews were undertaken with senior nurse manager res-pondents who were identified from the postal questionnaire as having 'pieces of information' which clearly described a working experience between the community psychiatric nursing service and local psychiatrists, both positive and negative. These were drawn from quite disparate geo-graphic locations in England (drawn from within the East Anglian, Trent, Yorkshire, North West (two) and South West Regional Health Auth-orities). The interviews were conducted in the light of exemplar advice provided by McCrossan (1984) and Galtung (1967). Three question areas were pre-chosen by the researcher within which the respondents were allowed a good deal of freedom:

1. The explanation of the change in the proportion of referrals from psychiatrists over time. Why and how had this been achieved?

2. The extent and nature of psychiatrist influence on the developments of the community psychiatric nursing service.
3. The strategies for dealing with such experience.

Such interviews sought to move away from the inflexibility of formal methods, yet allowed the interview a set form and ensured that all topics were discussed. The researcher was therefore free to choose how and when to put questions and how much to explore and probe whilst keeping within the framework imposed by the topics to be covered.

The sampling frame was the Community Psychiatric Nurses' Association Directory (CPNA, 1985a). It was argued that since the 1984 fieldwork, the introduction of general management to the National Health Service (Griffiths, 1983) was likely to have meant changes to the list of published personnel. A covering letter to explain the purpose of the study and the survey instrument were, therefore, sent to the senior nurse manager of each community psychiatric nursing service listed in the Directory. A reminder letter was posted four weeks after the first mail-out.

Data collected from both the postal questionnaire and the transcribed interviews were mostly coded retrospectively and handled on the PRIME computer system at the University of Surrey and, later, on the VAX system at Brighton Polytechnic. At both establishments, the Statistical Package for the Social Sciences (Norusis, 1983) was employed for the quantitative analyses.

A guarantee of confidentiality through anonymity was provided to each respondent and regional health authority was treated as the smallest unit of analyses for that purpose. The present study was not considered to contain an ethically contentious dimension, though informal ethical advice was sought. Some changes have been made to the interview transcriptions when specific mention was made of gender. In every other respect, the material here has been presented verbatim.

SELECTED FINDINGS

Of the 192 questionnaires posted to each community psychiatric nursing service in all district health authorities in England, 135 were returned following one reminder letter. Five were returned uncompleted. Therefore, 130 questionnaires were available for analysis, a response rate of 67.7%. The distribution of responses is shown in Table 9.1.

The total resident population served by respondents was 32.5 million. The mean average resident population per health district was 251.5K with a standard deviation (s.d.) of 114.7K. Fifteen services (11.5%) were located in mainly rural settings and compared with 39 (30%) in urban locations, 76

Table 9.1 Distribution of response to questionnaires by regional health authorities

Regional health authority	No. of health districts	No. of respondents	Response (%)	Sample (%)
Northern	16	8	50	6.2
Yorkshire	17	13	76.5	10
Trent	12	7	58.3	5.4
East Anglian	8	6	75	4.6
NW Thames	15	8	53.3	6.2
NE Thames	16	9	56.3	6.9
SE Thames	15	11	73.3	8.5
SW Thames	13	11	84.6	8.5
Wessex	10	9	90	6.9
Oxford	8	5	62.5	3.8
S Western	11	6	54.5	4.6
W Midlands	22	17	77.3	13.0
Mersey	10	8	80	6.2
N Western	19	12	63.2	9.2
Total	192	130	67.7	100

(58.5%) were described as both. The mean average geographic area per health district was 297.5 miles^2.

It was observed that services began between 1954 and 1984. In keeping with a previous study (CPNA, 1981), the early to mid-1970s were the important growth years, which peaked in 1974 when 1 in 6 of all existing services were established. The mean average age of an English community psychiatric nursing service at the end of 1986 was therefore 11.5 years (standard deviation (s.d.) 4.3). Both median and modal values were 12 years, within the range 2–32 years. For rather more than a quarter of CPN service respondents (26.2%), the manpower planning targets were un-specified. For the 93 services (71.6%), that reported explicit targets the distribution into ratio bandings was as shown in Table 9.2.

Based on the results of the present study the actual ratio, England-wide at the end of 1986, was 1:19000 (18952, s.d. 14529). Almost three-fifths of the sample were aiming at a target of 1:12000 or less; by the end of 1986, it was observed that a quarter (24.8%) had achieved such ratios; 96.9% of community psychiatric nursing services in England had yet to achieve the ratio of 1:7500 promulgated through the CPNA (Butterworth, 1987) and critically examined elsewhere (White, 1987, 1989a).

Each community psychiatric nursing service in England began most frequently with one or two members of staff in post, indeed 85 services

Table 9.2 Distribution of manpower planning ratios

Manpower planning target	Community psychiatric nursing services		
	no.	*%*	*Cumulative %*
Less than 7 500	14	10.8	11.0
7 500– 9 999	24	18.5	29.9
10 000–11 999	38	29.2	59.8
12 000–13 999	11	8.5	68.5
14 000–21 000	5	3.8	72.4
More than 21 000	1	0.8	73.2
Unspecified	34	26.2	100.0
Missing data	3	2.3	
Total	130	100	

(65.4%) began in such a way. By 1981, the mean average number of CPNs in post per service was 7.1 (s.d. 4.3). In 1985 the numbers had grown to a mean of 12.5 (s.d. 6.1). By 1986, the mean had grown to 15.5 (s.d. 7.3). The growth of community psychiatric nursing services is shown in Table 9.3.

Analysis showed that the mean percentage increase between 1981 and 1986 was 261.2%, s.d. 127.5. The observed range was between services which had doubled in numbers (100%) and those which had grown by 750%. A distinction was drawn on the percentage increase of the 5-year period (1981–1986), at the modal point of 200% (that is, services that had grown less than 200% over the preceding 5 years and those that had grown by more than 200%) and it was observed that 58.8% of the study cohort had achieved numeric growth of 200% or more. Twenty-three of the urban services (63.9%) had achieved more than 200% growth, compared with 13 (36.1%) that had not. Services that had been established since 1974 had a higher proportion (65.3%) of achieving more than 200% increase over 5 years, than the 44 services which were established before 1974 (47.7%). Of the services that did not have specified manpower planning targets, 58.1% had not achieved the arbitrary 200% growth threshold.

In common with several studies (for example Griffiths and Mangen, 1980; CPNA, 1981), the empirical evidence here has shown that the conventional organizational arrangement for community psychiatric nursing services, when each was first established, was for almost all the patient clientele to be referred by psychiatrists. The mean average of the referral volume that emanated from psychiatrists for all services in the study at inception was 93.6% (s.d. 16.8). Table 9.4 shows that almost

Table 9.3 Service growth in the study sample, over time

		Service inception	*1981*	*1985*	*1986*
Total CPNs in post		288	843	1602	2019
Mean		2.3	7.1	12.5	15.3
S.d.		1.5	4.3	6.1	7.3
Median		2	6	11	15
Mode		1	6	7	12
Range	Lowest	1	1	3	4
	Highest	10	30	36	53

Table 9.4 Proportion of referrals from psychiatrists at the inception of community psychiatric nursing services

Psychiatrist referrals	*Community psychiatric nursing services*	
%	*no.*	*%*
0	1	0.8
10	1	0.8
20	1	0.8
30	—	—
40	—	—
50	3	2.3
60	2	1.5
70	2	1.5
80	5	3.8
90	15	11.5
100	97	74.6
Missing data	3	2.3
Total	130	100

three-quarters (74.6%) of services, at their outset, had a psychiatrist-only referral system. By 1986, the proportion of referral volume each service received from psychiatrists had changed markedly, as shown in Table 9.5. The difference in the national position between the inception of the community psychiatric nursing services and 1986 are shown in Table 9.6. Therefore, the mean average reduction in the proportion of referrals from

Table 9.5 Proportion of referrals from psychiatrists at the end of 1986

Psychiatrist referrals %	Community psychiatric nursing services	
	no.	%
0	1	0.8
10	8	6.2
20	11	8.5
30	19	14.6
40	20	15.4
50	16	12.3
60	15	11.5
70	16	12.3
80	10	7.7
90	8	6.2
100	5	3.8
Missing data	1	0.8
Total	130	100

Table 9.6 Change in psychiatrist referrals between community psychiatric nursing service inception and 1986

	Service inception	1986
% of service with psychiatrist-only referral system	74.6	3.8
% of referrals from psychiatrists		
Mean	93.6	50.5
Median	100	50
Mode	100	40

psychiatrists per community psychiatric nursing service in England was 42.9%, over an average of 11.5 years to the end of 1986.

Almost half (47.7%) the study cohort received a contribution from Social Services to the planning process of community psychiatric nursing services, with two other sources each contributing to almost a quarter of the services *viz.* psychologists and general managers. While the categories may not be mutually exclusive, psychiatrists were the predominant contributors to such activity (86.2%). However, variation was observed in the extent to which local psychiatrists were reported to have been involved, see Table 9.7.

Analysis showed that the extent to which psychiatrists were involved with CPN service development plans was significantly associated with the percentage reduction in psychiatrist referral. Services with little or no involvement were observed to more frequently report a 40% plus reduction in the proportion of psychiatrist referrals up to 1986, than those with which the psychiatrist was more involved. Whereas those services with a greater involvement more frequently reported less than a 40% reduction, than those with little or no psychiatrist involvement (χ^2 =7.79, df 1, $p \geq$ 0.005). However, the extent of psychiatrist involvement was not systematically associated with service growth when separated into those services that had achieved less than a 200% increase in staff between 1981 and 1986 and those that had grown by more than 200%.

A ratio of less than 3:10 community psychiatric nursing services (29.2%) reported that local psychiatrists, in general, were in sympathy with the services own ambitions. Fifty-five services (42.3%) reported that psychiatrists were not in sympathy, while it was unclear for a further 35 services (26.9%). The sympathy of the local psychiatrists with the ambitions of the CPN services was not shown to have been significantly related to numeric growth. Only 1 in 7 services (13.8%) reported a positive memorable experience (Flanagan, 1954) of the influence that a local psychiatrist had on community psychiatric nursing service development. While some respondents described having unclear, or no, memorable

Table 9.7 Reported extent of psychiatrist involvement in community psychiatric nursing service development

Extent of psychiatrist involvement	Community psychiatric nursing services		
	no.	%	Cumulative %
Not at all	17	13.1	13.2
A little bit	48	36.9	50.4
Moderately	31	23.8	74.4
Quite a bit	20	15.4	89.9
Extremely	13	10.0	100
Missing data	1	0.8	
Total	130	100	

experience to report, a proportion of services (42.3%) provided accounts of negative experience.

Over three-quarters (78.2%) of the negative memorable experience was related to the movement of community psychiatric nursing services toward a closer identification with GPs.

> In 1980, we (CPNs) stopped being Consultant attached so that we could deliver a more fairer service which was not medically dictated. We had CPNs coming back from the (CPN) course who were not prepared to be an injection service, or purely a support network for the Consultants. We felt our skills should be utilised more efficiently. The other thing we did in 1980, was to break away and sectorise ourselves, because the Consultants were not sectorised. We aligned ourselves with Social Service districts. The psychiatrists were not very happy at all, but they did not do anything to keep things as they were because by the time they realised what we'd done, it was too late and fully operational. We did not consult them. It was to do with the nursing service. Nurses were organising nurses. That was the decision we took – not lightly. We realised that there would be repercussions. But we know from our experience of the Consultants, we would never achieve it if we didn't take an independent decision to do it.
>
> (Trent Regional Health Authority)

The account above embraced many of the recurrent features involved in such a move. A single-minded determination to establish and maintain working practices that satisfied CPNs, based on a reasoned case of need, appeared crucial.

> I said to them (Consultants) the Community Psychiatric Nursing Service was, in itself, a profession; that we had an approach to make to the local community which was not necessarily tied in with the expectations of the Consultant Psychiatrists. We would note their objections; we would note their anxieties and their apprehensions. But we had a service to provide as we saw it. And that service would be provided.
>
> (East Anglian Regional Health Authority)

The apparently captive nature of the relationship between CPNs and consultant psychiatrists was illustrated by an account of one community psychiatric nursing service that, despite a determined ambition similar to that described in the account above, had remained organizationally unchanged for 15 years.

> I wasn't prepared to risk my job (to lead the CPN Service toward a closer identification with General Practitioners). That would have been

on the line. I would have been going against my senior's directive and they were not prepared to give me the OK. Nobody was prepared to take the Consultants on. And nobody was prepared to argue as strongly in our (CPNs) favour, to do that. We feel, up to now, that the Consultants have got away – for a long time – with being very powerful; dictating how nurses work. I feel this is very unfair. We can't dictate how doctors work. I feel very strongly that nurses are a professional group of people. They have learnt skills during their training and should be able to use these skills to care for mentally ill people in the community.

We have endeavoured to bring to the knowledge of the GPs the political situation. I think they are quite aware of the battles we have been having over the years. We have said to them that 'there is no way we can open up our service to you. We will provide you with some service, but you must understand our situation.'

(North West Regional Health Authority)

Even for those services that had successfully chosen to broaden the scope of their work practices, the cooperative management of patients clearly remained an issue.

In the early stages of development of our service, a Psychiatrist stated that if GPs referred directly to the CPN without his involvement, he would refuse to be involved at a later date, if the GP subsequently referred the patient to him.

(South East Thames Regional Health Authority)

Because the psychiatrists were not sectorised that meant that they were travelling all round the city, which meant that on a long road as many as ten Consultants with patients on the same road. This meant that even though you (CPNs) were operating in a geographical area we could still have to relate to all Consultants. So what we actually did, because it was impossible to attend all the ward rounds, was to invite the Consultant to be available for an hour, or half an hour, on a certain day of the week to discuss patients. So we organised our own ward rounds, if you like. The ones (psychiatrists) who were, I won't say 'pro-CPN', but the ones who didn't want to influence the way we operated, they were very co-operative. They continued this and still do. The psychiatrists who were not 'pro-CPN', they referred the people who it was impossible to deal with. The minute you went back to discuss them, they would say 'well, its not my problem. You're the CPN. What do you expect me to do about it?'

(Trent Regional Health Authority)

The referral of such 'people who it was impossible to deal with' has been reported by White (1983) as a strategy also employed by GPs as a means of influencing the development of the CPN potential. Despite the apparent uncooperative posture that it was not uncommon for psychiatrists to adopt, examples were observed of gradual reconciliation to new organizational arrangements.

> When we moved out of hospital into a community base, the Consultants were against this move. Then they demanded our attendance whenever they wanted. And we said 'no'. After a lot of flack and threats, we are stronger. They are now coming out to join us.
>
> (West Midlands Regional Health Authority)

For community psychiatric nursing services that chose not to take unilateral action to change the organization of CPN working practices, the formal planning processes were engaged. The same single-minded determination to achieve objectives, commonly held by the community psychiatric nursing team, were present though debated in the more public planning arena. Conventional, institutionalized dialogue between psychiatrists and community psychiatric nursing service managers was reported to demonstrate that a competence existed in the latter and exercised to planned effect.

> Consultants play games in any planning, in that they seem to opt out any real planning strategy. And then when the strategy has been agreed they then butt in 'Ahh yes, but you haven't consulted us; we haven't agreed to this; you haven't notified us; you haven't informed us, we've played no real part in this.' I say to them 'you had every opportunity to be involved; it was of your choosing that you didn't want to be involved and this is the end result and this is what will happen.' But I am not a very popular person. I don't want to appear openly negative towards them, and I do try to encourage them to take part, but at the end of it if they choose not to be part of it then decisions are made and, as far as I am concerned, they're abided by.
>
> (South West Regional Health Authority)

> Consultants within this District could have led this District forwards themselves, in leaps and bounds, and got the full support of the District and the Region. No trouble at all. They could have had everything they wanted here. Built a social empire for themselves to work in and kept their working practices to suit themselves. I think, however, they would rather bury their heads than be involved in anything creative. Its like they're saying 'I'm too clinically busy to be involved in planning'. But when the planning comes along, they're prepared to sit and write long letters criticising it because they don't want it, or it doesn't suit their idea of what the framework should be.
>
> (North Western Regional Health Authority)

The examples of apparent organizational prowess of the community psychiatric nursing services was not only observed in an absolute sense, but also relative to the apparent unwillingness of psychiatrists to take the initiative, previously discussed by Sturt and Waters (1985).

> When the (Consultants) meet with one another, they can only agree at a very superficial level. They can't agree because there is so many new Consultants and old Consultants and different models of working, they can never get together and unite. In all the Districts I've worked in, I have never known a group of Consultants to be cohesive. I have never seen them actively get together to plan anything. I have never known it, quite honestly. That's where the Consultants have fallen down. They don't work with the Team. They see themselves above the Team. The Team is something that functions, runs about, for them rather than with them. They have to learn to take people with them, then they'll go forward and they'll control the Service. They have lost the chance to do that at the moment and I don't see them getting it back because I don't think they have the power, or the willpower, to change their image. Consultants haven't yet learnt to be leaders and that's their major failing. When they learn to be leaders, God help the managers.
>
> (North Western Regional Health Authority)

These data above tend to lend support to the notion that in a number of district health authorities:

> . . . development of Community Psychiatric Nursing Services has been in spite of, rather than because of, the psychiatrists.
>
> (West Midlands Regional Health Authority)

DISCUSSION

The origins and historical development of community psychiatric nursing have been well accounted since the first experimental secondment of two 'out-patient nurses' to extramural duties in the London Borough of Croydon in 1954 (for example Hunter, 1959,1974; Moore, 1961; May, 1965; Greene, 1968; Griffith and Mangen, 1980). During the intervening years, a national network of separate community psychiatric nursing services has developed, although in what Parnell (1978) observed to have been in a local and rather fragmentary way.

From 1974 onwards, the availability of a nationally recognized, academic year-long course (English National Board, 1987) has grown to 24 centres in England (White 1989b). The prevailing educational model has lent itself to the development of a CPN's role popularly characterized by Barker (1981), within which the role has been argued to contain four elements: assessor and therapist to patients and relatives, consultant to other professionals and clinician to monitor the wide range of psychotropic drugs. Jones, Brown and Bradshaw (1978) have suggested that the 1960s community care policy relied chiefly on the effect of the then 'new' range of psychotropic drugs introduced in the mid-1950s. White (1983) observed that the administration of such preparations had long been regarded as the *sine qua non* of community psychiatric nursing and provided an indicator of the predominant client group, referral source and operational base with which CPNs have been historically linked – previously hospitalized individuals with disorders alleviated by the regular injection of such substances, particularly those with schizophrenia as a diagnosis, the psychiatrist and the psychiatric hospital, respectively.

In 1980, 77% of all CPNs worked in services which were based in a psychiatric hospital or a psychiatric unit of a district general hospital. By 1985 the proportion who worked from such an arrangement had fallen to 56.4%. It has been suggested (CPNA, 1985b) that, in general terms, community psychiatric nursing services' resources were therefore being diverted from traditional hospital bases (−20.5% change between 1980 and 1985), to locations that were more community oriented (+23.1% change between 1980 and 1985). However, it has yet to be established, that the base from which a community psychiatric nursing service was provided has been, of itself, the single determinant of service style, especially in terms of the referring agencies and/or the clientele so referred. Indeed, a counter-intuitive observation has been made (Brooker and Simmons, 1985) to show that referrals, from psychiatrists and other ward based staff, to a health clinic attached team of CPNs, were higher than to a CPN based in a day hospital. Moreover, as Skidmore (1986) found, in an examination of CPN services based in three distinctly different settings, the base location appeared irrelevant to the effectiveness of CPN teams.

The present study has shown that the movement of community psychiatric nursing service bases from hospital to non-hospital locations to be, in part, symbolic. For CPNs there was the sense in which being resited outside hospital was, of itself, a liberating experience, despite the caution implied by White (1986) that a change of master is no freedom. More pertinently, there is some evidence that such a movement has not been generally welcomed by local psychiatrists, with over three-quarters of all negative memorable experience recalled by senior nurse managers being related to the closer identification of CPNs with GPs.

Moreover, the present study has also shown that the proportion of referrals from psychiatrists to community psychiatric nursing services, even to services that have not been resited outside a psychiatric hospital base, have been substantially reduced from the inception of services. The picture that has thus emerged from the findings of the present study is that psychiatrists accounted for something less than half of client-referral volume to CPNs in England. The other half of CPN work-load was generated by other agencies, including GPs.

It has been suggested (A.C. Brown, personal communication) that, although the proportion of referral volume from psychiatrists has clearly reduced, absolute numbers of referrals from psychiatrists may have remained constant. Thus, the observed change might be explained by additional CPN recruitment to services being deployed to primary care settings. Brown's suggestion had been in support of an argument that the influence of psychiatrists, in absolute terms, had not diminished. His observation might also suggest, therefore, that the level of community psychiatric nursing service provision to patients with chronic mental illness (patients commonly referred by psychiatrists), while having not benefited from the additional human resources, had not received less attention. Goldberg (1985) had properly cautioned that that might have been the effect 'as CPNs drift away from the hospital based service', although Wolsey (1984) had established in one regional health authority that clients with schizophrenia still constituted 50% of generic CPN case-loads.

Goldberg (1985) had also asked for the sort of central policy statement which would 'insist' that CPNs were part of multidisciplinary community care teams with access to supervision of their work from both psychiatrists and clinical psychologists. Such an organizational arrangement, he argued, would acknowledge the unique contribution that CPNs could make to primary and secondary care services, but would emphasize strongly the importance of community work with the chronic mentally ill. Therefore, his call was a reaffirmation of the Royal College of Psychiatrists' 1980 policy position in relation to community psychiatric nursing and, five years on, was a call for a realignment in the organizational arrangements which had fast shifted ground over that period. Since 1985, when Goldberg presented his paper to a joint Department of Health and Social Security/Royal College of Psychiatrists' conference, the 1980 policy position of the Royal College of Psychiatrists has remained unchanged. Moreover, the Royal College of Psychiatrists has yet to specifically encourage the practice of direct referral from GPs to CPNs as proposed by the Social Services Committee on Community Care (1985). The Committee acknowledged that psychiatrists were 'not only entitled, but obliged to resist' policies which harm the quality of medical care and to alert policy makers and the public where 'their patients interests may be damaged'.

The literature on the sociology of the professions has shown that professional influence means that, on many issues, decisions are made which serve the professional as well as the public interest. As Freidson (1973) observed:

Quite apart from the development of a profession, however, the maintenance and improvement of the profession's position in the market place, and in the division of labour surrounding it, requires continuous political activity. No matter how disinterested its concern for knowledge, humanity, art or whatever, the professional must become an interest group to at once advance its aims and protect itself from those with competing aims.

It was, therefore, theoretically consistent for the present study to find that community psychiatric nursing services with little or no involvement of psychiatrists significantly reported a reduction in the proportion of psychiatrist referrals of more than 40% more frequently, than those services with greater psychiatrist involvement. This finding suggested that the nature and extent of the influence of psychiatrists on the style of the community psychiatric nursing service provided was both in keeping with the policy position of the Royal College of Psychiatrists in particular and theoretical predictions concerned with the concepts of power and control and the division of labour in general.

Crossman (1972) argued that the National Health Service was a consultant-dominated service and it was the consultants who decided the direction of development of the service through their power over allocation of resources. Furthermore, Heller (1978) argued that a switch of resources to primary care and services for Cinderella groups 'cannot take place given the present power structure within the Health Service. The switch will be resisted by those powerful factions that have already distorted the system into its present shape'. Of those community psychiatric nursing services that reported negative memorable experience in the present study, four out of five understood it in terms of psychiatrists' largely unsuccessful attempts to acquire and/or maintain power and control of the work practices of CPNs.

Qualitative data presented here tend to support the impressions, reported both in the medical press and in evidence provided to the Social Services Committee on Community Care, regarding the inter-professional tensions arising out of attempts to develop a network of community psychiatric services. The Audit Commission (1986) also acknowledged the 'potential conflict of interests' of CPNs whose roles straddled both primary and secondary services and noted that these tensions led to delay in developing community care. The Commission further noted that there had been delay by professionals who felt that their interests, and the interests of clients and patients were threatened. The picture that thus emerged from the literature suggested that:

... decision-making is typically incremental rather than rational and its focus parochial rather than systems wide; organisations are primarily motivated by maximisation or defence; of sectional interests rather than altruistic pursuit of common goals; and conflict, competition or the avoidance of interaction are more likely than consensus ...

(Winstow and Webb, 1985)

The present study has made a further empirical contribution to such literature, upon which the summary above was based, and has illustrated ways in which CPN managers have encountered such 'conflict, competition and avoidance of interaction'. Goldie's (1977) analysis of the division of labour among the medical and paramedical workers in mental health has shown that it was not possible to treat each occupation as homogeneous and that the segmentation, which thus arose, generated certain types of accommodation to the problem of securing professional status without power or autonomy. Goldie argued that in each occupation some groups defined their situation as one of ancillary workers to the psychiatrist, where they had a distinct but subordinate part to play under medical leadership. Others defined their situation as one of complementing the psychiatrists, where the boundaries of appropriate occupational work were blurred and doctors were assigned a coordinating rather than directive role. Finally, others adopted an anti-psychiatry position, opposed to the whole notion of any hierarchical division of labour.

Elements of all three positions have been illustrated here, in particular, examples of independent and steadfast nursing action, to bring about a desired change to an existing organizational arrangement of community psychiatric nursing, which appeared necessary in anticipation of psychiatrists' objections. Such unilateral action, while claimed as a nursing solution, also held the potential for becoming, of itself, part of the interdisciplinary problem (Watzlawick, 1968). This, because CPNs risked the charge of not having engaged the conventional planning processes, for abandoning the Rules of Engagement, and so contributing to a cycle of acrimony. For some community psychiatric nursing services such a risk was seen to be sufficient grounds not to embark on unilateral change, while for others the ramifications were predicted and set in the risk/benefit equation before the venture was planned and undertaken.

Whatever the nature of the relationship with local psychiatrists, and evidence has been provided to show that some were very difficult (indeed, even relationships reported as being positive were often reported to have difficult underlying tensions), growth in the CPN work-force nationally was observed to be systematically independent of the present nature of such relationships, when examined over the most recent five-year period. When set against another finding, reported earlier, that services with greater involvement from psychiatrists achieved significantly lower percentage reductions in the proportion of referrals from them, the following observation can be made.

Psychiatrists have, in the past, been firm advocates of CPN growth, especially, as Brooker (1985) remarked, in specialisms where psychiatrists were keen for CPNs to 'mirror their own organizational practices'. Organizational practices have been observed here to be more likely maintained with greater psychiatrist involvement and influence. The mechanism for direct involvement and influence has been through the referral process and a substantial reduction in the proportion of referrals from psychiatrists has also been observed here. The reduction has been observed to be indicative of a movement of community psychiatric nursing services from psychiatrists towards a closer identification with GPs, from hospital to community. Thus, opportunities for psychiatrist organizational practices to be mirrored have similarly reduced. It could be argued, therefore, that given such important changes, early public advocacy from psychiatrists for community psychiatric nursing service development might become weaker in the future. That is, psychiatrists' original patronage of CPNs may have been conditional upon the development of a particular style of community psychiatric nursing service provision.

CONCLUSION

While growth in the number and size of community psychiatric nursing services has been considerable, and yet more urged, the conditions under which it occurred were particular to a set of assumptions about service delivery that were relevant, arguably, only until the early 1980s. From then onwards, the context within which negotiations have taken place have changed, for example: district health authorities have announced psychiatric hospital retrenchment or closure plans; the introduction of general management to the National Health Service eager to examine existing work practices; British research (to add to previous American and Canadian work) to show CPNs in a very favourable light when compared with routine psychiatric out-patient care from psychiatrists (Paykel and Griffith, 1983).

The basis upon which CPNs gain access to their clientele, not only defined what they were able to do with people so referred, but also determined the extent to which their performance was judged by others. Referral processes, Goldie (1977) argued, could be considered to provide at least an outline of the structure of relationships between medical and lay occupations. Analysis of the quantitative data in the present study has shown that, broadly, the proportion of referrals received by CPNs from psychiatrists has halved over the last decade or so. Such a finding was indicative of a closer identification of CPNs with GPs, which psychiatrists found largely unwelcome. The majority of psychiatrists were reported not to be in general sympathy with the ambitions of local community psychiatric nursing services and positive relationships with psychiatrists were a minority finding.

Data presented here have provided examples of apparently successful strategies for dealing with psychiatrist influence on community psychiatric nursing service development. Open conflict with psychiatrist colleagues was occasionally reported by senior nurse managers with high expectations of making a significant contribution to patient care, while lacking any preparation for, or skill in, 'playing the game' according to the traditional handmaiden rules described by Stein (1978). Thus, the present study has provided information about the influences on and tensions arising from developments in community psychiatric nursing and shown how CPNs have encountered them.

On the basis of empirical evidence provided here and reported elsewhere, together with consistent indications drawn from the theoretical literature of the power relations that exist between occupational groups, the recent call from an organ of the medical establishment was clearly significant. The *Lancet* leader (Anon., 1985) urged psychiatrists to avoid the prophetic rearguard action, by ensuring that their speciality 'emerge from its torpor, cease its self-flagellation and take on the mantle of leadership again'. Should action eventually manifest from either direction, both might test the robustness of the recent accomplishments claimed by CPNs and reported here, beyond first-order changes (Watzlawick, 1974). The stage has been set.

<h2 style="text-align:center">REFERENCES</h2>

Anon. (1985) Psychiatry – a discipline which has lost its way. *The Lancet*, 20 March, 731–732.
Audit Commission (1986) *Making a reality of community care*, HMSO, London.
Baker, A.A. *et al.* (1985) *The changing pattern of care in psychiatry*, National Health Service Health Advisory Monograph, Department of Health and Social Services, London.
Barker, C. (1981) Into the community. *Health and Social Services Journal*, **20**, 315–318.
Baruch, G. and Treacher, A. (1978) *Psychiatry Observed*, Routledge and Kegan Paul, London.
Beeby, N. (1986) *The social construction of psychiatric knowledge*, MSc Thesis, University of Wales, Aberystwyth.
Brook, L. (1982) Postal survey procedure, in Hoinville, G. and Jowell, R. (eds) *Survey Research Practice*, Heinemann, London.
Brooker, C. (1985) *The 1985 National Community Psychiatric Nursing Survey Update: Implication of the findings for the evolution of a survey methodology.* MSc Thesis, City University, London.
Brooker, C. and Simmons, S. (1985) A study to compare two models of community psychiatric nursing care delivery. *Journal of Advanced Nursing*, **10**, 217–223.

Butterworth, C.A. (1987) Mandatory training for CPNs: An interim report. *Community Psychiatric Nurses Journal*, May/June, 22–25.

Carr, P.J. (1979) *To describe the role of the nurse working in a psychiatric unit which is situated in a district general hospital complex*, PhD Thesis, University of Manchester, Manchester.

Carr, P.J., Butterworth, C.A. and Hodges, B.E. (1980) *Community Psychiatric Nursing: Caring for the mental ill and handicapped in the community*, Churchill Livingstone, London.

Cartwright, A. (1978) Professionals as responders: variations in, and effects of response rates to questionnaires, 1961–1977. *British Medical Journal*, 18 November, 1419–1421.

Community Psychiatric Nurses' Association (1981) *Community Psychiatric Nursing Services Survey*, CPNA, Bristol.

Community Psychiatric Nurses' Association (1985a) *Community Psychiatric Nursing Services Directory*, CPNA, Bristol.

Community Psychiatric Nurses' Association (1985b) *The 1985 CPNA National Survey Update*, CPNA, Bristol.

Corrigan, J. and Soni, S. (1977) Community Psychiatric Nursing: an appraisal of its impact on community psychiatry in Manchester, England. *Journal of Advanced Nursing*, **2**, 347–354.

Corser, C.M. and Ryer, S.W. (1977) Community Mental Health Care: a model based on the primary care system. *British Medical Journal*, **2**, 936–938.

Crossman, R.H.S. (1972) *A politician's view of health service planning*. University of Glasgow Press, Glasgow.

Department of Health and Social Security (1975) *Better Services for the Mentally Ill*, White Paper, Cmnd 6223, HMSO, London.

Dingwall, R. (1983) *The sociology of the professions*, Macmillan, London.

du Sautoy (1985) Evidence submitted by Under Secretary, Association of County Councils to the Social Services Committee on Community Care with special reference to adult mentally ill and mentally handicapped people, Volume III, HMSO, London.

Dunnell, K. and Dobbs, J. (1982) *Nurses working in the community*, HMSO, London.

English National Board (1987) List of institutions approved to run post basic clinical course number 811 – Nursing Care of Mentally Ill People in the Community, ENB, London.

Flanagan, J. (1954) The critical incident technique. *Psychological Bulletin*, **51** (4), 327–358.

Freidson, E. (1970) *Professional Dominance*, Atherton, New York.

Freidson, E. (1973) *The Professions and their Prospects*, Sage Publications, London.

Galtung, J. (1967) *Theory and Methods of Social Research*, George Allen and Unwin, London.

Goldberg, D. (1985) *Implementation of Mental Health Policies in Lancashire*, paper presented at a joint DHSS/Royal College of Psychiatrists Conference on Community Care, Gaskell, London.

Goldie, N. (1977) The division of labour among the mental health professionals – a negotiated or imposed order? in Stacey, M. *et al.* (eds) *Health and the division of labour*, Croom Helm, London.

Greene, J. (1968) The psychiatric nurse in the community. *International Journal of Nursing Studies*, **5**, 175–183.

Griffith, J.H. and Mangen, S.P. (1980) Community psychiatric nursing: a literature review. *International Journal of Nursing Studies*, **17**, 197–210.

Griffiths, R. (1983) NHS Management Inquiry: Letter to Rt Hon Norman Fowler MP., Secretary of State for Social Services, Department of Health and Social Security, 6 October.

Harker, P., Leopoldt, H. and Robinson, J.R. (1976) Attaching community psychiatric nurses to general practice. *Journal of the Royal College of General Practitioners*, **26**, 170.

Hart, N. (1983) Medical Profession, in Mann, M. (ed) *Sociology*, Macmillan, London.

Heller, T. (1978) *Restructuring the Health Service*, Croom Helm, London.

Horrocks, P. (1985) Memorandum to Social Services Committee on Community Care with special reference to adult mentally ill and mentally handicapped people, on behalf of the NHS Health Advisory Service. HMSO, London.

Hughes, E. (1958) Men and their work, Free Press, Glencoe.

Hughes, E. (1963) Professions, *Daedalus*, **92**, 4.

Hunter, P. (1959) The changing function of professional staff in the mental hospital, in *Ventures of Professional Co-operation*, Association of Professional Social Workers, London.

Hunter, P. (1974) Community psychiatric nursing in Britain: an historical review. *International Journal of Nursing Studies*, **2**, (4), 223–233.

Jones, K., Brown, J. and Bradshaw, J. (1978) *Issues in Social Policy*, Routledge and Kegan Paul, London.

Joseph, K. (1971) Written answer to question by Dr Stutterford, Hansard 879, December, 280–281.

Leopoldt, H. (1975) GP attachment and psychiatric domiciliary nursing, *Nursing Mirror*, February 13, 82–84.

Marsh, C. (1982) *The Survey Method: the contribution of surveys to sociological explanation*, George Allen and Unwin, London.

May, A.R. (1965) The psychiatric nurse in the community. *Nursing Mirror*, 31 December, 409–410.

McCrossan, L. (1984) *A handbook for interviewers*, Office of Population Censuses and Surveys, Social Survey Division, HMSO, London.

McNeill, P. (1985) *Research Methods*, Tavistock, London.

Moore, S. (1961) A psychiatric out-patient nursing service, *Mental Health Bulletin*, **20**, 51–54.

Morrison, A. (1985) Psychiatry in decline – a personal view. *Bulletin of the Royal College of Psychiatrists*, **9**, 4–7.

Moser, C.A. and Kalton, G. (1971) *Survey methods in social investigation*, Heinemann, London.

Norusis, M. (1983) *SPSS-X, Introductory statistics guide*, SPSS Inc., Chicago.

Oppenheim, A.N. (1966) Questionnaire design and attitude measurement, Gower, London.

Parnell, J. (1978) *Community Psychiatric Nurses: abridged version of the report of a descriptive study*, The Queen's Nursing Institute, London.

Parsons, T. (1951) *The Social System*, Free Press, Glencoe.

Paykel, E.S. and Griffith, U.H. (1983) *Community Psychiatric Nursing for Neurotic Patients: the Springfield Controlled Trial*, Royal College of Nursing, London.

Petroyiannaki, M. and Raymond, M.J. (1978) How one community psychiatric nursing service works. *Journal of Community Nursing*, February, 21.

Royal College of Psychiatrists (1980) Community Psychiatric Nursing: a discussion document. *Bulletin of the Royal College of Psychiatrists*, August, 114–118.

Royal College of Psychiatrists (1985) Memorandum submitted by the RCP to the Social Services Committee on Community Care with special reference to adult mentally ill and mentally handicapped people, Volume II, HMSO, London.

Sencicle, L. (1981) Which way the CPN? *Community Psychiatric Nurses' Journal*, January/February, 10–14.

Shaw, A. (1975) CPN attachment to group practice, *Nursing Times*, **73** (12), 9–14.

Simmons, S. and Brooker, C. (1986) *Community Psychiatric Nursing: a social perspective*, Heinemann, London.

Skidmore, D. (1986) The effectiveness of community psychiatric nursing teams and base locations, in Brooking, J. (ed) *Psychiatric Nursing Research*, Wiley, Chichester.

Sladden, S. (1979) *Psychiatric nursing in the community*, University of Edinburgh Monograph Number 6, Churchill Livingstone, Edinburgh.

Social Services Committee on Community Care (1985) *Community care with special reference to adult mentally ill and mentally handicapped people*, Second Report, Volumes 1–3, HMSO, London.

Stein, L. (1978) The doctor–nurse game in Dingwall, R. and McIntosh, J. (eds) *Readings in the Sociology of Nursing*, Churchill Livingstone, Edinburgh.

Sturt, J. and Waters, H. (1985) Role of the psychiatrists in community based mental health care, *The Lancet*, **i**, 507–508.

Watzlawick, P. (1968) *Pragmatics of human communication: a study of interactional patterns, pathologies and paradoxes*, Faber and Faber, London.

Watzlawick, P. (1974) *Change.* Norton, Cranfield.

White, E. (1983) '*If its beyond me . . .*' Community Psychiatric Nurses in relation to General Practice. MSc Thesis, Cranfield Institute, Cranfield.

White, E. (1986) Factors influencing general practitioners to refer patients to community psychiatric nurses, in Brooking, J. (ed.) *Psychiatric Nursing Research*, Wiley, Chichester.

White, E. (1987) *Psychiatrist influence on community psychiatric services planning and development, and its implications for community psychiatric nurses*, MSc Thesis, University of Surrey, Guildford.

White, E. (1989a) Chinese Whispers: the folklore of community psychiatric nursing manpower planning targets. *Journal of Advanced Nursing*, **14**, (5) 373–375.

White, E. (1990) The historical development of the educational preparation of community psychiatric nurses, in Brooker, C. (ed.) *Community Psychiatric Nursing: a research perspective*, Chapman and Hall, London.

White, E. and Mangan, J. (1981) *Community Psychiatric Nursing: Roots to Branches*, Report to Chief Nursing Officer, Department of Health and Social Security, CNO–80–7.

Williamson, F., Little, M. and Lindsay, W. (1981) Two CPN services compared, *Nursing Times*, **77**, 105–107.

Winstow, G. and Webb, A. (1985) *Studies in central-local relations*, Allen and Unwin, London.

Wolsey, P. (1984) *Is there a case for training community psychiatric nurses in social interventions with families of schizophrenic patients?* MSc Thesis, University of Birmingham, Birmingham.

World Health Organization (1967) *The psychiatric hospital as a centre for preventive work in mental health*, Fifth Report of the Expert Committee on Mental Health, WHO, Geneva.

CHAPTER TEN

The training needs of CPNs in relation to work with schizophrenic clients

Phil Wolsey

SUMMARY

This chapter contains an account of a piece of research on the training needs of community psychiatric nurses (CPNs) who work with people who suffer with schizophrenia and their families. It was carried out as part of an MSocSc course at the University of Birmingham between 1982 and 1984 (Wolsey, 1984).

BACKGROUND

From the author's point of view, the research served a number of purposes. After some years working in child and family psychiatry, it presented an opportunity for review and update in a mainstream psychiatric subject area. It was also an opportunity to examine and evaluate family treatment approaches with a particular client group, people suffering from schizophrenia, and thus to build on six years experience of working as a family therapist.

The publications of the Medical Research Council's (MRC) Social Psychiatry Unit seemed to offer a bridge between family therapy and mainstream, conservative adult psychiatry. Family therapy adherents were seen to some extent as pariahs, certainly by British psychiatrists, because the founding fathers of the family systems approach had long held the view that families caused schizophrenia by the way they communicated with their offspring (Bateson *et al.*, 1956; Clare 1976; Palazzoli *et al.*, 1978).

Here then, as a counter to these ideas was a line of research being pursued as a mainstream MRC project. Whilst these workers held that the family had an impact on the course of the illness which could either be benign and supportive, or unhelpful and problematic, they also acknowledged, for instance, a genetic contribution to the aetiology of the illness, and saw the family as a potential resource and not necessarily a handicap to the sufferer.

Family therapy is not the only technique deployed by these research teams. However it was the spark that lit the torch of the author's interest and effort.

Aims of the study

Broadly, the aims of the study were:

1. To summarize the development of the concept of expressed emotion.
2. To present details of the research into developing interventions designed to reduce stress in families and the sufferer and hopefully reduce relapse.
3. To present the author's findings about the training needs of CPNs, elicited by:
   (a) comparing the current state of our knowledge concerning the management of people suffering from schizophrenia and living with their relatives, with the actual management practices and state of knowledge of CPNs in the West Midlands Region.
   (b) examining the current training of CPNs with a view to discovering whether or not this training is adequate to deal with this client group and if not, to argue the case for further training.

Expressed emotion and schizophrenia

In 1965, Dunham showed convincingly that the accumulation of people with schizophrenia in central roominghouse areas in the city of Detroit was due not to inner city areas making their indigenous populations vulnerable to schizophrenia, but to the movement into the area of people in a pre-schizophrenic state during the preceding five years (Leff, 1976). This has begged the question: Why does someone with this illness leave his or her family and move into such areas? In attempting to answer this, one obvious line of investigation was to compare two groups, those patients who lived with relatives and those who did not. There now exists a solid body of work that has 'achieved a level of prediction unparalleled in psychiatry' (Birchwood, Hallett and Preston, 1988).

Brown, Carstairs and Topping (1958) attempted to ascertain outcome for long-stay patients discharged from hospital, and to look for factors in their history and subsequent social experiences which were associated with their level of adjustment in the community. A total of 229 patients were studied, 156 of them schizophrenic. In a subsequent paper, Brown (1959) analysed the schizophrenic sub-group data in detail; 31.6% of the group were failures (defined as re-admission to hospital within one year of discharge). Clinical state on discharge was related to outcome. Superior pre-admission achievement was related to post-hospital success, even when clinical state at discharge was taken into account. Patients who returned to parents, wives, or hostels relapsed significantly more in the first year than those who returned to lodgings. Those who did succeed while living with parents had significantly *lower* social adjustment scores. If the schizophrenia sufferers or their parents were away at work for part of the day, they were more likely to succeed than if they were in close contact.

Brown concluded that the differences were due to interaction with the environment rather than differences in the severity of the patients' clinical state on discharge. If the group rated as 'relieved' at discharge are separated from those labelled 'recovered' and 'not improved' then those of the relieved group who returned to parents were found to have the greatest degree of behavioural disturbance compared to those of this group who went elsewhere.

Brown *et al.* (1962) extended the 1958 work and improved the research design by making it a prospective study of (mainly) short-stay male schizophrenics. In view of the 1958 result, i.e. that deterioration seemed related to close contact with relatives, two hypotheses were tested:

1. That a patient's behaviour would deteriorate if he or she returned to a home in which, at the time of discharge, strongly expressed emotion, hostility or dominating behaviour was shown towards him or her by a member of the family.
2. That even if a patient returned to such a home, relapse could be avoided, if the degree of personal contact was small.

Of the 128 patients studied, 53 (41%) returned to hospital in the year after discharge.

Forty-two per cent of the combined 'no mental state symptoms at discharge' and 'minimal disturbance' group and 64% of the combined 'moderate' and 'severe' disturbance group deteriorated in behaviour (statistically significant). A total of 55% of the sample deteriorated in the year, three-quarters of whom were readmitted. Of the five scales used to measure emotional involvement, the degree of emotional expression and the degree of hostility shown by the key relative towards the patient were predictive, substantial and useful.

Of patients returning to high emotional involvement homes 76%

deteriorated, in contrast to 28% of those returning to low emotional involvement homes (statistically significant).

Patients who were moderately or severely disturbed at discharge and who returned to high emotional involvement homes, deteriorated less frequently when personal contact with the key relative was less than 35 hours per week. For patients in the two least disturbed mental state categories and those living in low emotional involvement homes, low contact was not associated with a lower deterioration rate.

In approximately one-third of cases, the high emotional involvement was probably due to the effects of the past or present behaviour of the patient. In about another third, the ratings of emotional involvement seemed probably due to the characteristic behaviour of the relative. In the remainder of cases, it was suggested that some complex interplay between the key relative and the patient was responsible for the rating. The nature of these relationships were subsequently teased out and will be presented later.

This work still had some way to go in terms of research design. In the years between the publication of the 1962 study and the Brown, Birley and Wing, 1972 study, much work was done by the team to refine the ratings of expressed emotion (the Camberwell Family Interview, Brown and Rutter, 1966; Rutter and Brown, 1966), and to standardize the diagnosis (Present State Examination, Wing, Cooper and Sartorius, 1974). The hypothesis to be tested was: a high degree of expressed emotion is an index of characteristics of the relatives that are likely to cause a florid relapse of symptoms, independently of other factors such as length of history, type of symptomatology or severity of previous disturbance.

A total of 101 patients diagnosed schizophrenic (53 female and 48 male) were selected for the study. The Camberwell Family Interview was used to measure the following:

1.   number of critical remarks about someone else in the home;
2.   hostility;
3.   dissatisfaction;
4.   warmth;
5.   emotional over-involvement;
6.   overall index of relatives' expressed emotion (EE).

High expressed emotion was defined as seven or more critical comments, marked over-involvement of parents, and hostility; all measures chosen for their relationship with relapse. Parents were assigned to a high EE and a low EE group based on this index.

Measures were also made of the patient's behaviour before and at the time of admission including work impairment, disturbed behaviour and social withdrawal. Relapse was of two types: Type I involved a change from a 'normal' or non-schizophrenic state to a state of schizophrenia; Type II involved a marked exacerbation of symptoms.

It was found that 58% of patients with parents from the high EE group relapsed and 16% of those with parents from the low EE group relapsed (p=0.001). The EE ratings of the patients themselves did not relate to relapse. The greatest reduction in the number of relatives' critical comments occurred with respect to those patients who had markedly improved (or, put another way so as not to infer the direction of this relationship at this stage, those patients who markedly improved lived in families who showed the greatest reduction in critical comments). This was measured at follow-up and reflected an overall reduction in critical comments between admission and follow-up after discharge.

Work impairment and disturbed behaviour were related to relapse. Statistical analysis supported the hypothesis that EE independently contributes to relapse because:

1. when impairment and behavioural disturbance are controlled, the association between EE and relapse is little reduced;
2. the association between impairment/disturbance and relapse is greatly decreased when EE is controlled;
3. the association between impairment/disturbance and relapse is weaker than that between impairment/disturbance and EE or between EE and relapse.

Type of clinical condition was not associated with EE and was independently related to relapse.

This study bears out the crude results of the earlier studies. The research design was adequate and had produced findings '... of such theoretical and practical importance for the study of schizophrenia, that it was considered essential to attempt to replicate them' (Leff, 1976).

Vaughn and Leff (1976) using the same basic research design, compared a group of schizophrenics with a group suffering from reactive depression – both groups diagnosed using the Present State Examination (PSE).

The hypothesis to be tested was the same as for the Brown, Birley and Wing, 1972 study. Twenty-one patients were assigned to a high EE group, sixteen to a low EE group; 48% of the high EE group and only 6% of the low EE group relapsed. The marital status and sex differences were replicated, the relapse rate for schizophrenic men was double that for women and the relapse rate for the unmarried significantly greater than that for the married. The relationship between EE and relapse was independent of the patient's behaviour disturbance during the three months before admission and in this study, maintenance drug therapy was shown to have a significant protective effect, as did low face to face contact for the high EE group. Vaughn and Leff pooled the 1972 study data with that of their own, similarity in research design making this possible. Additive effects were found, which are reproduced in Figure 10.1.

These results point the way to strategies for influencing the course of schizophrenic illness. We now know that people with schizophrenia living in high EE homes with face-to-face contact of more than 35 hours per week and without medication, show a 92% rate of relapse compared to those in high EE homes with low face-to-face contact and with medication, whose relapse rate, 12%, compares with that of low EE groups for whom drugs and face-to-face contact seem irrelevant (but see below).

In a two year follow-up of their 1976 study, Leff and Vaughn (1981) traced 25 out of the 26 patients who had not suffered a relapse at the nine-month follow-up. They reported that the relapse rate of patients in high EE homes had slowed down considerably but was still almost double that in the low EE group, that the significant advantage for high EE group patients on maintenance drugs at nine months had disappeared at the end of two years and that, contrary to the nine month result, a significant protective effect of maintenance therapy for the low EE group had emerged.

The conclusion that the protective effect of maintenance drugs for the high EE group is lost at two years may well be a statistical artefact: at nine-month follow-up the relapse rate is 25%, at two years it is 43%, but this is a cumulative figure arrived at by calculating what proportion the same three original relapses are of a sample reduced by four because these four discontinued their drugs. In fact, none of the high EE patients who stayed on regular maintenance therapy relapsed nor indeed did any of the low EE group who stayed on regular medication. It was the second result – that a significant protective effect of maintenance therapy had emerged at the two year point – which prompted publication.

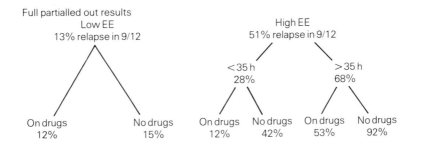

Figure 10.1 Nine month relapse rates of a group of 128 schizophrenic patients. *Source*: adapted from Vaughn and Leff (1976).

Leff and Vaughn go on to speculate that even in a supportive environment, medication may protect patients from, or moderate the impact of, life events. Brown and Birley (1968) and Birley and Brown (1970) distinguished between independent events outside the control of the subject and possibly independent events which were not so clearly out of his or her control. Forty-six per cent of the schizophrenics studied had experienced an independent life event in the three weeks prior to relapse. Leff *et al.* (1973) investigated the relationship between maintenance therapy and life events, extending the critical period from three to five weeks and found a significantly greater occurrence of life events for those who relapsed on medication, compared to those who remained well. Leff and Vaughn (1980) state:

> Episodes of schizophrenia in patients living with high EE relatives are not preceded by an excess of life events, whereas those in patients from low EE homes are. Thus the onset or relapse of schizophrenia is associated either with high EE or with an independent life event.

Conclusion

The EE concept appears to be robust but requires, for unequivocal vindication, a controlled experiment in which it is manipulated. It can be seen that a clinically useful programme might include attempts to lower EE and/or reduce face to face contact, a neuroleptic drug regime and strategies for helping patients to negotiate stressful life events.

Before going on to consider these issues, it is perhaps important to emphasize a few points. Other stressors besides family tension are implicated in relapse: schizophrenic symptoms may still manifest themselves in low EE families, but the relatives' response tends to be cool and measured (Vaughn and Leff, 1981). Wing and Brown (1970) showed that an impoverished social environment leads to an increase in negative symptoms, suggesting that the planned use of social withdrawal as a strategy for lowering stress has drawbacks. Creer and Wing (1974) found that three-quarters of schizophrenic patients living at home did not attend any sort of day centre and had nothing to do all day. Finally, EE is not necessarily a measure of pathological relationships. Wing (1978) has stated: 'The role of the relative is a very difficult one, since it is unnatural to acquire the degree of detachment and neutrality required'.

SOCIAL INTERVENTIONS: LITERATURE REVIEW

In the studies I propose to review, a pragmatic approach to schizophrenia is taken, in which the condition is viewed as an illness whose course is affected by stress; one of the stressors may, but does not necessarily have to be, unhelpful family relationships. The evidence that heredity plays a part in schizophrenia is compelling (Tsuang and Vandermey, 1980). As Wing (1978) puts it: 'one has to be strongly motivated if one wishes to avoid the conclusion that heredity is important in schizophrenia.'

However, there is at present, no evidence to suggest that schizophrenia is a transactional or interactional phenomenon embedded in the matrix of family relationships, although there is evidence that certain types of family atmosphere and life events can exacerbate the condition.

Study A

The work of Goldstein *et al.* (1978) marks the beginning of a series of research efforts whose results show great promise in the prevention of relapse. Goldstein *et al.* randomly assigned 104 acute young schizophrenics to one of four groups, in a 2×2 factorial design which had two levels of maintenance phenothiazine (high dose and low dose) and two social therapy conditions (present or absent). The diagnosis was confirmed using a standardized interview, 69% of the patients were first admissions. Previous work at this centre had shown that, of the patients discharged from it, 45% were readmitted for substantial periods within six months of discharge and that the majority of readmissions occurred within three to four weeks. It was decided, therefore, to use crisis oriented family therapy of six sessions duration.

Goldstein and Kopeikin (1981) relate aspects of this approach in more detail. Clearly mindful of the British work on EE, they suggest that therapists must actively intervene to prevent criticism and to redirect discussions into a transactional, problem solving mode or, when the family find this impossible, to limit contact between the patient and significant others outside the sessions. They have often found it necessary to attempt to modify unrealistic expectations about the length of recovery time, informing the family that it may be at least six months and possibly a year before genuine recovery of social functioning can be observed. Their approach then, is a problem solving, stress reduction model.

None of those patients receiving the higher dose and family therapy relapsed within six months. Forty-eight per cent of those receiving low dose and no family therapy relapsed within six months. The other two groups had intermediate relapse rates.

Those therapy cases in which the goal of anticipatory planning of future crisis management was achieved did significantly better at six-month follow-up (King and Goldstein, 1974). Unfortunately, at three-year follow-up, the effects of therapy seemed to have dissipated completely (Goldstein and Kopeikin, 1981).

Overall, this is an exciting piece of work that suggests that it is possible to discharge schizophrenic patients after an extremely short stay in hospital and work with them and their families whilst the patient is still quite disturbed.

Study B

Anderson, Hogarty and Reiss (1980, 1981), after reviewing the evidence, concluded that the vulnerability-to-environmental-stress model seemed the most well substantiated. In their approach, the family is first seen before the patient leaves hospital. They argue that sessions with an acutely psychotic patient are unhelpful, so the patient is usually excluded, except for one session before discharge. Following the creation of a therapeutic alliance with the family, four or five complete nuclear families are convened for a one day educative workshop covering aspects of the illness, medication, and management of the patient and his or her family life at home. Family sessions with the patient present are then resumed and occur every week, then every two to three weeks for six months to one year. The two main themes are reinforcing family boundaries and the planned resumption of responsibilities by the patient. Later, either an agreement is made to continue treatment in depth on unresolved issues or maintenance sessions of gradually decreasing frequency are instituted. In addition, this group was also using social skills training with the individual patient.

In a recent publication, Hogarty *et al.* (1986) report the one year results of a four cell design in which 103 young patients (mean age 27 years, two-thirds male) were assigned to groups with (a) family treatment only, (b) social skills training (for the patient) only, (c) family treatment and social skills combined, and (d) supportive individual psychotherapy. All four groups were taking medication. Diagnosis was standardized, EE ratings used and the definitions of relapse (i.e. Type I and II) conformed to those of the UK research teams. Nineteen per cent of the family treatment only group relapsed; 20% of the social skills training only group relapsed; *none* of the combined family treatment and social skills training group relapsed; 41% of the medicated only controls relapsed.

In this study, family therapy is used judiciously, much more emphasis being placed on the provision of formal education about the disorder and on strategies for managing more effectively, thus framing relatives as allies rather than antagonists. It remains to be seen whether relapse is prevented or only delayed by these interventions. Nevertheless, the result is impressive and the research design competent.

Study C

A research group (UCLA-Camarillo, based in the US) have described the development and piloting of their early ideas for working with families and sufferers using social skills training, a token economy programme for the patient when in hospital and then an education programme, symptom management strategies, and problem solving techniques for the patient and family (Liberman *et al.*, 1981); Wallace and Liberman, 1985).

Drawing on this early experience, the same research centre has reported on a home based family therapy approach using the social skills, problem solving techniques mentioned above and integrating it to some extent with a systems approach (Boyd, McGill and Falloon, 1981; Falloon, Boyd and McGill, 1981, 1984; Falloon *et al.*, 1985). This meets a number of objections to the previous work. Firstly, as Liberman *et al.* (1981a) freely admit, behavioural approaches have been criticized on the grounds that they have a tendency not to generalize to other situations. Whilst the early work meets this objection to some extent by setting homework assignments and by having the schizophrenic and his or her family work together on specific areas, the new work has the family *in situ*, which necessitates the discharge home of the patient. Secondly, incorporating a systems approach meets the objection that family behaviours, including those of a patient behaving incompetently, may be functional for the family i.e. that there may be a family contingency that rewards unskilled or disturbed behaviour. Thirdly, this is a less time intensive approach – if good results can be achieved with less than the 300 hours of therapy required in the early work the advantages are obvious.

Forty patients who met the DSM III (Diagnostic and Statistical Manual of Mental Disorders: Third edition) criteria for a diagnosis of schizophrenia (this closely correlates with the PSE) and were rated as members of high EE families or families showing other observable evidence of major family deficits in coping behaviour, were randomly assigned to receive home based family therapy or clinic based supportive individual therapy with an experienced psychotherapist – the intention being to compare the experimental clinical intervention with the best alternative community care available. Treatment consisted of weekly sessions for three months, fortnightly sessions for six months and monthly follow-ups for 15 months.

The goals of the family intervention were the prevention of relapse and rehospitalization, the promotion of improved social functioning (Boyd, McGill and Falloon, 1981) and to teach the family to overcome sources of stress with specific interventions for dealing with high EE (Falloon, Boyd and McGill, 1981). The approach advocated the continued use of neuroleptic medication and employed an educational approach combined with family training in verbal and non-verbal skills and problem solving skills as previously described. In addition, other behavioural strategies such as time out, limit setting, contingency contracting, social skills training (for any member of the family) were used and the families were offered a 24-hour crisis facility.

The experimental group showed fewer symptoms over 24 months and significantly fewer were admitted to hospital. During the 15-month follow-up phase, there were six major relapses in the experimental group compared to 31 in the individual-management condition. This seemed to relate to the fact that the families were able to recognize impending deterioration and took active steps to remedy these episodes.

An unpublished pilot study on a portion of the sample revealed that only the family therapy group showed a significant drop in personal criticism, guilt induction and intrusiveness at the three month post therapy follow-up.

The research design is basically sound and the interventions are well described. Birchwood, Hallett and Preston (1988) have drawn attention to the fact that given that the interventions went beyond the family itself to looking at stress reduction strategies in relation to external events impinging on the family, it is not clear how much the resolution of intra-familial stress was responsible for the treatment effect.

This study seems particularly relevant to community psychiatric nursing. The treatment is home based and the interventions are operationalized and teachable. Longer term follow-up will reveal whether this approach prevents or merely delays relapse. In view of its possible efficacy in overcoming life events stressors, it may be suitable for wider application, for example in preventing relapse in low EE families.

Study D

The final study returns us to this side of the Atlantic and the MRC Social Psychiatry Unit in London. In this study, Leff *et al.* (1982) linked the basic research on EE to their applied research in the following way:

> A causal relationship between high EE and relapse, and low EE and patients staying well, can only be demonstrated convincingly by an experiment in which relatives' EE is manipulated and patients' relapse is monitored. The same argument applies to the possible protective nature of low face-to-face contact, which can only be established beyond doubt by an experimental approach.

Twenty-four families (assessed as high EE using the Camberwell Family Interview) and their schizophrenic relatives (diagnosed using PSE and Catego) were randomly assigned to either an experimental or control group in equal numbers. The experimental group were given a package of social interventions involving lectures for the relatives, on the causes, course, management and treatment of schizophrenia, family or marital therapy sessions for the patient and his or her family or spouse, and a relatives group which included in its membership, relatives rated as low EE and perhaps therefore, with ideas about the management of a schizophrenic relative which they could pass on to the high EE members.

Vaughn and Leff (1981) found that the most striking characteristic of the low EE relatives generally was that they held the view that the patient was suffering from a legitimate illness whilst high EE relatives exerted considerable pressure on the patient to behave as a normal individual might be expected to. Information about the schizophrenics' vulnerability to stress and emotional tension in the home was tactfully and supportively spelt out in the education phase.

The relatives group is more fully described in Berkowitz *et al.* (1981). The purpose of the group was to encourage those who had critical, hostile or over-involved attitudes to learn to be more like the low EE members. The group methods were eclectic: modelling; role playing problem situations; group problem solving; reiteration of information about schizophrenia; and family therapy type strategies to encourage parents to go out together, find solutions together and as a parental unit, separate from their adult offspring. The group was also able to support various members simply through the cathartic discharge of feelings. In this climate of support, experience and solutions were shared.

In view of the limitations on what could be talked about in the group, joint interviews were held at home. The first session included the patient. In subsequent sessions, the patient was not always present. The therapy could be individual therapy with the relative, or marital therapy with the parents of the patient. Again, the aim was to reduce EE and/or social contact using techniques ranging from dynamic interpretation to behavioural intervention. It was usually explicitly stated that it would be better if the relatives and the patient spent less time together as this was better for the patient.

Five experimental relatives changed from high to low criticism, three others showed some decrease. Only three critical relatives remained virtually unchanged. Two relatives in the control group changed spontaneously from high to low. A drop in the mean over-involvement score failed to reach statistical significance. Face-to-face contact fell below 35 hours per week in five experimental families. During the nine-month follow-up period only one experimental patient relapsed compared to six in the control group. All were Type I relapses. In the eight families who achieved one or both of the goals of the intervention, not one relapsed. (This figure subsequently became nine following the publication of outcome of a patient who entered the programme late, making the result even more significant).

At the two-year follow-up, (Leff *et al.*, 1985) in those experimental families where relatives' EE and/or face-to-face contact was lowered, the relapse rate was 14% compared with 78% for control patients on regular medication. This is an exciting result. The research design was more than adequate, the measurement tools tried and tested. All the patients in the trial had a high risk of relapse making the results that much more impressive. The respective relapse rates resembled those one would have predicted from Vaughn and Leff's (1976) figures.

It is not clear from this particular design, which of the interventions if any, carries the most weight. It is interesting that the work failed to have much impact on over-involvement. On occasion, attempts to reduce face to face contact locked emotionally over-involved families even more firmly together (Berkowitz *et al.*, 1981). Vaughn analysed the interaction patterns of families with a schizophrenic relative and found, *inter alia*, that high emotional involvement and high criticism were most often found in two-parent households where there was considerable conflict between an over-involved mother and a critical father over the patient, usually a son. Little attention appears to be paid to the functional nature of some of the problems that are presented and I would speculate again that an approach that assumes that people behave problematically solely because of cognitive, knowledge based deficits may fail because it is over-simplistic. Tarrier and Barrowclough (1986) have proposed an educational model that takes into account the patient's and relatives' perceptions and focuses on the patient's specific symptomatology rather than trying to give an academic presentation of the whole field. Tarrier *et al.*, (1988, 1989) have also reported good nine-month and two-year results from their package of behaviourally based social interventions.

The British study of Leff *et al.*, (1985) is the most convincing of the social interventions reviewed. When very little community psychiatric nursing practice is research based, there is a *prima facie* case for training CPNs in the application of the techniques described.

Conclusion

In drawing the strands of this literature review together for the purposes of using it as a guide to one's own clinical practice, there seems to be a case for education about the illness, advice on how to deal with positive and negative symptoms, social skills training and problem solving techniques for the patient and family. The education should be delivered in a strategic manner, taking account of the idiosyncratic needs of a particular family. Over-involvement may well respond to mainstream family therapy techniques which address the possible functional nature of the over-involvement.

It should be clear that for the most part the outcome research is very recent and its conclusions tentative. Where policy and practical application are concerned, Frude (1980) argues that we need only have a reasonable assurance about effectiveness: 'Few would claim that a therapy ought not to be practised until its effectiveness has been demonstrated beyond doubt.' The research cited certainly appears to offer a reasonable assurance of effectiveness.

The field application of this research should not merely be restricted to patients with a rigorous diagnosis of schizophrenia living in families with high EE. The various packages have elements that apply to schizophrenics living in other residential settings. Schizophrenics in low EE families who are at risk from life events can be taught coping skills which might protect them. Patients with borderline diagnoses or even entirely different diagnoses (for example reactive depression) might benefit from the approach. Wards, landladies, and supervised group homes might also find the concepts useful.

THE FIELD RESEARCH

The broad aims of the research were stated in the introduction to this chapter. In order to achieve them, the following questions were posed.

1. To what extent are CPNs aware of the evidence on the role of social factors in the course and outcome of schizophrenics who live with their relatives?
2. What role do CPNs feel they play in the management of this group?
3. What training do CPNs receive in the skills that might enable them to manage this group in a way that is consistent with the current state of our knowledge?
4. How does the literature on the theory and practice of community psychiatric nursing compare with my own findings?

The whereabouts of every CPN team in the West Midlands Regional Health Authority (WMRHA) was established and 18 CPN teams were sent a postal questionnaire. My initial hypothesis was that CPNs have little knowledge of social interventions in the families of schizophrenics or of the role of social factors on the course and outcome of people suffering from schizophrenia, and that their training does not equip them to carry out these interventions even if they are made aware of this knowledge. I therefore based my questionnaire on the null hypothesis that:

CPNs have adequate knowledge of social factors and social interventions and the necessary skills to intervene in the families of schizophrenic people.

The questionnaire sought information in six categories:

1. general information: name, place of work, hours of work, years of service, educational qualifications;
2. post-registration training experiences;
3. details of case-load with particular reference to schizophrenics living with their families;
4. CPN's knowledge of the particular concepts of life events, expressed emotion, face to face contact and their relationship to schizophrenia;
5. the CPN's role in managing schizophrenic patients who live with their relatives. The CPN's assessment of their skill level;
6. an inventory of skills extracted from the literature on social interventions with families of schizophrenics.

It was my intention to try and build a complete picture of community psychiatric nursing by adding the information gleaned from my questionnaire to my literature search, examining the various training course syllabuses for CPNs and the job descriptions I had requested from nursing officers when I sent out my questionnaire.

Results

A total of 120 questionnaires were sent to CPNs that had been identified by their nursing officers as carrying a case-load which included people suffering from schizophrenia. Of these 78 (65%) replied, despite efforts to improve this figure. Moser (1969) states:

> There is much evidence in the survey literature that respondents and non-respondents differ in important respects ... any success in correcting for non-response bias hinges on the possibility of gaining some knowledge, however meagre, about the non-respondents.

Some knowledge of non-responders was gained and will be presented.

Fifty-three (68%) of my respondents were charge nurse/sister grade. Three of the clinical teams who returned all the questionnaires sent out were charge nurse/sister only teams. This suggests that the basic post is charge nurse/sister with perhaps a staff nurse training post (or posts) in some areas. A total of five teams completed *all* the questionnaires sent out. Within those five teams there were 18 charge nurses/sisters and deputy charge nurses/sisters, three staff nurses, two SENs and two nursing officers. Sixty-six per cent of the nurses who replied had been CPNs from one to six years, suggesting a sizeable core of experience in the community.

In Question 18 of my questionnaire, I listed every English National Board (ENB) course that seemed remotely connected to community psychiatric nursing, group, marital, family or behavioural therapy techniques. Respondents were asked to tick those they had attended: 72 (92%) of respondents had not attended an ENB course; 5 (7%) had attended the one-year full-time course ENB – clinical course number 810 (now ENB c.c.no. 811).

In keeping with my null hypothesis, my questions were designed to give CPNs every opportunity to give an account of their training, experience and skills, so that I could compare them with the skills and techniques outlined in the literature on social interventions in the families of schizophrenics.

Training courses.

Thirty-one CPNs (40%) had completed courses in counselling, ranging from one-day to six-months day release. The bulk of them (20) lasted from two to five days.

Ten (13%) CPNs had completed courses in behavioural methods, again of varying duration, the shortest was one day and the longest was six months – total hours of instruction was not stated.

Thirteen (17%) CPNs stated that they had attended courses in family therapy, 5 of these were on a one-year part-time course organized by the Midlands Branch of the Association for Family Therapy.

Twelve (15%) CPNs had completed courses in group work of varying types, 10 (13%) had completed anxiety management courses ranging from 4 to 7 days duration.

Work experience.

16 (20%) CPNs stated that they had acquired skills in group methods through work experience.

4 (5%) CPNs stated that they had acquired family therapy skills.

3 (4%) CPNs stated that they had acquired skills in behavioural methods through work experience.

11 (14%) CPNs stated that they had acquired counselling skills through work experience.

2 (3%) CPNs stated that they had acquired anxiety management skills through work experience.

If we sum the two sets of figures to see, for example how many nurses have done courses in counselling or have acquired skill through work experience, we get the results shown in Table 10.1.

It can be seen that even when the figures are inflated by our either/or formula, there does not appear to be an homogenous community psychiatric nursing profession trained in using family, group and behavioural methods – the core of the social interventions package. The major investment in fact appears to have been in non-directive individual counselling

Table 10.1 Combined sum of courses completed or skills acquired through work experience

Course	no.	%
Group methods	24	31
Family therapy	15	19
Behaviour therapy	12	15
Counselling	36	46
Anxiety management	10	13
Community psychiatric nursing	20	26

which, valuable though it is, appears to me to be at odds with the context in which CPNs work as opposed to say, hospital based nurses whose concern *is* the identified patient. CPNs, on the other hand, are visiting group homes, seeing families and marriages, and working with clients who may have a complex professional network encrusted around them which the CPN needs to take account of. In other words they see families in their social context (Simmons and Brooker, 1986). This surely indicates a need for group or family skills, with training priorities influenced accordingly.

a) Case-load details. These are summarized in Table 10.2. On average, 48% of the CPN's case-load falls into the schizophrenic diagnostic category. This compares with Parnell's (1978) figure of 45% drawn from a much larger sample of 453 CPNs. My figures can only be an estimate of course – they hardly represent the PSE classification, but they do give some indication that CPNs are actually working with the population I am interested in and that according to them, two-thirds of this population are living with their families.

b) CPNs' knowledge of life events, expressed emotion, and face-to-face contact in the families of schizophrenics. CPNs were asked to indicate their views about the role these factors played in relapse. In order to ascertain their knowledge of the literature, no attempt was made to define the terms. Relapse was defined according to the definition used by Brown, Birley and Wing (1972) and Vaughn and Leff (1976). The results are summarized in Table 10.3. Only thirty per cent of my sample were able to answer all four of the stress factor questions correctly. The high 'did not know' figures relative to the 'incorrect' figures suggests that CPNs answered the questions honestly. The figures suggested that CPNs as a body are not familiar with the work on life events and family factors.

Table 10.2 Case-load details

	Generic case-load	Total schizophrenic case-load	Schizophrenics living with relatives case-load
Total no. patients	2874	1404	920
Mean CPN and s.d.	42 + or −	21 + or −	14 + or −
	s.d. 16.617	s.d. 15.382	s.d. 10.004
Range	103	88	53
Sample size of CPNs	67	68	68
No reply	4	3	3

Table 10.3 CPNs knowledge effects of life events, expressed emotion, and face-to-face contact in the families of schizophrenics

	Positive life events and relapse		Negative life events and relapse		Expressed emotion and relapse		Face-to-face contact and relapse	
	no.	%	no.	%	no.	%	no.	%
Correct	52	66	52	66	45	58	32	41
Incorrect	5	7	8	10	4	5	3	4
Did not know	13	17	8	10	21	27	34	43
Did not reply	8	10	10	14	8	10	9	12
Totals	78	100	78	100	78	100	78	100

c) The CPNs' role in managing schizophrenic patients who live with their relatives. The CPNs' self-assessment of their skill level. Respondents were asked:

Please describe in your own words, your role in the management of your schizophrenic patients who live with their relatives.

Most CPNs wrote in general terms about their role, 55 (70%) describing their role in terms of advising, counselling, educating, observing, assessing the patient and monitoring medication. The bulk of the replies described a number of useful roles (advisor, counsellor, observer, etc.) but rather imprecisely. They could be describing an extremely sophisticated approach in a very general way.

In order to try and discover if CPNs had a more specific approach, respondents were asked:

Do you take special measures to deal with schizophrenic patients you have identified as having a high risk of relapse? If yes, state briefly what those measures are.

The answers were: yes, 60 (70%); no, 9 (11%); 9 (11%) did not reply; 44 (56%) said they would increase their visits; 24 (30%) described their role in terms of increased visits, adjustment of medication, and referral back to either GP or consultant psychiatrist. This suggested to me that an interpretation I had not intended was put on the question i.e. I was seeking comments on preventive measures to be taken before relapse was in any way manifest, whilst the CPNs had interpreted my question in terms of measures to be taken once relapse was imminent or under way. However, the information is useful in that it suggests that deterioration or exacerbation is thought by some 24 CPNs to be the firm province of doctors.

Fifty-five (71%) CPNs again couched their replies in general terms, for example increased support, monitor more closely, look for early signs. Nine (12%) CPNs made suggestions which would get the patient away from home for periods of time, for example 'day care', 'days out', 'take the patient out', etc.

d) Non-respondents. I attempted to glean some information about the non-respondents. Seven out of 17 CPN teams made a 100% return. I gained further information about five teams whose returns were less than 100%, giving me some information on a total of 12 teams in all. This was achieved by identifying those members of the family therapy course for CPNs that I am involved in, who were also members of these incomplete teams, and interviewing them. This meant that I had information on a total of 100 CPNs or 83% of the population under study.

These CPNs were asked to speculate about why their colleagues had decided not to complete a questionnaire. Their comments suggest that concern about confidentiality was an important constraint. For reasons of convenience and economy, I requested that the nursing officer in each team collect and post back to me in one pre-paid envelope, all the questionnaires returned. It seems that many CPNs were reluctant to give their nursing officer the opportunity to have sight of their completed questionnaire because they felt that some of the information requested was of a personal nature. One CPN felt that the other CPNs in his team who had not responded had failed to do so because the emphasis on training and skills highlighted their own inadequate training and preparation, and made them feel threatened.

The trends highlighted by the supplementary information that was

received seemed to point to the non-respondents having similar characteristics to the respondents in the following important respects:

1. The questions did not turn up a plethora of CPNs who had completed
    the course ENB 810 or courses in family therapy.
2. The questions revealed that a high proportion of the CPNs were of
    charge nurse/sister grade, a finding consistent with the *respondents'*
    replies.

A tentative conclusion might be that the non-respondents are either
similar to the respondents in their characteristics or perhaps slightly more
inadequately trained. Finally, if these data are biased, a reasonable suspicion might be that CPNs are even less adequately trained than the results
suggest, particularly as skills gained from work experience are very difficult
to validate.

Implications for the training and practice of CPNs

The literature on the skills and clinical training of CPNs remains very scant
(however, see Chapter 11).
Sladden (1979) conducted a PhD research study into the work of a team
of five CPNs in order, *inter alia*:

> To identify the nurses' activities in relation to individual patients and
> families – the skills and techniques employed – and to relate them to a
> simple breakdown of diagnostic categories.

She identified a trend in psychiatry as being 'to regard the family group,
rather than the 'sick' individual as the locus of disturbance' and decided,
therefore, to look also at the nurses' work with the family as a whole.
Sladden found that disturbed relationships in the patient's family or marriage were the most prominent among the social problems reported by the
CPNs. However, clinical procedures were reported comparatively infre-
quently but:

> ... clinical assessment and observation received pride of place ... the
> emphasis placed on clinical observation approximates more closely to
> the idea of the nurse as ancillary medical worker than to that of a ther-
> apist whose core function rests in interaction with the patient.

When the patients' condition deteriorated, the CPNs tended to look for
precipitants in medication and treatment factors rather than to family
relationships or the social environment. This is consistent with my findings
that most CPNs volunteered increased visits, adjustment of medication,
referral back to GP or consultant and close monitoring as their role in the
management of the patients' deterioration, and that those who volunteered

more operationally defined approaches, lacked the methodology to back them up. Sladden states:

> Where relationship difficulties existed (and they were reported for more than half the sample cases) ... the nurses showed that they were well able to identify and describe such situations ... but the researcher gained the impression that they were often at a loss as how to deal with them.

These relationship problems evoked feelings of 'anxiety, helplessness, anger, frustration, inadequacy and guilt'. She concludes that there is little in current systems of CPN training that enables the CPN to intervene constructively in family relationship problems. This paper only studied five CPNs so generalization is hazardous in the extreme. However, my own data and that of others begins to form a picture of CPNs valiantly carrying out difficult work with inadequate preparation and training.

As recently as 1980, Carr, Butterworth and Hedges identified four ideologies used in mental health: Freudian theory, behaviourism, humanistic psychology and medicine. Gurman and Kniskern (1978) exhaustively reviewed outcome in behavioural and non-behavioural family and marital therapies and concluded that these approaches were as effective or more so than other psychotherapies. The systems/cybernetics model of family therapy is an important omission from the Carr, Butterworth and Hedges analysis. Amongst much discussion of group-work, social psychology and behavioural methods, family therapy is briefly mentioned and then virtually passed over.

Attempts have been made by Skidmore and Friend (1984), Woofe *et al.* (1986) and Wolsey (1984) to detect differences in the clinical practice of ENB c.c.no.810/811 trained CPNs and others. No differences have been found. Skidmore and Friend in an article appropriately entitled 'Muddling Through' concluded that 'because of their lack of skills, they (CPNs) tended to manage encounters with patients by trial and error'. However, contrary findings are reported by Brooker in Chapter 11 of this book.

Woofe, Goldberg and Fryers (1988) and Woofe and Goldberg (1988) further confirmed the biomedical ideology of most CPNs in a small study of CPNs and mental health social workers (MHSWs) in Salford. They found that MHSWs were as concerned with clients' interactions with family and community networks, as they were with symptoms. CPNs, on the other hand, focused mainly on psychiatric symptoms, treatment arrangements and medications. For CPNs, there was a tendency to see the client on their own whether seen at home or in a clinic. The arrangements for the clinical supervision and case-load management of MHSWs was superior to that of CPNs. It should be stressed that this was a small local study so making a generalization is fraught with difficulty.

Should CPNs carry out social interventions in the families of schizophrenic patients?

A question not yet considered, concerns which professional group or groups is the most appropriate to carry out the approaches reviewed in this work. The most obvious candidates would appear to be social workers whose *basic* training, unlike nursing, reflects a concern with the client's family and social context. Historically, the numbers of CPNs rose rapidly after the demise of the mental welfare officer following the Seebohm report (HMSO, 1968; Hunter, 1980). Their passing was widely grieved by psychiatrists (Clare, 1976). In the present economic climate, the evidence suggests that social work is more preoccupied with children than the needs of the mentally ill (Hunter, 1980). The impact of the Approved Social Worker under the new Mental Health Act (1983) remains to be assessed. The current evidence suggests that patients visited by CPNs see little of social workers (Hunter, 1978; Sladden, 1979). Creer and Wing (1974) found that the relatives' chief complaints were that little advice was given by professionals on the specific management of difficulties of their schizophrenic relatives. The Royal College of Psychiatrists (1980) caution that it is important that two workers are not duplicating the same work with one individual or family and state that:

> Further work is needed to determine the circumstances in which the CPN would assist the social worker and/or psychiatrist in carrying out crisis assessments and short-term family therapy.

Whilst there are many isolated examples of good training and practice by CPNs, it has to be said that the recent introduction of the 1983 Registered Mental Nurse syllabus was in recognition of the poor basic training offered by the previous syllabus.

An infrastructure that includes psychiatric nurse tutors with the necessary clinical credibility (they too had this poor clinical training, a situation which is not helped by the fact that most of them are currently removed from the clinical area) and that also includes a trained workforce able to offer good role models to students is going to be some time in coming.

CONCLUSION

The research efforts reviewed in this chapter are beginning to filter through. Whitfield *et al.* (1988) has described a training scheme in Southampton for CPNs, social workers, an occupational therapist, a clinical psychologist and a senior registrar. The results of the Manchester based experimental training programme for CPNs in social interventions (Brooker, 1990) are awaited with keen interest. If the study does demonstrate that it is possible to teach CPNs these skills then the implications for community based mental health services are potentially enormous. First because reduced relapse in CPNs' schizophrenic clients will reduce pressure on in-patient beds and be more economic. Second, because CPNs might be encouraged to reorient their focus of intervention away from the 'worried well' to people with severe long-term problems. Finally, one would hope that carers of clients with schizophrenia will be offered a much improved service.

In 1988 the first of a series of three-day national workshops on social interventions was organized by myself and the Community Psychiatric Nurses' Association. The event was well received and over-subscribed – evidence of the tremendous interest shown by CPNs in working with this client group.

Wolsey and Betts (1988) have discussed the problems of training student nurses in working in the community. Given that it is now theoretically possible 'to map out a course of training for an RMN learner that over three years involves only 9 months placement in in-patient settings' (Simmons and Brooker, 1986), the ENB c.c.no.811 must increasingly be superseded by changes in basic training to prepare nurses for their likely deployment in the community. In future, it is likely that many of the training needs of CPNs will be met in basic training, including the training needs of CPNs in relation to schizophrenic patients and their families.

In my own district, we have been experimenting with a student clinic. Students are initially given workshops in family therapy, individual counselling and group-work by myself and service colleagues. These students then see new referrals whilst being supervised live via a telephone link to me, a colleague and the other students. This team is behind the one-way screen in a video suite and the session is videotaped for later analysis. When the trainer is able to move with the students from the classroom to the clinical area the benefits are obvious. It is now possible to arrange this experience for all our RMN student groups for a period of one day per week for 20 consecutive weeks and it represents a powerful (and surprisingly popular!) resource for training students in the acquisition of clinical skills. Project 2000 offers the prospect of the supernumerary student taught by graduate tutors who are encouraged to carry out research and to retain their clinical practice. This is an exciting time to be a psychiatric nurse.

REFERENCES

Anderson, C.M., Hogarty, G.E. and Reiss, D.J. (1980) Family treatment of adult schizophrenic patients: a psycho-educational approach. *Schizophrenia Bulletin,* **6** (3), 490–505.

Anderson, C.M., Hogarty, G.E. and Reiss, D.J. (1981) The psycho-educational family treatment of schizophrenia, in Goldstein, M.J. (ed.) *New Developments in Intervention with Families of Schizophrenics,* Jossey-Bass, San Francisco.

Bateson, G., Jackson, D.D., Haley, J. and Weakland, J. (1956) Toward a Theory of Schizophrenia. *Science,* **1**, 251–264.

Berkowitz, R., Kuipers, L., Eberlein-Vries, R. and Leff, J. (1981) Lowering Expressed Emotion in the Relatives of Schizophrenics, in Goldstein, M.J. (ed.) *New Developments in Intervention with Families of Schizophrenics,* Jossey-Bass, San Francisco.

Birchwood, M., Hallett, S. and Preston, M. (1988) *Schizophrenia. An Integrated Approach to Research and Treatment,* Longman, London.

Birley, J.L.T. and Brown, G.W. (1970) Crises and life changes preceding the onset or relapse of schizophrenia: clinical aspects. *British Journal of Psychiatry,* **121**, 241–258.

Boyd, J.L., McGill, C.W. and Falloon, I.R.H. (1981) Family participation in the community rehabilitation of schizophrenics. *Hospital and Community Psychiatry,* **32** (9), 629–632.

Brooker, C. (1990) The application of the concept of expressed emotion to the role of the community psychiatric nurse. *International Journal of Nursing Studies,* in press.

Brown, G.W. (1959) Experiences of discharged chronic schizophrenic mental hospital patients in various types of living group. *Millbank Memorial Fund Quarterly,* **37**, 105–131.

Brown, G.W. and Birley, J.L.T. (1968) Crises and life changes and the onset of schizophrenia. *Journal of Health and Social Behaviour,* **9**, 203–214.

Brown, G.W., Birley, J.L.T. and Wing, J.K. (1972) Influence of family life on the course of schizophrenia disorders: a replication. *British Journal of Psychiatry,* **121**, 241–258.

Brown, G.W., Carstairs, G.M. and Topping, S. (1958) Post-hospital adjustment of chronic mental patients. *The Lancet,* **ii**, 685–689.

Brown, G.W., Monck, E.M., Carstairs, G.M. and Wing, J.K. (1962) Influence of family life on the course of schizophrenic illness. *British Journal of Preventive Social Medicine,* **16**, 55–68.

Brown, G.W. and Rutter, M. (1966) The measurement of family activities and relationships. A methodological study. *Human Relations,* **19**, 241–263.

Carr, P.J., Butterworth, C.A. and Hedges, B.E. (1980) *Community Psychiatric Nursing: Caring for the Mentally Ill and Mentally Handicapped in the Community,* Churchill Livingstone, Edinburgh.

Clare, A. (1976) *Psychiatry in Dissent,* Tavistock, London.

Creer, C. and Wing, J.K. (1974) *Schizophrenia at Home,* National Schizophrenia Fellowship, Surbiton.

Dunham, H.W. (1965) *Community and Schizophrenia. An Epidemiological Anal-*

ysis, Wayne State University Press, Detroit.

Falloon, I.R.H., Boyd, J.L. and McGill, C.W. (1981) Family management training in the community care of schizophrenia, in Goldstein, M.J. (ed.) *New Developments in Interventions with Families of Schizophrenics*, Jossey-Bass, San Francisco.

Falloon, I.R.H., Boyd, J.L. and McGill, C.W. (1984) *Family Care of Schizophrenia*, Guilford Press, New York.

Falloon, I.R.H., Boyd, J.L., McGill, C.W., Williamson, M., Razani, J., Moss, H.B., Gilderman, A.M. and Simpson, G.M. (1985) Family management in the prevention of morbidity of schizophrenia: clinical outcome of a two-year longitudinal study. *Archives of General Psychiatry*, **42**, 887–896.

Frude, N. (1980) Methodological problems in the evaluation of family therapy. *Journal of Family Therapy*, **2** (1) 29–44.

Goldberg, S.C., Schooler, N.R., Hogarty, G.E. and Roper, M. (1977) Prediction of relapse in schizophrenic out-patients treated by drug and sociotherapy. *Archives of General Psychiatry*, **34**, 171–184.

Goldstein, M.J. and Doane, J.A. (1982) Family factors in the onset, course and treatment of schizophrenic spectrum disorders an update on current research. *Journal of Nervous and Mental Diseases*, **170** (11), 692–700.

Goldstein, M.J. and Kopeikin, H.S. (1981) Short and long-term effects of combining drug and family therapy, in Goldstein, M.J. (ed.) *New Developments in Intervention with Family of Schizophrenics*, Jossey-Bass, San Francisco.

Goldstein, M.J., Rodnick, E.H., Evans, J.R., May, P.R.A. and Steinberg, M.R. (1978) Drug and family therapy in the aftercare of acute schizophrenics. *Archives of General Psychiatry*, **35**, 1169–1177.

Gurman, A.S. and Kniskern, D.P., (1978) Research on marital and family therapy. Progress, perspective and prospect, in Garfield, S.L. and Bergin, A. (eds) *Handbook of Psychotherapy and Behaviour Change: An Empirical Analysis*, 2nd edn. Wiley, New York.

HMSO, (1968) *Report of the Committee on Local Authority and Allied Personal Social Services*, Chairman F. Seebohm, Cmnd 3703, HMSO, London.

HMSO (1989) Caring for people. Community Care in the next decade and beyond. Cmnd 849, HMSO, London.

Hogarty, G.E., Anderson, C.M., Reiss, D.J., Kornblith, S.J. *et al.* (1986) Family psychoeducation, social skills training and maintenance chemotherapy in the aftercare treatment of schizophrenia. *Archives of General Psychiatry*, **43**, 633–643.

Hunter, P. (1978) *Schizophrenia and Community Psychiatric Nursing*. National Schizophrenia Fellowship, Surbiton.

Hunter, P. (1980) Social Work and Community Psychiatric Nursing. A Review. *International Journal of Nursing Studies*, **17**, 131–139.

King, C.E. and Goldstein, M.J. (1974) Therapist ratings of achievement of objectives in psychotherapy with acute schizophrenics. *Schizophrenia Bulletin*, **5** (1), 118–129.

Leff, J.P. (1976) Schizophrenia and sensitivity to the environment. *Schizophrenia Bulletin*, **2**, 566–574.

Leff, J.P. (1983), Social interventions in the families of schizophrenics: addendum (letter) *British Journal of Psychiatry*, **142**, 311.

Leff, J.P., Hirsch, S.R., Gaind, R., Rohde, P.D. and Stevens, B.C. (1973) Life events and maintenance therapy in schizophrenic relapse. *British Journal of Psychiatry*, **123**, 659–660.

Leff, J.P., Kuipers, L., Berkowitz, R. and Sturgeon, D. (1982) A controlled trial of social interventions in the families of schizophrenic patients. *British Journal of Psychiatry*, **141**, 121–134.

Leff, J.P., Kuipers, L., Berkowitz, R. and Sturgeon, D. (1985) A controlled trial of social intervention in the families of schizophrenic patients: two year follow-up. *British Journal of Psychiatry*, **146**, 594–600.

Leff, J.P. and Vaughn, C.E. (1980) The interaction of life events and relatives' expressed emotion in schizophrenia and depressive neurosis. *British Journal of Psychiatry*, **136**, 146–153.

Leff, J.P. and Vaughn, C.E. (1981) The role of maintenance therapy and relatives' expressed emotion in relapse in schizophrenia. A two year follow-up. *British Journal of Psychiatry*, **139**, 102–104.

Liberman, R.P., Wallace, C.J., Vaughn, C.E., Snyder, K.S. and Rust, C. (1981), Social and family factors in the course of schizophrenia, in Bowers, M. and Downey, R.W. (eds) *The Psychotherapy of Schizophrenia*, Guilford Press, New York.

Moser, C.A. (1969) *Survey Methods in Social Investigation*, Heinemann, London.

Palazzoli, M.S., Cecchin, G., Prata, G. and Boscolo, L. (1978) *Paradox and Counter-Paradox: A New Model in the Treatment of the Family in Schizophrenic Transaction*, Jason Aaronsen, New York.

Parnell, J.W. (1978) *Community Psychiatric Nursing: A Descriptive Study*, Queens Nursing Institute, London.

Royal College of Psychiatrists (1980) Community psychiatric nursing. A discussion document by a Working Party of the Social and Community Psychiatry Section. *Bulletin of Royal College of Psychiatrists*, August, 114–118.

Rutter, M. and Brown, G.W. (1966) The reliability and validity of measures of family life and relationships in families containing a psychiatric patient. *Social Psychiatry*, **1**, 38–53.

Simmons, S. and Brooker, C. (1986) *Community Psychiatric Nursing: A Social Perspective*, Heinemann, London.

Skidmore, D. and Friend, W. (1984) Muddling through. *Nursing Times*, 9 May, 179–181.

Sladden, S. (1979) *Psychiatric Nursing in the Community: A Study of a Working Situation*, London, Heinemann.

Tarrier, N. and Barrowclough, C. (1986) Providing information to relatives about schizophrenia: some comments. *British Journal of Psychiatry*, **149**, 458–463.

Tarrier, N., Barrowclough, C. and Vaughn, C. (1988) The community management of schizophrenia: a controlled clinical trial of a behavioural intervention with families to reduce relapse. *British Journal of Psychiatry*, **153**, 532–542.

Tarrier, N., Barrowclough, C., Vaughn, C., Bamrah, J.S., Porceddu, K., Watts, S. and Freeman, H. (1989) Community management of schizophrenia: a two year follow-up of a behavioural intervention with families. *British Journal of Psychiatry*, **154**, 625–628.

Tsuang, M.T. and Vandermey, R. (1980) *Genes and the Mind*, Cambridge University Press, Cambridge.

Vaughn, C.E. and Leff, J.P. (1976) The influence of family and social factors on the course of psychiatric illness. A comparison of schizophrenic and depressed neurotic patients. *British Journal of Psychiatry*, **129**, 125–137.

Vaughn, C.E. and Leff, J.P. (1981) Patterns of emotional response in relatives of schizophrenic patients. *Schizophrenia Bulletin*, **7** (1), 43–44.

Wallace, C.J. and Liberman, R.P. (1985) Social skills training for patients with schizophrenia: a controlled clinical trial. *Psychiatric Research*, **15**, 239–247.

Whitfield, W., Taylor, C. and Virgo, N. (1988) Family care in schizophrenia. *Journal of the Royal Society of Health*, **1**, 3–5.

Wing, J.K. (1978) *Reasoning about Madness*, Oxford University Press, Oxford.

Wing, J.K. and Brown, G.W. (1970) *Institutionalism and Schizophrenia*, Cambridge University Press, Oxford.

Wing, J.K., Cooper, J.E. and Sartorius, N. (1974) *Measurement and Classification of Psychiatric Symptoms*, Cambridge University Press, Cambridge.

Wolsey, P. (1984) *Is There a Case for Training CPNs in Social Interventions in the Families of Schizophrenic Patients?* MSocSc Thesis, University of Birmingham, Birmingham.

Wolsey, P. and Betts, A. (1988) What can we do with the learners? *CPN Journal*, February 5–12.

Woofe, K. and Goldberg, D.P. (1988) Further observations on the practice of community care in Salford: differences between community psychiatric nurses and mental health social workers. *British Journal of Psychiatry*, **153**, 30–37.

Woofe, K. Goldberg, D.P. and Fryers, T. (1988) The practice of community psychiatric nursing and mental health social work in Salford: some implications for community care. *British Journal of Psychiatry*, **152**, 783–792.

CHAPTER ELEVEN

A six-year follow-up study of nurses attending a course in community psychiatric nursing

Charles Brooker

SUMMARY

Since the mid-1970s an approved post-registration education course has been available for community psychiatric nurses (CPNs). The outline curriculum was originally prepared by the Joint Board of Clinical Nursing Studies (JBCNS) and latterly by the English National Board (ENB). Unlike courses on health visiting or district nursing the course is not mandatory and it has been estimated that 22% of all CPNs nationally have been awarded the certificate to date. There has been little research undertaken which has evaluated the consequences of completing the training. This is problematic at a time when the financial situation in many health authorities has led some managers to question its value. This study employs a longitudinal survey design to follow up six cohorts of students who have undertaken the community psychiatric nursing course at Sheffield Polytechnic between the years 1981–1987. The results indicate that course attendance has a significant impact in the following areas: clinical skills, attitudes to clients and knowledge base. In addition, two-thirds of the sample initiate important changes in practice on return to their seconding authority, an observation corroborated by a second data set obtained from seconding health authority managers. The course does not fulfil all the students' major expectations, a finding which is discussed in relation to the implementation of the new outline curriculum (ENB clinical course number 811 'Nursing mentally ill people in the community'). In conclusion, the paper argues that the post-registration education of CPNs is a crucial activity that requires constant refinement in relation to the needs of seconding health authorities and demands a coherent funding strategy.

INTRODUCTION

The role of the CPN was first established in the mid-1950s and early 1960s (Peat and Watt, 1984; May and Moore, 1963). From its inception community psychiatric nursing has been a readily accepted and constantly expanding feature of community mental health services (Brooker, 1987). However, the fact that CPNs, unlike their district nurse and health visitor colleagues, do not need a mandatory qualification to practise has long been controversial (Butterworth, 1987).

The first pilot training programme for CPNs was established in London and lasted for 13 days (Rawlings, 1970). Today, many more course centres exist nationally and are approved by the national board for the country concerned. Recently, there has been growing concern that the future of post-registration education for CPNs is not secure, and a number of factors have contributed to this general feeling of anxiety. Firstly, now that the course lasts 36 weeks, it is perceived as costly, both in terms of course fees and time lost from the service by the seconded student. In the current climate of the National Health Service, there is much evidence that when financial savings are demanded one of the first areas hit is post-registration education. Secondly, health service managers rightly pose the question, given the high cost of the course, and the fact that the qualification is not mandatory, what do I get for my money? Unfortunately, until now, there have been no systematic studies which have attempted to answer this question. Finally, there are a number of commentators (Brooking, 1985) who have argued that the introduction of the 1982 revised basic Registered Mental Nurse (RMN) curriculum has obviated the need for a community psychiatric nursing course at all. Supposedly, the new RMN syllabus is sufficiently 'clinical skills' and 'community experience' oriented to replace ENB c.c.no.811 in community psychiatric nursing.

These are all bleak arguments largely built upon untested assumptions (and predominantly resource-led) which this study was set up to examine by looking closely at the discernible value of attendance on the CPN course. The study looked at the following areas specifically:

1. What are the characteristics of students attending the course?
2. How do they and their managers assess its value – at least one year after course completion (see section on 'sample')?
3. What changes occur in services after students return?
4. What happens to the careers of students after they obtain the qualification?

BACKGROUND

The first experimental post-registration course for CPNs was established at Chiswick Polytechnic in 1970. The content of the course has been described by one of its first participants (Cole, 1971). It is perhaps not surprising that, given community psychiatric nursing's stage of development at that particular time, much of the course-work involved defining the parameters of a CPN's role.

The first formal outline curriculum ('Community psychiatric nursing for registered nurses' – JBCNS c.c.no.800) was prepared several years later. The curriculum was organized in relation to the specific skills, knowledge and attitudes that would be required to achieve the following objectives:

1. The nurse will be skilled in assessing the needs of the psychiatric patient and his or her family; and in care, treatment, training and education leading to optimum habitation or rehabilitation.
2. The nurse will be able to promote liaison and cooperation with other relevant services in the patient's and family's interest and be able to give help and advice to colleagues.
3. The nurse will be skilled in organizing and assessing priorities in the day-to-day management of his or her work.
4. The nurse will be able to give information to the patient and his or her family on health care and social resources in the community, and will be able to pass on effectively knowledge and skills to students.
5. The nurse will have an appreciation of research and its contribution in the field in which he or she is working.

In 1979, this initial outline curriculum was revised (JBCNS c.c.no.810, 'The nursing care of the mentally ill in the community') and although objectives 1, 3 and 4 remained essentially the same, objective 2 talked about the importance of developing a therapeutic relationship with patients and their families, and objective 5 was extended to include not just an appreciation of research but the ability to facilitate research itself.

In 1985, when a third revision to the outline curriculum was made (ENB c.c.no.811, 'Nursing care of mentally ill people in the community'), significant further changes were discernible. The course was still two-thirds practise based, and one-third theory related (out of a total of 36 weeks), but the content altered. Objective 1 was similar, but additionally couched in terms of the four stages of the nursing process. Objective 2 remained essentially unchanged. Objective 3 had become more orientated towards service management and stated that 'the nurse will be able to contribute to the planning and development of psychiatric services in the community'. Finally, objectives 4 and 5 relating to teaching and research were more fully developed in Occasional Publications One and Five (ENB, 1985).

Other noteworthy changes that occurred include the statement for the first time of the following:

1. knowledge of local cultural problems and ethnic groups;
2. the nurse's role as an advocate for the patient (although the outline curriculum's title includes the phrase 'mentally ill people' for some reason inside the document the word 'patient' persists);
3. principles of health education and the role of the nurse as health educator;
4. social and psychological factors which predispose towards mental health.

All in all, between 1973 and 1985 a period of just 12 years, the content of the outline curriculum changed dramatically as did thoughts about the role of the psychiatric nurse. Correspondingly, the calls for mandatory training, noted earlier, became increasingly strident. In parallel with these advances, it is important to note that during the period 1980–1985 the CPN work-force itself grew at the dramatic rate of 65% (see Community Psychiatric Nurses Association, 1985). *Ipso facto*, the proportion of CPNs attending the course declined. Table 11.1 demonstrates the marked regional variation in the number of qualified CPNs in 1985, ranging from just 6.0% in the West Midlands Region to 33.0% in the Wessex Region. The national average for course completers within district health authorities (DHAs) at this time was 22%.

In recognition of this variation the ENB resolved, early in 1985, the following:

1. Education Officers were to support the implementation of a new revised curriculum (ENB c.c.no.811, 'Nursing mentally ill people in the community') and the development of new such courses.
2. The ENB were to give financial support for tutor appointments in four new centres and help develop a distance learning approach through a project in the North West Region.
3. The ENB allocated special development monies to reimburse health authorities during the period 1986–1988. A total of £500000 was provided over a three-year period.

Today, the ENB initiatives outlined above, combined with an increased willingness (and recognition of the need) to run the ENB c.c.no.811 within health authorities, has led to a proliferation of both course centres and the number of places available (see Table 11.2).

Historically, the provision for and content of CPN educational courses has significantly advanced since 1970 when a pilot programme, lasting a mere 13 days, was set up. The course is now nine months in duration and run at 24 approved course centres with 420 places available and already

Table 11.1 Proportion of trained CPNs within DHAs by region in England, 1985 (from CPNA, 1985)

Regional health authority	Trained %	Response by DHAs in original survey %
Yorkshire	17.0	94.0
Northern	31.0	94.0
Trent	30.0	83.0
East Anglia	11.0	75.0
NW Thames	23.0	93.0
NE Thames	23.0	81.0
SE Thames	23.0	93.0
SW Thames	23.0	100.0
Wessex	33.0	100.0
Oxford	26.0	100.0
S Western	23.0	82.0
W Midlands	6.0	91.0
Mersey	11.0	100.0
N Western	30.0	100.0
Total	22.0	86.5

Source: CPNA (1985)

Table 11.2 Increase in course centres/places for ENB c.c. no. 811 in England by year

	1985	1986	1987	1988
No. of courses	10	16	20	24
No. of course places	218	293	350	420

these figures are under-estimates. However, the qualification obtained by students is not mandatory and the outcome of attending the course has rarely been evaluated. One possible exception is a four-year study undertaken at Manchester Polytechnic during the period 1979–1983 (Skidmore and Friend, 1984; Skidmore, 1986). The project's initial brief was to examine the effectiveness of CPN intervention in relation to work-base, i.e. hospitals, primary health care and a combination of the two. A number of services (n=12) were selected at random with a total of 120 CPNs interviewed by the research team. Forty per cent of these CPNs had undertaken the CPN course (*n*=48) allowing some comparisons of trained versus untrained CPNs' effectiveness to be included in the final publication. In one of the reports (Skidmore and Friend, 1984), the authors state:

> It quickly became apparent that there was no significant difference between the teams or in the effectiveness of nursing care by those with the ENB certificate as opposed to those without it.

It is unfortunate that the study gives no clue as to how 'effectiveness' in this context was measured. In the second published study (based on the same research programme), similar claims are made about the comparability of CPNs who are trained and those who are not. Skidmore (1986) states:

> Seventy per cent of this sample maintained that they were inadequately trained for their 'community' role even after they had completed the 810 course.

Again, however, there is no indication given as to the precise measures of effectiveness that were employed. Despite the uncertainty involved in understanding which specific analyses were used on which to base the sweeping assertions given above, Skidmore's conclusion that CPNs require a more skills-based training is largely accepted. It is intended that the establishment of the new curriculum (ENB c.c.no.811) has gone some way to meeting this need. This issue will be discussed further later in the chapter.

To summarize, CPNs education has developed significantly in terms of curriculum content, course length and course availability. However, there is little research to date that has looked systematically at the outcomes of CPN course completion.

METHOD

The samples

The CPN student sample consisted of every student who successfully completed ENB cc.no.810 at Sheffield Polytechnic between the years 1980–1986 (*n*=87). The sample of community psychiatric nursing service managers consisted of every manager from a health authority who had ever seconded a student to the ENB c.c.no.810 at Sheffield Polytechnic (*n*=26).

Survey method

Although there are well reported advantages and disadvantages in the conduct of postal surveys (see Hoinville and Jowell (1978) for such a discussion) economic constraints primarily determined this choice of research method. A major problem with mail questionnaires can be non-response which leads to the introduction of certain biases. To improve response to the survey the following strategies were therefore adopted: a stamped addressed envelope was included; a covering letter explaining the survey aims was enclosed; a reminder letter was sent out six weeks after initial mail-out; the United Kingdom Central Council (UKCC) were approached and agreed to redirect questionnaires to non-responders using their up-to-date address lists. It seemed reasonable to suppose that after seven years had elapsed, a number of the early student cohorts' addresses would be out of date. Similar tactics were employed to enhance response from the service managers although the UKCC were not approached. For purposes related to the Sheffield course administration, an up-to-date list of service managers' names and base addresses was already available.

Questionnaire design

The student questionnaire had five main areas: the student's 'status' pre- and post-course, brief personal details, views on course outcome and plans for the future. A mixture of closed and open questions were included. The questionnaire was piloted with a group of CPNs not included in the sample and consequently modified slightly.

The questionnaire directed to the seconding managers of individual services was designed in two parts. Firstly, to obtain basic details about the service and its commitment to CPN education. Secondly, to elicit the views of managers of the value, or otherwise, of CPNs returning to the authority on completion of the course.

Copies of both survey instruments are available on request from the author.

Analysis

The data was analysed using the Statistical Package for the Social Sciences (SPSS) at Sheffield Polytechnic. All aspects of this exercise from data coding through to actual analysis were carried out by an independent research worker.

Response

The response for the 'manager' set of data overall was 81.0%. This varied slightly according to each regional health authority, 75% ($n=9$) in Trent, and 85% ($n=11$) in Yorkshire. There was also one respondent from the Northern Region.

The CPN student response in total was 74% ($n=64$). It was interesting to note that response did not improve as a function of time as one may have expected in a longitudinal study design (See Table 11.3).

The overall response rate was high when compared with that of other studies of this nature. For example, Everest, Richards and Hanrahan (1979) followed up nurses trained at the Maudsley Hospital over a period of 11 years and achieved a 47.6% response. Rogers and Powell (1983) examined a range of JBCNS course attenders for a period of three years and attained a 64.0% response, and Brooker and Brown (1986) looked at nurse therapists who had been trained for up to four years and obtained a response rate of 77%. As mentioned earlier, the strategy which undoubtedly improved response significantly was the use of the UKCC register. Figure 11.1 demonstrates the impact of both a reminder letter and UKCC register on overall response through time – an increase in response from 42% to 74%.

RESULTS

Characteristics of the services seconding students to the course

These data were obtained from the questionnaire distributed to service managers and therefore relate to DHAs within the Trent and Yorkshire Regional Health Authorities. Services had been established just over a decade ($\bar{x} = 10.2$ years), the number of CPNs within services was approximately 18 ($\bar{x} = 17.7$ w.t.e.) of whom 4.5 had completed the course ($\bar{x} =$ mean and w.t.e. = whole time equivalent). Therefore, the overall figure for those qualified within teams was 25.4% (slightly above the last known national average, see Table 12.1). The referral patterns for seconding services are given in Table 11.4 and compared with the national position in

Table 11.3 Students' response rate by cohort

Cohort no.	Response %	N
1	50	5
2	93	13
3	57	8
4	87	13
5	71	10
6	79	15
Total	74	64

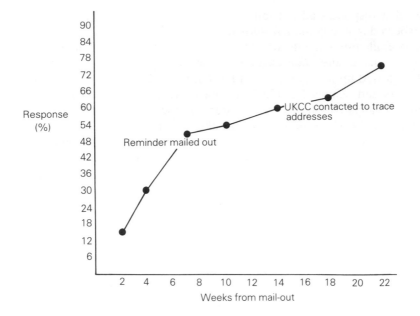

Figure 11.1 Response rate for student sample through time.

Table 11.4 Referral patterns of seconding CPN teams compared with the national figures for 1985

Referral agent	1987 Seconding service %	1985 National services %
Psychiatrist	45.6	59.15
GP	36.0*	23.3
District nurse/health visitor	8.0	5.0
Social services	3.5	3.2
Self/family	5.6	2.2
Other	1.3	7.15
Total	100.0	100.0

*It is worthwhile noting that a significant positive correlation was observed between the number of course completers within DHAs and the percentage of GP referrals ($r=0.475$, $p > 0.003$).

1985. The noted trend for a decline in the percentage of psychiatrist referrals and increase in GP referrals to CPN teams (White, 1987) seems to be reflected here.

Service managers were asked details of the DHA's post-basic education budget and the amount of money allocated to this fund. Thirty-three per cent of managers (*n*=7) knew what the actual amount allocated to post-basic training was, the mean amount given by this group was £4114. Further, 39.0% (or £1620) of this budget is routinely given to fund CPN training. Although 95% of the responding health authorities stated that by 1992 the community psychiatric nursing service would increase in size by an average of 5.6 wtes, no service was able to state that there were plans to increase the post-registration education budget accordingly.

The vast majority of managers (90.5%), however, felt that post-registration CPN education should be mandatory but that CPNs should be paid the same amount after training as before. A small proportion of the sample (30%), found it hard to retain CPNs after completion of the course and this point along with others is developed further with the student data.

Seconding managers' views on CPN training

Sixty-six per cent of the manager sample observed positive differences in CPNs' work practice after the completion of training. Examples of these differences are given in Figure 11.2 under the broad headings of attitudes, knowledge and skills.

In addition to these differences in work practice, managers provided many examples of changes that students initiated on their return from the course. Some examples of these changes include: developing a counselling clinic in a health centre; setting up community groups in stress management; reviewing the services operational policy in the light of broad organizational change; development of a model for in-service training; a redesign of the service's evaluation package; and the initiation of GP attachment. This section is also further expanded when the student data is examined.

It should also be noted that some managers (28%) noted areas of disappointment in students on their return to the service. A number of the remarks made in this section are outlined below.

Course was only used for the individual's benefit not the service as a whole.

CPN wanted to make major changes which the Health Authority was too inflexible to allow.

There was no change in attitude or skills.

The student still wanted to work from a hospital base.

Attitudes to clients

- now see clients as individuals with their own responsibilities
- more aware of their own limitations
- assessment is deeper and more systematic
- more likely to use client's strengths therapeutically
- client is given more choice

Attitudes to colleagues

- more questioning and supportive
- share their new skills with colleagues
- higher self-esteem rubs off on others
- more enthusiastic in promoting colleagues' professional development

Attitudes to referring agents

- more appropriately assertive in communicating CPNs' capabilities
- greater understanding of other agencies' contribution
- better able to justify interventions
- improved liaison and communication
- a greater empathy in regard to the referrer's position

Knowledge base

- greater understanding of nursing process and care evaluation
- more ability to understand overall service machinery
- improved understanding of research based practice
- strong development of the concept of community
- better informed about theoretical models of practice

Clinical skills

- more aware of a range of skills that they might develop
- more confidence in trying new tactics
- increased willingness to identify supervision needs
- much better at prioritizing and planning case work
- far more appreciation of clients' families needs

NB The above are all direct quotations elicited from the open questions in the questionnaire.

Figure 11.2 Examples of positive differences in CPN work practice observed by managers on CPNs' return to service.

Characteristics of the students attending the course

These findings refer to 74% of the total population of ENB c.c.no.810 students attending Sheffield Polytechnic between the years 1980–1986. The mean age of students on completion of the course was 33.6 years, although this varied from 30.5 years for cohort 4, to 37.0 years for cohort 3. A reduction in mean age by cohort was expected but not observed. The sex ratio was even, with men and women each constituting 50% of the total sample. On average, CPNs attending the course had worked as unqualified CPNs for 2.1 years (ranging from 3 months to 15 years). The majority of the students had been formally educated up to 'O' level standard as Table 11.5 demonstrates. In addition to being on the Register for the mentally ill (the formal course entrance qualification), 49% of the students were also Registered General Nurses (RGNs).

In an effort to explore the effect of attending the course on the students' careers two questions were included which ascertained the sample members' pay grade before starting the course compared with the pay grade that they were on at the time of this study. The results are presented in Table 11.6.

It is perhaps an encouraging finding that of the total sample 97% (n=59) were engaged full-time in clinical practice when the course began and that for 60% (n=35) this is still the case, of the remaining 40% (n=24) the majority have become managers of services with a smaller proportion going into nurse education. These findings corroborate the data obtained earlier from the service managers, namely that it is not difficult retaining CPNs once they return from the course.

The students' views on the value of the CPN course

a) Clinical skills. The sample was asked to state whether or not attending the course has improved their individual skills. The results by

Table 11.5 Student sample by level of education at entry to the course

Qualification	Students %
Up to CSE level	15.7
Up to 'O' level	44.9
Up to 'A' level	27.0
Degree	1.1
None of the above	11.3
Total	100.0

Table 11.6 ENB c.c. No. 810 students' pay grade before and after the course by cohort

Cohort	Staff nurse		Charge nurse grade 2		Charge nurse grade 1		Senior nurse grade 7		Senior nurse grade 6	
No.	Pre	Post	Pre	Post	Pre	Post	Pre	Post	Pre	Post
1	—	—	80.0	40.0	20.0	20.0	—	40.0	—	—
2	—	—	83.0	23.0	8.3	23.0	—	15.0	—	12.5
3	13.0	—	87.0	12.5	—	50.0	—	12.5	—	—
4	23.0	—	77.0	54.0	—	15.0	—	15.0	—	—
5	—	—	100.0	89.0	—	—	—	—	—	—
6	—	—	100.0	93.0	—	—	—	—	—	—
Total										
%	6.5	—	89.0	55.6	3.2	15.8	—	11.1	—	1.5
No.	4		57	35	2	10	—	7	—	1

NB 4.8% ($n=3$) became senior nurse grade 5
    1.6% ($n=1$) became tutor
    1.6% ($n=1$) became senior tutor
    7.9% ($n=5$) constitute an 'other' category

cohort are given in Table 11.7. The students who indicated that an improvement in clinical skills had occurred were invited to give examples. Figure 11.3 lists a number of such areas of improvement. It is interesting to note that on average, just under two-thirds of the students (62.5%) believed that their clinical skills improved but that this varied between cohorts, for example in cohort 2, 77% stated that there were improvements whereas in cohort 5 this was true for only 40%.

b) Knowledge base. The sample was asked to indicate whether or not there had been an improvement in the acquisition of a knowledge base on which to base practice. The results are given by cohort in Table 11.8. It can be seen that for a very large proportion of the sample (95.3%) the course improves the knowledge base on which it is built. There is little variation in this assessment by cohort. Examples of improvements in the area of knowledge base are given in Figure 11.4.

c) Attitudes to clients. The students were asked to assess whether or not the course had improved their attitudes to clients. The results are given by cohort in Table 11.9. The whole sample's response to the question of the course improving attitudes is similar to the earlier one concerning clinical skill, in that just over half rate the attitudinal area as one which

Table 11.7 Students' response to the course improving their clinical skills

Cohort no.	% 'Yes'	% 'No'
1	60.0	40.0
2	77.0	23.0
3	75.0	25.0
4	54.0	46.0
5	40.0	60.0
6	66.6	33.3
Total %	62.5	37.5
n	40	24

- become aware of different models of assessment which improved my practice
- changed from being a doctor's assistant to being an autonomous independent nurse
- recognized for the first time the CPN role with family members not formally designated as having a problem, e.g. informal carers
- listening and verbal communication skills improved
- stimulated to adopt the advocacy role for clients
- gained confidence to actually experiment with new skills which I learned about on the course. (This was made possible by working with a small case-load with expert clinical supervision)
- learned to accept for the first time the need for access to credible clinical supervision
- case-load management skills improved drastically meaning I had more time with each client and interventions had more depth

Figure 11.3 Examples given by respondents of improvements in clinical skills.

Table 11.8 Students' response to course improving knowledge base on which practice is built

Cohort no.	% 'Yes'	% 'No'
1	100.0	0.0
2	92.3	7.7
3	100.0	0.0
4	100.0	0.0
5	90.0	10.0
6	93.0	7.0
Total %	95.3	4.7
n	6	3

- provided me with a knowledge base beyond that given by the basic RMN course
- gave me background knowledge of other people from different ethnic/racial backgrounds
- sociological/social policy theory very important in understanding the nature of communities in which people live and experience problems
- awareness of a social model of health as opposed to the medical model which was the only model my RMN training gave me
- left the course with a greatly improved awareness of the theories behind alternative therapies/intervention strategies
- gained my first understanding of the term 'health education'
- started acquiring my own conceptual framework for practice based on research from many fields
- learned a great deal from my peers and my alternative service placement about how CPN service mechanics can be improved
- knowledge gained from 'research' module inspired me to look in greater depth at aspects of service evaluation

Figure 11.4 Examples given by respondents of improvements in knowledge base.

Table 11.9 Sample's response to course improving attitude to clients

Cohort no.	% 'Yes'	% 'No'
1	60.0	40.0
2	61.5	38.5
3	75.0	25.0
4	38.0	62.0
5	80.0	20.0
6	40.0	60.0
Total %	56.3	43.8
n	36	28

improved. However, the variation by cohort is markedly different. Cohort 5 estimated that 80% improved their attitudes to clients, whereas this figure for cohort 4 was the lowest, i.e. 38%. This may indicate that the respondents do not see improvements to clinical skills as related to improved attitudes to clients. Examples of cited improvements in attitudes to clients are given in Figure 11.5.

d) Initiation of changes in practice. The students were asked if, as a direct result of completing the course, they initiated positive changes in community psychiatric nursing practice on their return to their own health authorities. The results are given in Table 11.10.

- less tendency to take over responsibility for clients' life, now encouraged to make their own decisions
- altered my institutional perspective – less inclined now to 'label' clients
- more accepting of the clients' broad range of attitudes and values
- became more aware and empatic, understanding my personal prejudices with more effect
- I now call 'clients' the 'people I see' (before the course I called them 'patients')

Figure 11.5 Examples given by respondents of change in attitudes to clients.

Table 11.10 Sample's response to course initiating change in practice on return to seconding health authority

Cohort no.	% 'Yes'	% 'No'
1	100.0	0.0
2	46.0	54.0
3	87.5	12.5
4	61.5	38.5
5	70.0	30.0
6	60.0	40.0
Total %	65.6	34.4
n	42	22

An important finding is that two-thirds of the sample (65.6%) did manage to initiate positive changes in practice on their return from the course – a finding endorsed earlier by the findings reported from the 'service manager' data set. Again, there is enormous variation which seems difficult to account for – ranging from 100% in cohort 1 to 46% in cohort 2. The examples of change reported by the students are presented in Figure 11.6. It should be pointed out that a number of the changes that course attenders cite may seem today, in 1990, to be activities that all services should be engaged in. However, as the study is longitudinal, these new projects were being introduced into services in the Trent and Yorkshire Regional Health Authorities as early as 1982, i.e. one year after the first cohort completed the course.

e) The students' major expectations. Finally, the sample was asked to indicate whether or not the course fulfilled the students' major expectations. The results are given by cohort in Table 11.11. Just over half the sample (56.3%) reported that the course met their major expectations. The least satisfied cohorts were numbers 2 and 4, with the

Clinical initiatives

- started on social skills group
- introduced new assessment format
- started evening groups for anxiety management
- set up a group for problem drinkers in a health centre
- relocated depot clinic and systematically reduced levels of prescribed injections in liaison with the consultant

Liaison initiatives

- moved from 'closed' to 'open' referral system
- initiated a monthly meeting for all workers at a health centre
- devised a role in conjunction with local 'accident and emergency' clinic

Organizational initiatives

- formulated the first written operational policy for the team since the service was set up ten years ago
- implemented a self-directed learning package for basic RMN learners
- initiated a research project to examine service development based on users' and carers' needs
- established community support teams for the elderly and their carers
- reduced excessive case-load numbers
- planned the sectorization of the team

Figure 11.6 Examples of changes in practice initiated on returning to seconding health authority.

Table 11.11 Students' response to the course fulfilling major expectations

Cohort no.	% 'Yes'	% 'No'
1	80.0	20.0
2	46.0	54.0
3	50.0	50.0
4	46.0	54.0
5	80.0	20.0
6	53.0	47.0
Total %	56.3	43.8
n	36	28

best satisfied cohorts being 1 and 5. It may have been expected that 'overall satisfaction' declined over time as students observed other developments occurring in psychiatric nursing, such as the introduction of the 1982 basic RMN curriculum, but this does not appear to be the case. In Figure 11.7 the minority sub-sample makes some observations about the ways in which the ENB c.c.no.810, during the period 1980–1986, did not meet their major expectations.

The survey's results pinpoint significant areas of satisfaction and disappointment with the course from both the seconding managers and the students themselves. The following section will discuss these areas in more depth and highlight ways in which the course has developed under the aegis of the ENB c.c.no.811 curriculum to address major causes of dissatisfaction.

DISCUSSION

Although the results presented in the previous section relate entirely to the ENB c.c.no.810 offered at Sheffield Polytechnic they do have, arguably, wider implications both for the delivery of current ENB c.c.no.811 courses and, indeed, its successor. It is at this stage that the discussion crucially needs development within the context of the wider debate about the future of nurse education as a whole, and the arguments for the development of the CPN's role to the level of the specialist nurse practitioner, as outlined in the Project 2000 proposals, will be addressed towards the end of this section. However, first the implications for the 'here and now' of CPN post-registration education will be examined in relation to the study's original aims.

- the course as a whole contained little that an RMN should not have covered in basic training, as such the experience was little more than 'revision'
- needed sessions to upgrade skills for already practising therapists especially counselling skills
- allocation of supervisors is an arbitrary affair, all former course members are far more clinically expert
- too much on assessment not enough on actual intervention
- not enough recognition for all the hard work the course entailed, on return to my health authority the course was under-valued and no opportunity given to put new ideas into practice
- no emphasis on relevant CPN research as a basis for practice
- special groups for clients were ignored, particularly the elderly and people with schizophrenia
- the course was just too knowledge based and not at all skills oriented

Figure 11.7 Ways in which the course did not fulfil students' major expectations.

The professional and personal profiles of CPN students

There are noteworthy comparisons to be made in terms of the professional/personal profiles of the Sheffield CPN cohorts, trained nurse therapists (Brooker and Brown, 1986) and other JBCNS psychiatric course completers (Rogers and Powell, 1983).

In a major survey of all JBCNS course attenders, Rogers and Powell (1983) did not report the mean age of sub-samples, but Brooker and Brown (1986) established that nurse therapists' mean age was 33.2 years, a very similar figure to the 33.6 reported here for the CPN sample. It was expected that the more recent a cohort in the Sheffield data the younger the mean age would be but this was not corroborated. CPN course students are not, it would seem, becoming younger although with the enormous growth in services in the last five years, one may have expected this to be the case.

Table 11.12 demonstrates that similar proportions of all three samples possess the RMN certificate course but that a much higher proportion of the Sheffield sample are doubly qualified, i.e. RMN and RGN. This may well be because many more women than men qualify as RGNs as Table 11.13 indicates. In Sheffield at least, CPN students are far more likely to be

Table 11.12 The proportions of the three study samples by statutory qualifications obtained

	Nurse therapist		Sheffield CPNs		All other JBNCS course completers	
	%	n	%	n	%	n
RGN/RMN	33	17	48	31	35	53
RMN only	48	25	50	33	42	49

Table 11.13 A comparison of male/female sex ratios in psychiatric nursing

	Sex ratio		
	Male		Female
All qualified psychiatric nurses	1	:	3
The Sheffield CPN sample (1980-86)	1	:	1.12
All qualified nurse therapists	2	:	1
All other post-basic psychiatric course takers (Rogers, 1983)	1.8	:	1

women than are either nurse therapists or other JBCNS post-registration course completers.

There are two main reasons why a consideration of the CPN student sex ratio is important. Firstly, men have traditionally perceived post-registration education as a route to career progression. Whilst, of course, possession of the CPN certificate does not automatically guarantee career advancement this is far more likely if the CPN is qualified. It is therefore reasonable to assume, on paper at least, that women could compete in equal numbers for managerial positions within the area served by the Sheffield course. The second area in which the finding assumes significance relates to the concept of consumer satisfaction. Munton (1988) in unreported pilot research, has shown that consumers are not only aware of their CPN's sex but would like far more choice in the sex of the CPN working with them. Services should be, and do seem to be locally, aware of findings such as these when making decisions about which CPN should be seconded onto the course. This would result in more of a balance being achieved in the sex ratios of trained, as opposed to untrained, CPN personnel within districts.

Students' and managers' perceptions of the value of the course

Figure 11.7 presents a series of comments on ways in which the ENB c.c.no.810 course at Sheffield did not meet some students' major expectations. The remarks appear to support other trends in these data. For a little over a third of students overall, the 810 course did not reflect adequately the emphasis on clinical skills acquisition, although as Table 11.7 demonstrates, there was marked variation in this aspect of student assessment ranging from 23% for cohort 2 to 60% for cohort 5 stating: 'No, the course did not improve my clinical skills'. There was, however, a high general agreement that the course was very good at providing a knowledge base on which to build.

In a sense these findings are somewhat difficult to reconcile. As Table 11.11 shows, 44% of students stated that the course did not fulfil their major expectations, with the single most important criticism being lack of focus on clinical skills. However, as already stated, the majority of students do report improvements in skills, which is a finding re-enforced by clinical initiatives promulgated by students on their return to seconding health authorities; an activity also endorsed by service managers (see Figure 11.6).

As we have seen, students reports of improvements in knowledge base are consistently very high but there does appear to be an association between a declining trend by cohort in relation to improvements in clinical skills and the overall measure of course satisfaction. One plausible explanation for the incongruity is that students' clinical skills are improved, but not to the extent that they may have ideally expected.

There is also a strong argument that one of the desirable effects of the Sheffield CPN course has been to facilitate a move, on the part of seconding health authorities, to primary health care. This seems to be a national trend which has been extensively discussed elsewhere (see Simmons and Brooker, 1986; White, 1987 for fuller reports). The study provides evidence for this assertion in terms of both its quantitative and qualitative data.

Firstly, Table 11.4 indicates quite clearly that seconding services' medical referrals have changed dramatically when compared with the national picture in 1985. Although it is not possible to identify specific referral rates by psychiatrists and GPs in Trent and Yorkshire, Table 11.14 does help to augment the evidence more precisely. Although the 1987 data derived from this survey are a combined Yorkshire/Trent figure there is strong evidence for an equalization between GP and psychiatrist referrals. At this stage it is worthwhile mentioning again the highly significant positive correlation reported as a footnote to Table 11.4. This analysis it will be recalled, correlated the number of ENB c.c.no.810 course completers within DHAs with the percentage of GP referrals.

Secondly, extracts from the qualitative data also highlight ways in which the students believe the course reoriented their conceptual thinking and attitudes in a manner which opened up the possibility of the CPN having a meaningful role in primary health care. A selection are extracted below:

I changed from being a doctor's assistant to being an autonomous independent nurse

Table 11.14 Percentage of medical referrals to CPN teams in Trent and Yorkshire, 1985 and combined for 1987

	1985*		1987	
	Consultant psychiatrist %	GP %	Consultant pyschiatrist %	GP %
Yorkshire	73.5	14.3	45.6	36.0
Trent	56.6	28.8		

*Source: 1985 CPNA Survey Update

Awareness of a social model of health as opposed to the medical model which was the only model my RMN training gave me

Altered my institutional perspective, I was less inclined to 'label' clients

I now call 'clients' 'the people I see' (before I called them 'patients').

The final corroboration for the premise that the 810 course released CPNs from viewing clients entirely within the confines of the medical model may be gauged from Figure 11.6. From this it is also worth selecting several examples of the changes in practice that students initiated on their return to seconding health authorities. One student reports setting up a group for problem drinkers in a health centre, whilst another cites the movement away from a 'closed' to an 'open' referral system. Readers will be able to select more examples from the lists provided in other Figures.

To recapitulate, the ENB c.c.no.810 at Sheffield during the period 1980–1986 assumed an important role in the education of CPNs from the Yorkshire and Trent Regions. CPNs rated their knowledge base for practice much improved and they (and their managers) stated that they initiated a broad spectrum of positive changes when they returned to the service. Whilst these data relating to changes in clinical skills are more difficult to interpret, it is suggested here that clinical skills do improve but maybe not to the ideal level students expected. More generally, the course has been instrumental in facilitating a change in community psychiatric nursing service style and, as CPNs have discovered, their role with the frankly mentally ill may be usefully combined with a preventive remit in the primary health care setting.

As has been frequently emphasized, the results obtained in this survey relate to Sheffield Polytechnic, during the years 1980–1986 and, perhaps most importantly, to the ENB c.c.no.810. The old '810' outline curriculum has now been superseded and in its place the ENB c.c.no.811 syllabus is present in at least 24 course centres nationally. Most centres have planned their new courses taking serious account of what consumers have reported their shortcomings to be. For example at Sheffield the course has become far more skills oriented with significant timetabling allocated to counselling, the use of Heron's six categories and behaviour therapy. All the assessed course-work relates theoretical perspectives, such as the published research on the social origins of depression and high expressed emotion in the families of schizophrenics, to practical case-work. Finally, each student now undertakes a major piece of work such as a pilot research project, the design of a health education package or an extended care study. It is too early to evaluate the effects of these course changes but this is seen as an important ongoing exercise. What is crucial to communicate is that the course as it develops is fluid enough to respond to changing needs of the seconding health authorities.

Such is the interest in community psychiatric nursing education both within Sheffield and elsewhere in the country that Charles Irving recently directed a question in the House of Commons to the Secretary of State for Health and Social Services which asked what measures the Government was taking to arrest the decline in the proportion of trained CPNs. Mrs Edwina Currie replied as follows:

> With the rising number of nurses working in community psychiatric nursing, we have already made clear to health authorities and professional bodies our concern that all staff should be properly prepared for this specialized area of work ... We use every opportunity to encourage staff to undertake the formal post-basic clinical course in community psychiatric nursing care ... We will shortly be discussing with regional nursing officers what the deficiencies now are and the ways they may be rectified.
>
> (Parliamentary Question 2716/1986/87 – Hansard, 9 March 1987)

The UKCC through the vehicle of the Project 2000 document has spelt out a vision for the future of nurse education generally (UKCC, 1986). In recommending the concept of a specialist practitioner with a recordable qualification in community psychiatric nursing the Project 2000 team envisaged a role as follows:

> We see the specialist practitioner role as combining teaching with practice and this suggests that shared learning for some specialist practitioners could be appropriate. Some specialist practitioners will also undertake a management function but it is vital that a caseload is maintained.

Further on in the Project paper strong arguments are made for the need for post-registration education for CPNs (and other nurses) with the CPN specialist practitioner acting as a team leader and supporting the registered practitioner.

At regional level, the Trent Health Authority, has recently reviewed the provision of post-registration nurse education within its boundaries and stated in relation to CPN post-registration education:

> The preparation of trained community psychiatric and mental handicap nurses is considered to be of increasing significance as emphasis on services for these two care groups moves from hospital to community.
>
> (Trent RHA, 1988)

The report continued that the Region should plan an *additional* centre for the 811 course (on top of the two that currently exist) and although one short course in community psychiatric nursing (ENB c.c.no.992) exists, that no more short courses should be planned as:

... it is felt the greater priority in this sphere of care is for nurses to be soundly prepared by attending the long clinical course [i.e. ENB c.c.no.811].

Whilst the groundswell of professional and ministerial opinion seems to strongly support the continuance of a post-registration education for the CPN, and at a time when the number of course centres have doubled in the past two years, CPN educationalists are confronted by two problems.

Firstly, the funding of post-registration CPN education is giving urgent cause for concern. Whilst this is an anxiety shared with other colleagues in different branches of nursing, the fact that the CPN course is not yet mandatory for practice makes the issue even more vexed. The cost of the course fees and travelling expenses are confounded by the cost of 'replacing' the seconded student for nine months. Alternative funding arrangements should be explored and solutions include nationally or regionally protected monies.

A second difficulty is that unit general managers when making tortuous decisions about savings are being attracted to examine 'the value for money' the community psychiatric nursing course represents by the publication of recent reports. Wooff, Goldberg and Fryers (1988) for example have recently suggested that in one health authority in the North Western Region, trained and untrained CPNs are alike in a number of respects. The study, which examines differences in the context and content of both CPNs and mental health social workers' (MHSWs) roles, reports that:

CPNs focused mainly on psychiatric symptoms, treatment arrangements and medications and spent significantly less time with individual psychotic patients than they did with patients suffering from neuroses.

and that, in addition:

CPNs primarily applied a biological model of care and allowed or encouraged ventilation of problems while MHSWs mainly applied a psychosocial model – a likely reflection of the different basic training of the two professions.

On the basis of small, incomparable sub-group analysis within the CPN group, Wooff also asserts that no significant differences were demonstrable in the work of 'trained' as compared with 'untrained' CPNs. In the discussion section of this paper the authors imply that these findings can be generalized to the total population of trained CPNs but this is inaccurate given such small sample sizes.

Further, Gourney and Brooking, holders of a Department of Health research grant, are examining the effectiveness of CPNs in primary health care. Pilot research has already been conducted in this study and is soon to be reported. In advance of publication, Gourney has already stated that:

> The skills based training in psychiatric nursing is woefully inadequate
> and I think we learn mainly by chinese whispers. The first problem is
> that there are too many treatment approaches in a one year (ENB 811)
> training course, and the movement towards having CPNs working
> generically will dilute their effectiveness.
>
> Nursing Times (1988)

What is tending to be the result of the type of research cited above is
that, rather than being examined in detail for what it has to say about the
relevance of CPN education offered today, it is leapt upon by budget
holders as justification *not* to spend on the course at all. Thus, a tension is
created by an alienation of practitioners, service managers and educationalists on the one hand, and those who ultimately hold the purse-strings on
the other. The other consequence of studies such as Skidmore's, Wooff's,
Gourney's and indeed the paper presented here, is that there is a very real
danger of over-generalization from what in fact are small, local studies.
Curiously, Professor Butterworth's MCs thesis (Butterworth, 1987b) which
described welcome 'discernible differences' in JBCNS c.c.no.800 course
completers, and benefitted from a national random sample, is scarcely
recalled in the current economic climate.

CONCLUSION

In the six years that the ENB c.c.no.810 in community psychiatric nursing
ran at Sheffield Polytechnic (1980–1986) the students seconded to the
course benefitted in many ways. This was the view of both seconding
managers and the students themselves. There were reports of the course
not fulfilling students' major expectations which concerned the emphasis
within the course on skills training. These conflicted with other findings but
could be explained, inasmuch as students did leave the course more skilled
but perhaps not to the extent they may have ideally expected. The ENB
c.c.no.811 outline curriculum has allowed a number of changes to be made
that enhance the opportunity for students to acquire skills. Changes in the
curriculum have essentially been effected on the basis of seconding
managers' views of changing needs in local community based mental health
services.

There is strong evidence that during the period of the reported study the
810 course facilitated the process of community psychiatric nursing
services moving into the arena of primary health care. This in turn has
exposed CPNs to other models of care rather than the limiting use of the
medical model. As a consequence there has been a trend towards the
equalization of GP and psychiatrist referrals, that suggests at least in one

way that CPNs are offering a more balanced service.

Whilst a variety of official and professional sources strongly endorse the continued necessity for the post-registration evaluation of CPNs this is being seriously threatened by the lack of a coherent post-registration educ-ation funding strategy. One recommendation suggested here is that if this cannot be worked out at a regional level, with protected top-sliced funding, then the Department of Health should facilitate such a strategy nationally by recommending the minimum level of trained CPNs within district health authorities that they are willing to accept. The English National Board for Nursing (and other national boards) have a key role to play in medi-ating any such planning.

That further research is required in this substantive area is self-evident. Such work is necessary not only because of the economic concerns but also because there are compelling educational arguments for so doing.

ACKNOWLEDGEMENTS

I should like to thank the UKCC for facilitating the study's response rate through their list of registered nurses' addresses; Joanne Jackson, who compiled the student sampling frame; Joan Symonds for all her patient word processing; but the greatest thanks of all go to Ted White for all his encouragement and comments on the first draft of this chapter.

REFERENCES

Anon (1988) CPN training too narrow to be effective. *Nursing Times*, May 11, 6.

Brooker, C. (1987) An investigation into the factors influencing variation in the growth of community psychiatric nursing services. *Journal of Advanced Nursing*, **12**, 367–375.

Brooker, C. and Brown, M. (1986) National survey of practising nurse therapists, in Brooking, J. (ed.) *Readings in Psychiatric Nursing Research*, Wiley, Chichester.

Brooking, J. (1985) Advanced psychiatric nursing education in Britain. *Journal of Advanced Nursing*, **10**, 495–498.

Butterworth, A. (1987a) Mandatory training for community psychiatric nurses – a final report. *Community Psychiatric Nursing Journal*, **7** (6), November/December, 33–42.

Butterworth, A. (1987b) *Assessment and Evaluation of Patients by Community Psychiatric Nurses*. MSc Thesis, University of Aston, Birmingham.

Cole, E. (1971) Community Psychiatric Nursing Course. *Nursing Mirror*, 14 May, 16.

Community Psychiatric Nurses' Association (1985) *The National CPNA Survey Update*, CPNA, Bristol.

English National Board (1988) *Community Nursing Courses in the Mental and Mental Handicap Nursing Fields, EDG/ECW*, 8 January.

Everest, R., Richards, E. and Hanrahan, M. (1979) What happens to Maudsley nurses? A follow-up study. *International Journal of Nursing Studies*, **16**, 253–266.

Hoinville, G. and Jowell, R. (1978) *Survey Research Practice*, Heinemann, London.

May, A. and Moore, S. (1963) The Mental Nurse in the Community. *The Lancet*, **i**, 213–214.

Munton, R. (1988) *What Aspects of Community Psychiatric Nursing does the Client Find Satisfactory*? Project Paper, Sheffield Polytechnic, Sheffield.

Peat, L. and Watt, G. (1984) The passing of an era. *Community Psychiatric Nursing Journal*, **4** (2), 12–16.

Rawlings, J. (1970) Course in community psychiatry. *Nursing Mirror*, 26 June, 20.

Rogers, J. and Powell, D. (1983) The Career Patterns of Nurses who have Completed a JBCNS Certificate. *Joint Board of Clinical Nursing Studies*, London.

Simmons, D. and Brooker, C. (1986) *Community Psychiatric Nursing – A Social Perspective*, Heinemann, London.

Skidmore, D. (1986) The effectiveness of community psychiatric nursing teams and base-locations, in Brooking, J. (ed.) *Readings in Psychiatric Nursing Research*, Wiley, Chichester.

Skidmore, D. and Friend, W. (1984) Muddling Through. *Nursing Times*, **9**, 179–181.

Trent Regional Health Authority (1988) English National Board Post-Basic Nurse Training Project, Sheffield.

United Kingdom Central Council (1986) *Project 2000: A New Preparation for Practice*, UKCC, London.

White, E. (1987) *Psychiatrist Influence on Community Psychiatric Services Planning and Development, and its Implications for Community Psychiatric Nurses*, MSc Thesis, University of Surrey, Guildford.

Wooff, K., Goldberg, D.P. and Fryers, T. (1988) The practice of community psychiatric nursing and mental health social work in Salford: some implications for community care. *British Journal of Psychiatry*, **152**, 783–792.

CHAPTER TWELVE

The historical development of the educational preparation of CPNs

Edward White

SUMMARY

Little has been written on the historical development of the educational preparation of community psychiatric nurses (CPNs) in the UK. The present documentary study is the first of its kind and will show how the absence of a tradition of further training for psychiatric nurses is explained, in part, by an early reluctance to allocate necessary funds. The study will unfold a short history characterized by a series of debates in which the educational considerations have been inexorably linked to material interests and will conclude that the requirement for clarity, commitment and investment has persisted.

INTRODUCTION

.... only a part of what was observed in the past was remembered by those who observed it: only a part of what was remembered was recorded; only a part of what was recorded has survived; only a part of what has survived has come to the historian's attention; only part of what has come to their attention is credible; only part of what is credible has been grasped; and only part of what has been grasped can be expounded or narrated by the historian.

(Gottschalk, 1962)

The single most important policy initiative in the provision of psychiatric care from the psychiatric institution to community locations in the UK was effected when Enoch Powell (1961), then Minister of Health, announced that the country's 150 000 mental illness beds would be reduced by half, by 1975. Such a prediction, based on Government statistics (Tooth and

Brooke, 1961), has since been acknowledged as overly optimistic, though hugely influential (Simmons and Brooker, 1986). Titmuss (1961) argued at the time that the new policy, which has since been reflected by Government enquiries connected with the health service (Department of Health and Social Security, 1975, 1976, 1981), was based on rather limited statistics of doubtful interpretation. He thought that the primary motive was economic and was doubtful of the Conservative Government's intentions: 'To scatter the mentally ill in the community before we have made adequate provision for them is not the solution; in the long run not even for Her Majesty's Treasury'. Further, that if there was no real intention to develop community care facilities, the care of the mentally ill would be from 'trained staff to untrained staff, or ill-equipped or no staff at all'.

The earliest reported developments in community psychiatric nursing, in 1954 and 1957 (Hunter, 1959; Moore, 1961), preceded by several years such changes to the settings in which care was to be delivered. Such was the avant-garde nature of community psychiatric nursing, that synchrony with both service and education has remained elusive, largely independent of geographic location. For example Bagley and Evan-Wong (1973) made an early claim that the use of:

> . . . specialist psychiatric community nurses seems most advanced in Scotland, where psychiatric nurses can successfully fill the gaps in community care following the abolition of the specific role of the mental health officer.

They concluded, however, that given the extending role of the psychiatric nurse in the community, training in sociology, social policy and social administration, as well as in techniques of counselling and psychological relationships, would be advantageous. Indeed, Pasker (1972) was 'amazed' that so many nurses were able to take up posts in the community services without special training.

In the USA, the Community Mental Health Centers Act of 1963 had a revolutionary impact on psychiatric nursing (Davis and Underwood, 1976). The new freedom to work away from the security of the bureaucratic state hospital system 'proved a frightening experience for many psychiatric nurses'. In the early days of community mental health, many psychiatric nurses had no educational preparation or specific experience in the field. Since 1963, a number of educational programmes have developed to prepare nurses for community mental health positions; however, all practising mental health nurses may not have had such preparation. In Italy, despite recent changes for all nurse training to become Infermiere Professionale (Registered Nurse) level, the present mainstream educational preparation of Italian nurses working in community psychiatric settings, has remained essentially out of sympathy with the needs of the new style services. In this, White (1989a) has argued, a parallel with the British context can be drawn.

The historical development of attempts at such educational preparation in the UK is relatively recent and, until the present publication, has yet to be chronicled. This work has been confined to the substantive course and relates entirely to the British context. It is argued here that such an account can offer a modest contribution to an important body of knowledge and thus form an additional explanative source of reference for the present situation.

METHOD

The author was given access to the Department of Health's records and their assistance is gratefully acknowledged. Access was also negotiated to similar types of records and reports held at the English National Board for Nursing, Midwifery and Health Visiting, London. In addition, copies of the minutes of the Education Committee of the Community Psychiatric Nurses' Association from 1974, were made available. Furthermore, professionals who, in some way, were instrumental in the early development of the educational preparation of CPNs were traced and invited to offer first-hand written accounts of their experience, together with other unpublished, though relevant, documents held in their private possession. All such assistance and contributions are gratefully acknowledged. With these unpublished accounts material derived from the published literature has been interwoven.

It is recognized here that records of most proceedings have often been compressed and otherwise edited, so that when they become agreed versions, they will have become somewhat idealized, become abstracts of what speakers meant to say, or subsequently wished they had said, rather than what actually transpired. Reports differ from records in that they are usually written after the event, they are often intended to create an impression rather than merely to aid the memory and they are less intimate. Reports are therefore intrinsically less reliable than records and often suggest a greater tidiness in the sequence of events than was actually experienced (Madge, 1953). Such is the case for the present work and as it was for the evidence upon which it is based.

An attempt has thus been made to examine and integrate documentary evidence from several sources into a single work, that has been organized to allow both a chronology to be derived and a discussion of the issues that flow from it. In so doing, it has been acknowledged that when an investigator has an interest in ascertaining broad trends or detecting a shift over time in the type of attention paid to a particular matter, the writings of others become, as it were, the original data of the integrator. In this, the problems of selection, coding, retrieval procedures and the reporting of the findings and such like, become as real for documentary research as for research in any other form (Feldman, 1971). It has been argued (Black and Champion, 1976) that whatever uses secondary data sources have for scientific activity, they will depend on the subjective ingenuity of the investigator in using them to make a point. Such a quality, present in all methodological approaches, is acknowledged here as both a strength and weakness. Ironically, an exemplar of documentary method (Abel-Smith, 1982), who studied the politics of nursing from 1800 onwards, almost entirely omitted mental nursing because it had a separate development.

THE CHRONOLOGY

In 1962, it was reported that the British psychiatric nurse had a three-year training leading to entrance to the Register for Mental Nurses and that, until recent times, the first part of that training led to the same intermediate examinations as the general nursing trained nurse (Nursing Outlook, 1962; see also Speight, 1978). Specialization followed in the second and third years of training. At that time, a new syllabus of nurse training was being implemented that placed more emphasis upon the study of psychological development and interpersonal relationships. This, it was claimed, was 'a reflection of the wind of change, blowing through our mental hospital service and a movement toward a therapeutic community'.

Even so, those concerned with the pioneering service-development of community psychiatric nursing, recognized that the syllabus (of 1964) for the Certificate of Mental Nursing would require still further radical change, if psychiatric nursing education was to remain in sympathy with the intended new-style service provision. For Hunter (1970 and personal communication), this meant the inclusion of syllabuses in sociology, social policy and administration and social and psychiatric research. His was a prophetic view of the emerging role of psychiatric nurses and of the educational preparation which was necessary to be synchronous with new work practices. A similar argument has been made by Gunn (1969) who described 'a need for a nurse trained in both district nursing and psychiatric nursing'; a national scheme for training 'home nurses' having been approved ten years earlier in 1959.

Increasing interest in the notion of psychiatric community care led the General Nursing Council, in 1971, to acknowledge the need to extend student nurses' learning experience beyond the hospital, by including periods of community experience in training syllabuses. For mental nurses in basic training, such experience was incalcated in the 1974 Registered Mental Nurse (RMN) syllabus. Then, although 'a radical revision of the Syllabus should not be attempted on this occasion' (General Nursing

Council, 1974), the opportunity was taken to give 'additional emphasis to those aspects of care and treatment which are the main functions of the nurse for the mentally ill and to introduce sections on sociology and community care'.

Concurrent with such developments in basic psychiatric preparation, the Joint Board of Clinical Nursing Studies (JBCNS) was originally set up in 1970, to regulate post-registration nursing courses. It was financed, for the first three years, by the King Edward's Hospital Fund for London and the Nuffield Provincial Hospitals' Trust, together with the central departments, i.e. the Department of Health and Social Security (DHSS) and the Welsh Office. The Royal College of Nursing handled the money. It was later reconstituted in 1973 to include the specialist aspects of community, as well as hospital, nursing in England and Wales.

Basic conditions for JBCNS approval of courses were drawn up and related to the following considerations: the number of student and pupil nurses and medical students already doing basic training in the unit; the number of trained nurses and doctors to give teaching and supervision; proper standards of nursing practice, equipment and facilities; and adequate accommodation and library facilities. Furthermore, each course was required to run regularly and start on specified dates, to be planned as a separate entity and be withdrawn should recruitment not fulfil the available spaces, and to conform to the relevant JBCNS syllabus.

In order to consider matters of detail concerning courses, the JBCNS set up panels of experts in each clinical specialty. These panels, which included doctors and nurses, advised on course content, length, admission qualifications and any other relevant matters. The first four panels to be appointed, because of 'a claim to priority' (Anon., 1971), were in general intensive care, special care babies, venereal diseases and psychiatry.

Some post-registration courses are excellent, others good but a minority of courses are organized for the recruiting of pairs of hands. The Joint Board will rationalize the situation.

(Anon. *Nursing Times*, 1972)

Such an unequivocal posture was welcomed by an independent working party of educational innovators, who had already begun curriculum development work under the auspices of the Faculty of Health and Social Studies, Chiswick Polytechnic, in advance of the inauguration of the JBCNS. The working party had met to study the role of the nurse in community psychiatry and to plan a short post-registration course specifically for such nurses. Accounts of their work (Rawlings, 1970 and personal communication; Cole, 1971) report of a 13-day experimental community psychiatric nursing course held over nine weeks between June and November 1970. Well over 100 applications were received for the 20 available places. This was deemed sufficiently successful to warrant the development of a further three-month full-time course, divided into two equal blocks (Corea, personal communication). The course included the principles and practice of community psychiatric nursing as they were then understood and aspects of social psychology, sociology and social administration. This, in turn, was developed into an academic year-long pilot, pre-JBCNS approved, course.

In August 1972, in tandem with the work of the Chiswick Polytechnic group, and in anticipation of its reconstitution in 1973 to include specialist aspects of community (as well as hospital) nursing in England and Wales, the JBCNS convened the first Community Psychiatric Nursing Specialist Panel, being derived from the Community Care Specialist Panel. The DHSS asked, at the time, that the JBCNS consult with the Panel of Assessors for District Nursing and the Council for the Education and Training of Health Visitors on any matter that may impinge on their field of activities. It was also regretted that there was no general practitioner (GP) on the Community Psychiatric Nursing Specialist Panel.

The membership of the first Community Psychiatric Nursing Specialist Panel reflected such interests and was chaired by a principal nursing officer (Health Visiting). The 14-member panel also included four doctors, a director of social services and a second health visitor. Two of the psychiatric nurse members of the panel had previously written in the substantive area (Hunter, 1959, 1962; Harries, 1970a, 1970b, 1971, 1972 and personal communication).

In January 1974, when the Chair of the Community Psychiatric Nursing Specialist Panel presented the resultant syllabus to JBCNS for approval, some members were of the opinion that this nurse's role (CPN) might overlap with that of the health visitor. The Chair, however, saw the roles as being different and that the CPN would continue treatment of discharged patients, while the health visitor's role was mainly preventive. A similar argument had been made three months earlier in relation to district nursing, when a consultant psychiatrist member of JBCNS made a distinction between the two occupational groups and stressed the importance of training, of a specialized nature, for community psychiatric nursing. It was argued that a general community nurse, however highly trained, would not necessarily be able to deal with all psychiatric cases in the community and that a core of 'consultant' psychiatric nurses, with advanced training, would be necessary.

By March 1974, the JBCNS had published the *Outline Curriculum in Community Psychiatric Nursing for Registered Nurses*, JBCNS clinical course number 800 (JBCNS, 1974). The aim of the 36–39-week course was:

... to prepare a Registered Mental Nurse (RMN) or a Nurse of the Mentally Subnormal (RNMS) to work effectively in a multidisciplinary team in order to give psychiatric nursing care and therapeutic and habilitative or rehabilitative support to the patient in the community, taking into account his family and all relevant contacts.

The Outline Curriculum, judged by contemporary guidance, was prescriptive and modelled around centrally-set behavioural objectives against which to measure the relative achievement of the aim. Not less than one-third of the course was to be devoted to the

planned teaching programme commencing with a preparatory course of at least five days, or a residential workshop of 72 hours, which challenges the nurse to explore critically her present attitudes toward her speciality and sets the framework of knowledge and understanding of the course.

An equivalent minimum of two days each week was to be spent in field-work placements, of which a continuous block of 12 weeks were to be spent 'within the nursing team of the community psychiatric service to which the nurse will be appointed following completion of the course'. Close supervision of the clinical practice was to be ensured by the designation of 'a skilled nurse' as a personal supervisor during each 'field attachment'. There was to be a progressive assessment of skills, knowledge and attitudes, rather than one final examination.

In application to JBCNS for course approval in May 1974, Chiswick Polytechnic (later to become the West London Institute of Higher Education, WLIHE) was able to draw on a wealth of working experience as a result of hosting the precursor courses and claimed that it proved to have had a profound effect on the attitudes of nurses on the then current course. In approving the course to run for four more consecutive years under its authority, the JBCNS noted the recommendation and acknowledged that it would be the first approved course to be based in a polytechnic, rather than a school of nursing. The course was to be led by the second health visitor-member of the JBCNS Community Psychiatric Nursing Specialist Panel.

Each course was one academic year in length and was structured such that the theoretical components which were engaged during polytechnic attendance, were put into practice during the proportionately longer field-work placement periods (Speight, 1976). It has been recalled (Corea, personal communication) that the 'rigid timetable' ran between 8.30 am and 4 pm with 'each slot filled with purposeful activity'. The course, ironically, was experienced as being 'based on a health visitor's model ... but that was not such a bad thing because it helped us focus more on mental health promotion'. About half the participants of the course had not previously worked in the community, while the remainder had up to five years experience (Parnell, 1974). A later report (Thain, 1976) described 'all but two, of the sixteen students, had been working in the community'.

By July 1977, JBCNS c.c.no.800 had been approved to run in four centres. In addition to WLIHE, applications had been approved for North East London Polytechnic (NELP) in March 1975; Manchester Polytechnic in September 1975 and Gwent College of Higher Education in August 1976. An application from Plymouth Polytechnic, in May 1975, was deferred because the two clinical placements which had been arranged were insufficient to accommodate all the course members. Plymouth Polytechnic had earlier attempted, in 1970, to combine basic and community psychiatric nursing training in a diploma course in community psychiatric nursing. However, this foundered because of lack of students (Hunter, 1974).

The Gwent JBCNS 800 course was the first to propose that all course members should be RMNs and not intended for RNMSs. In July 1977, the JBCNS received two letters from the course tutors of two centres offering the community psychiatric nursing course, in which it was asked for consideration to be given to the revision of the Outline Curriculum, so that it would be possible to offer separate courses for RMNs and Registered Nurses of the Mentally Handicapped. This, it was asserted, was because there were clear differences in the content of the nurse training courses needed. The Specialist Panel members were reluctant to support this suggestion. It was argued that to provide two different courses could prejudice the continued provision of any course in this specialty, as there was unlikely to be an adequate number of applicants for both. The Specialist Panel argued that there was too much common material to justify a separate course and that it would be more helpful to revise the content of the clinical objectives, so that the common core and specialist aspects of each discipline were more clearly defined. In October 1977, the membership of the reconvened 11-member Specialist Panel was agreed and set the task to reconsider the JBCNS c.c.no.800 Outline Curriculum in terms of the differing needs of the RMN and the RNMS. It was the first panel in which a JBCNS Certificate holder was included as a member, together with four psychiatrists and three health visitors. The reconvened panel first met in January 1978.

At broadly the same time, in November 1976, the Community Psychiatric Nurses' Association (CPNA) was formed (Roberts, 1977). After the first National Symposium at Warwick University in May 1977, the CPNA agreed the formation of an Education Sub-Committee to consider the 'educational needs within the CPNA and to plan for future developments' (CPNA, 1978).

By April 1979, JBCNS had published the *Outline Curriculum in the Nursing Care of the Mentally Ill in the Community*, JBCNS c.c.no.810

(JBCNS, 1979), the counterpart for RNMSs was the JBCNS c.c.no.805. Although each remained structurally similar to the original JBCNS c.c.no.800, in terms of the relationship between theory and practice placements, attention was given to strengthen the presence of 'nursing process' as an organizing method of therapeutic intervention in the new course requirements. This, even though the original JBCNS c.c.no.800 course completers showed 'discernable differences' from those CPNs who were without a post-registration educational preparation. Sources of assessment information were more likely to be all encompassing, and less specifically 'medical diagnosis' oriented, when collected by nurses with the CPN certificate. Such nurses were also found to take greater notice of social stratification and family opinion in overall assessments (Butterworth, 1979).

The new curricula for the two courses had been designed as a result of 'the rapid development and increasing specialization of the community nursing services in the care and treatment of mentally handicapped and mentally ill patients' (JBCNS, 1979). The clinical nursing content of the course had been divided into three sections. The first section contained the common core material, while the second and third section concerned more specific aspects of each speciality. The clinical nursing content which related to the mentally ill, focused on the special aspects of the young person and the elderly. For the mentally handicapped, the role of the nurse as an enabler was highlighted to assist the mentally handicapped person to develop self-help and social skills. The aim of the two new courses had been held constant, though changed from '... in order to give *psychiatric* nursing care ...' found in the 1974 Outline Curriculum, to '... in order to give *appropriate* nursing care ...' in the 1979 version. By September 1982, the JBCNS c.c.no.800 Outline Curriculum had been withdrawn in favour of the JBCNS c.c.no.810 successor.

The early 1980s were important for two reasons. Firstly, in September 1980, legislation created National Boards for Nursing, Midwifery and Health Visiting in Northern Ireland, Scotland, Wales and England (ENB), and assumed the double-running shadow responsibilities with JBCNS, until cessation in September 1983. During this period, the ENB began to adopt committee structures which were similar to those of the erstwhile JBCNS. The interests of psychiatric nurses were made plain to the ENB largely by the persistent lobby and a 6550-signature petition from the Psychiatric Nurses' Association (ENB, 1982a), though the structural arrangements have yet to match, in influence, those for other nursing disciplines.

Secondly, a new syllabus of training for RMNs was published in 1982 (ENB, 1982b). It provided a model upon which 'a skills-oriented curriculum' could be constructed and, unlike the 1974 syllabus that it replaced, it required students to 'develop the skilful use of the nursing process'. It has been argued since (Brooking, 1985) that basic psychiatric nursing education should prepare the nurse to work in all settings of care, including the community, thus, 'it might be more appropriate to restructure basic education rather than insist on compulsory post-basic education'. A competing argument has always been that, independent of similarity in content, the levels of preparation were quite different. The latter view has been powerfully endorsed since (UKCC, 1986).

In April 1985, cognizant of the content of the 1982 RMN syllabus, and ever mindful of an emerging hesitation by budget holders to devote economic resources to non-mandatory post-registration clinical nursing courses, the ENB published the Outline Curriculum for ENB c.c.no.811 (ENB, 1985). This brought the skill requirements nearer to contemporary community psychiatric nursing practice. Again, the structure of the educational preparation was largely held constant, though more flexibility was encouraged to focus the content toward therapeutic intervention techniques.

Three years later, in March 1988, the Specialist Panel was again reconvened to reconsider the needs of psychiatric nurses trained under the 1982 RMN syllabus for further training to undertake community psychiatric nursing. The subsequent guidance, approved in January 1989, though yet to be published and to be known as ENB c.c.no.812 (ENB, 1989b), will aim

> to produce a specialist practitioner, beyond initial training as a registered mental nurse, who is able to function autonomously and as a member of a team in providing mental health nursing care to people in community settings.

An explicit system of individually negotiated exemptions will be developed later by the ENB, to make possible a reduction in supervised field-work placement periods during the course for some experienced psychiatric nurses who hold alternative, though relevant, qualifications.

More recently still, to compound the increasingly complex inter-relationships between basic and post-registration psychiatric nurse education, a Working Group of the ENB was convened in October 1988, to develop guidance for the Mental Health Branch of Project 2000 courses. Such guidance, approved and published in January 1989 (ENB, 1989a), continued to underpin the trend toward the provision of psychiatric care outside traditional institutional settings and exploited the content of the prevailing 1982 RMN syllabus. The first Mental Health Branch course completers will, at the earliest, seek specialist practitioner preparation in community psychiatric nursing from September 1992. The future developments in the education of CPNs may, therefore, allow the ENB c.c.no.812 to bridge the intervening three-year gap before further reconsideration becomes necessary.

DISCUSSION

Much of the fifteen year history of the educational preparation of CPNs has been characterized by a series of difficult and essentially unsuccessful struggles to secure and protect adequate finance for an effective system of post-registration nurse education. The original mechanics of mounting courses and the agreed financial arrangements for the secondment of staff, dealt with in the first report of the JBCNS, was circulated to health authorities under cover HM(72)49. Briefly, this involved the course members being paid their full salary for the duration of the course. It was suggested that the method of sharing the payment of seconded nurses salaries on a 50/50 basis between the seconding health authority and the health authority mounting the course, be continued. The seconding health authority also paid for any student travelling and subsistence allowances. However, it was noted that such an arrangement was only suitable if the nurse was giving some service to the health authority mounting the course. It was not suitable, for example when seconding to a JBCNS course based in a college of further education, nor if the subject was such that very little or no service was given during the course. In such cases, as with JBCNS c.c.no.800 – the first JBCNS course to have been sited in a polytechnic, the full salary was to be paid for by the seconding health authority.

From the outset, therefore, community psychiatric nursing education was in an anomalous, vulnerable position and, although JBCNS frequently stated its belief about the relative adequacy of funding to the DHSS, the Psychiatric Panel eventually reported the following points to the JBCNS:

1. That there was no established tradition of further training for psychiatric nurses, except for admission to another part of the Register or the Roll.
2. That the cost of mounting a course was seen as prohibitive and 'in-service' training was an acceptable and cheap alternative.
3. That the cost of secondment to courses, whether they were Polytechnic or hospital-based, appeared too great even when the need for well trained nurses was clear and apparently accepted, as in community psychiatric nursing.
4. That the need of the service for well trained psychiatric nurses was rarely directed, or well presented to district management teams and that a low priority was, therefore, given to allocating funds for continuing education and training.

Twelve years later, such issues have retained a contemporary ring and still closely characterize the latter day discussions between the ENB and the Department of Health (ENB, 1989c). The work of the Standing Advisory Group for Community Psychiatric Nursing Education (White and Brooker,

1989), through concerns about the difficulties of securing adequate funds for student secondments, has recently enabled a confident intelligence function to emerge, which has made it possible to plan and publish work (Rushforth, 1988) on the strategic planning issues related to community psychiatric nursing education. Such work has shown that although recruitment to an increased number of community psychiatric nursing courses rose by 10% between 1987 and 1988, from 366 to 405, the number of applicants failing to get a course place more than doubled to 177 over the same period. Nevertheless, 23% of course places were unfilled in 1988, largely due to under-resourced post-registration nurse education budgets at district health authority (DHA) level.

The work of the CPNA (1985) showed that 22.4% of the national CPN workforce were ENB course completers, a proportion which was modestly smaller than the 24.2% found in 1980 (CPNA, 1980b). Concomitantly, therefore, the practical prospect of mandatory training for CPNs has become weaker, as the argument for it has become stronger (Joint Organizations Working Group, 1987). The present Conservative Government has confirmed (Currie, 1987) that it has

> already made clear to Health Authorities and Professional Bodies our concern that all staff should be properly prepared for this specialised area of [CPN] work ... We use every opportunity to encourage staff to undertake the formal post-basic clinical course ... We will shortly be discussing with Regional Nursing Officers what the deficiencies now are and the ways they may be rectified.

The 1990 National Quinquennial CPN Survey, presently in preparation (White, 1989b), will be sensitive to any reported dividends arising from such discussions.

Ten years ago, the JBCNS argued that while responsibility for funding continued to rest with DHAs, rather than at national or regional level, an additional reluctance to second students would persist. This is because, as one area nursing officer put it:

> ... once having gained the Certificate, the staff concerned rarely remain with us for more than a few months' and although she appreciated 'that looked at from a national point of view the valuable training and expertise gained by these nurses is not lost, but that is of small comfort to us and of little help to our patients and their families.

Such parochial economic interests and concerns have underscored the development of consortia arrangements between small numbers of DHAs. Within these arrangements, participating health authorities each contribute financially to the cost of mounting a local course. Similarly, isolated arrangements have been made to top-slice a budget at regional health authority level, as in South West Thames, to free DHAs from the year-to-year search for sufficient funds to second staff. Comparative studies to confirm their educational and financial integrity have yet to appear in the published substantive literature.

Indeed, the continued absence of a national strategy for the development of community psychiatric nursing course centres and a cogent method for making relative judgements about the quality and unit cost of different educational modalities, has left CPN education *per se* vulnerable to criticism about structure, content, presentation or efficacy (Anon., 1988). The revisions to the outline curricula, described earlier, can be seen in part as responses to such close observation. The training of nurse therapists, sometimes used as a comparator, has itself been exposed to similar criticism, though rarely referred to in reviews. For example Brooker and Wiggins (1983) found that three out of eight nurse therapists training at the Maudsley Hospital failed to significantly improve the condition of their patient group, which amounted to 32.5% of the study cohort of 251 patients. More recently, Barker (1989) asserted that 'many people, patients included, find the scientific view of [Marks] behaviour therapy unnecessarily limiting, if not dehumanising'. Notwithstanding such observations, recent evidence (Chapter 11) has shown that a sample of ENB 810 course completers had a significant impact on the acquisition of clinical skills, attitudes to clients and knowledge base. In addition, two-thirds of the sample initiated important changes in practice on return to their seconding health authority, an observation corroborated by a second data set obtained from seconding health authority managers.

Such has become the sensitivity of the consumer view of managers of educational programmes for CPNs, that an assurance was given to the Standing Advisory Group for Community Psychiatric Nursing Education that changes to the shortened substantive course 'were not made as a result of pressure from management' (ENB, 1987a). However, seven years earlier, the JBCNS had confirmed with the CPNA that 'with the cut back in funding available for the service and, therefore, for nurse training, requests to provide a short course have increased considerably' (JBCNS, 1980). The CPNA has remained implacably opposed to shortened substantive courses because secondment to them would then be likely 'for reasons of economy' rather than for compelling educational arguments (CPNA, 1980a).

In September 1987, an experimental distance learning package became available from one community psychiatric nursing course centre. It was approved by the ENB (1987b), though some eight years earlier the Specialist Panel in Community Psychiatric Nursing of the JBCNS had considered and welcomed the idea of providing distance teaching by developing learning packages. It was felt that the development of such a course 'should be encouraged because of the present difficulties Health Authorities experience in obtaining trained nurses' (ENB, 1986). Indeed, the benefits of such an arrangement have been claimed in the course publicity (Hughes, 1989) in terms of the simultaneous contribution to service which students continue to make during their training and how this is translated into cost effectiveness; 'there will not be a need for excessive purchasing of academic books, as course materials will refer to a limited recommended list'. Although here too, course evaluation reports have yet to appear in the published literature for close scrutiny, the format and the language of the course can be seen as a deft, pragmatic response to the prevailing economic and managerial climate in the National Health Service.

Indeed, given the present climate, the nature of CPNs' preparation is likely to become increasingly instrumentalist and in the clamour to command the moral high ground for lean and fit education, the risk of *reductio ad absurdum* to thin and week training might become evident. The absence of an unequivocal, nationally agreed, post-registration psychiatric nurse education strategy, supported by the necessary financial resources, has continued over the period covered by this present review, to place the service and education sectors of mental health service provision in impossibly difficult positions. This study has shown that the educational considerations remain inexorably linked to material interests and, self-evidently, the requirement has persisted for clarity, commitment and investment.

REFERENCES

Abel-Smith, B. (1982) *A History of the Nursing Profession*, Heinemann, London.

Anon. (1962) *Nursing outlook*, **10** (9), 605.

Anon. (1971) Joint Board of Clinical Nursing Studies. *Nursing Mirror*, 7 May, 13.

Anon. (1972) Joint Board of Clinical Nursing Studies. *Nursing Times*, 10 August, 1006–1011.

Anon. (1988) CPN training too narrow to be effective. *Nursing Times*, 11 May, 6.

Bagley, C. and Evan-Wong, L. (1973) The community psychiatric nurses' role and potential interest in psychiatric nursing in teenagers making career choice decisions. *International Journal of Nursing Studies*, **10**, 271–279.

Barker, P. (1989) Reflections on the philosophy of caring in mental health. *International Journal of Nursing Studies*, **26**, 131–141.

Black, J. and Champion, D. (1976) Methods and issues in social research, Wiley, Chichester.

Brooker, C. (1989) A six year follow-up of nurses attending the JBCNS/ENB course number 810 in community psychiatric nursing at Sheffield Polytechnic, in Brooker, C. (ed.) *Community Psychiatric Nursing: A research perspective*, Chapman and Hall, London.

Brooker, C. and Wiggins, R. (1983) Nurse therapist variability: the implications for selection and training. *Journal of Advanced Nursing*, **8**, 321–328.

Brooking, J. (1985) Advanced psychiatric nursing education in Britain. *Journal of Advanced Nursing*, **10**, 455–468.

Butterworth, C.A. (1979) Assessment and evaluation of patients by community psychiatric nurses. MSc Thesis, University of Aston, Birmingham.

Cole, E.J. (1971) Community psychiatric nursing course. *Nursing Mirror*, 14 May, 16.

Community Psychiatric Nurses' Association (1978) General Council Meeting minute No.9, 2 October, CPNA, Rossendale, Lancashire.

Community Psychiatric Nurses' Association (1980a) *Community psychiatric nurses' education, training and their needs*, a discussion paper prepared in response to the JBCNS consideration of a proposal to establish a shortened course for CPNs, April, CPNA, Bristol.

Community Psychiatric Nurses' Association (1980b) *National Survey of Community Psychiatric Nursing Services*, CPNA, Bristol.

Community Psychiatric Nurses' Association (1985) *The 1985 CPNA National Survey Update*, CPNA, Bristol.

Currie, E. (1987) Parliamentary Question 2716/1986/7, 9 March, Hansard, London.

Davis, A.J. and Underwood, P. (1976) Educational preparation for community mental health nursing. *Journal of Psychiatric Nursing and Mental Health Services*, March, 10–15.

Department of Health and Social Security (1975) *Better services for the mentally ill*, HMSO, London.

Department of Health and Social Security (1976) *Priorities for health and personal social services in England, a consultative document*, HMSO, London.

Department of Health and Social Security (1981) *Care in the community, a consultative document for moving resources for care in England*, HMSO, London.

English National Board (1982a) Minute 82.3(a) 26 January, English National Board for Nursing, Midwifery and Health Visiting, London.

English National Board (1982b) *Syllabus of training 1982, Professional Register – Part 3, Registered Mental Nurses*, English National Board for Nursing, Midwifery and Health Visiting, London.

English National Board (1985) *Course Number 811: Nursing care of mentally ill people in the community*, English National Board for Nursing, Midwifery and Health Visiting, London.

English National Board (1986) Minute 86/8, Applications and Approvals Committee, 20 March, English National Board for Nursing, Midwifery and Health Visiting, London.

English National Board (1987a) Minute 87/11, Approvals and Applications Committee, 19 March, English National Board for Nursing, Midwifery and Health Visiting, London.

English National Board (1987b) Minute 40.3.1 Approvals and Applications Committee, 16 July, English National Board for Nursing, Midwifery and Health Visiting, London.

English National Board (1989a) *Project 2000: a new preparation for practice*, Guidelines and criteria for course development and the formation of collaborative links between approved training institutions within the National Health

Service and centres of Higher Education, English National Board for Nursing, Midwifery and Health Visiting, London.

English National Board (1989b) *Course Number 812: Nursing care of mentally ill people in the community*, In Press, English National Board for Nursing, Midwifery and Health Visiting, London.

English National Board (1989c) Community psychiatric nursing (MNC(88)37 and 88/26 refer), 10 January, English National Board for Nursing, Midwifery and Health Visiting, London.

Feldman, K. (1971) Using the work of others: some observations on reviewing and integrating. *Sociology of Education*, **44**, 86–102.

General Nursing Council (1974) *Training syllabus, Register of Nurses, Mental Nursing*, General Nursing Council for England and Wales, London.

Gottschalk, L. (1962) *Understanding History*, McGraw-Hill, New York.

Gunn, M. (1969) District nursing and the mentally ill. *Nursing Times*, 17 April, 497.

Harries, C. (1970a) *Psychiatric nursing: the future and the problems*, conference paper, Royal College of Nursing 'Roadshow', Birmingham.

Harries, C. (1970b) *Sharing care: the psychiatric nurse and the social worker*, conference paper, Bedford College, London.

Harries, C. (1971) Rethinking psychiatric nursing care. *Nursing Mirror*, 23 July, 13–16.

Harries, C. (1972) *Psychiatric community care: the psychiatric nurse*, a discussion paper to JBCNS, September, Joint Board of Clinical Nursing Studies, London.

Hughes, R. (1989) *ENB Course No. 811: Distance Learning Course*, Warrington Health Authority, Cheshire.

Hunter, P. (1959) The changing function of professional staff in the mental hospital, in *Ventures in Professional Cooperation*, Association of Professional Social Workers, London.

Hunter, P. (1962) Aftercare for the mentally ill as a British Hospital provides it. *Nursing Outlook*, **10** (9), 604–606.

Hunter, P. (1970) The role of the psychiatric nurse: some thoughts on training. Briefing paper to the Clinical Services Committee of the National Association for Mental Health, London.

Hunter, P. (1974) Community psychiatric nursing in Britain: an historical review. *International Journal of Nursing Studies*, **11**, 223–233.

Joint Board of Clinical Nursing Studies (1974) *Course number 800: Outline curriculum in community psychiatric nursing for Registered Nurses*, JBCNS, London.

Joint Board of Clinical Nursing Studies (1979) *Course number 810: Outline curriculum in the nursing care of the mentally ill in the community for Registered Mental Nurses*, JBCNS, London.

Joint Board of Clinical Nursing Studies (1980) Correspondence between the Professional Officer, JBCNS and the Secretary, Community Psychiatric Nurses' Association, 14 February, JBCNS, London.

Joint Organizations Working Group (1987) Mandatory training for community psychiatric nurses – a final report. *Community Psychiatric Nursing Journal*, November/December, 33–42.

Madge, J. (1953) *Tools of social science*, Longman, London.

Moore, J. (1961) A psychiatric out-patient nursing service. *Mental Health Bulletin*, **20**, 51–54.

Parnell, J. (1974) Psychiatric nursing in the community. *Queens Nursing Journal*, May, 36–38.

Pasker, P. (1972) Nursing. *New Society*, June, 469–470.

Powell, E. (1961) In, *Emerging patterns for the mental health services and the public*, proceedings from a conference, March, National Association for Mental Health, London.

Rawlings, J.A. (1970) Course in community psychiatry, *Nursing Mirror*, **130**, 20.

Roberts, L. (1977) CPNs Unite. *Nursing Times*, 3 February, 153.

Rushforth, D. (1988) Market forces and community psychiatric nursing courses. *Community Psychiatric Nursing Journal*, **8** (6), 22–26.

Simmons, S. and Brooker, C. (1986) *Community Psychiatric Nursing: A social perspective*, Heinemann, London.

Speight, I.M. (1976) JBCNS course number 800 in community psychiatric nursing. *Nursing Mirror*, 5 August, ii–iii.

Speight, I.M. (1978) Nurse education – signposts for the future, in Leopoldt, H. (ed.) *Contemporary themes in psychiatric nursing*, Squibb and Son, Twickenham.

Thain, A. (1976) A course member's view. *Nursing Mirror*, 5 August, iv.

Titmuss, R. (1961) In; *Emerging patterns for the mental health services and the public*, proceedings from a Conference, March, National Association for Mental Health, London.

Tooth, G. and Brooke, E. (1961) Trends in the mental health population and their effect on planning. *The Lancet*, **i**, April, 710–713.

United Kingdom Central Council (1986) *Project 2000: a new preparation for practice*, United Kingdom Central Council for Nursing, Midwifery and Health Visiting, London.

White, E. (1989a) Italian community mental health services and nurse education. *Community Psychiatry: its management and practice*, **2** (1) 6–8.

White, E. (1989b) *The 1990 National Quinquennial Community Psychiatric Nursing Survey*, Department of Nursing, University of Manchester, (in preparation).

White, E. and Brooker, C. (1990) The Standing Advisory Group for Community Psychiatric Nursing: Grasping the Nettle? Nurse Education Today, February, 63–65.

Index